GOLDEN HOURS

Care of the Very Low Birth Weight Infant

GOLDEN HOURS

Care of the Very Low Birth Weight Infant

First Edition

Robin L. Bissinger, PhD, APRN, NNP-BC, FAAN
Associate Dean of Academics
Neonatal Nurse Practitioner
College of Nursing
Medical University of South Carolina
Charleston, South Carolina

David J. Annibale, MD
Chief, Division of Neonatology
Program Director, Fellowship in Neonatal-Perinatal Medicine
Children's Hospital, Division of Neonatology
Medical University of South Carolina
Charleston, South Carolina

THE NATIONAL CERTIFICATION CORPORATION
CHICAGO

The National Certification Corporation

676 N. Michigan Ave., Ste. 3600
Chicago, Illinois 60611

GOLDEN HOURS: CARE OF THE VERY
LOW BIRTH WEIGHT INFANT
© 2014 by National Certification Corporation.

ISBN: 978-0-9890198-1-1

All Rights Reserved. No part of this publication may be reproduced or transmitted by any means, electronic or mechanical, including photocopying, recording, or otherwise, without written permission from the publisher. For information, write National Certification Corporation, 676 N. Michigan Ave., Suite 3600, Chicago, Illinois 60611.

This book and the individual contributions contained in it are protected by copyright by the Publisher (except as noted herein).

Notices

While all reasonable effort has been made to assure both the accuracy and timeliness of the information in this publication, new evidence and research continually impact practice. The authors, editors, and publishers do not take responsibility for the accuracy or completeness of any of the information contained herein and it is expected that providers utilize the most current information, policies, and guidelines at their practice sites for the care of patients.

This book and the authors, editors, and publishers recognize that this publication contains information on health care that is intended for use as assistance only to the professional practitioner. The actual use of, and interpretation of, this information is solely the responsibility of the practitioner.

Any reference to any procedure, device, drug, or drug dosage (unless otherwise indicated in the text) is based on the generally accepted standards in effect at the time of publication and, if applicable, reflects the then current FDA-approved usages for drugs and devices. Since such standards and usages are subject to change and interpretation based on research and new information, it is the responsibility of any practitioner to check the applicable current standards and FDA usage recommendations prior to use in practice. The editors, authors, and publisher disclaim any responsibility for any adverse effects resulting from the suggested procedures, from any undetected errors, or from the reader's misunderstanding of the text.

Library of Congress Cataloging-in-Publication Data
Golden hours: care of the very low birth weight infant / [edited by] Robin L. Bissinger, David J. Annibale.
    p. ; cm.
    Care of the very low birth weight infant
    Includes bibliographical references and index.
    ISBN: 978-0-9890198-1-1 (pbk. : alk. paper)
1. Pediatrics—Newborn infants—Diseases and abnormalities—Low birth weight.
2. Pediatrics—Premature infants. I. Bissinger, Robin L. 1958- II. Title: Golden hours: care of the very low birth weight infant.
[DNLM: 1. Neonatology—Handbooks, Manuals, etc. 2. Infant, Newborn, Diseases—Handbooks. 3. Intensive Care, Neonatal—Handbooks. 4. Neonatology—methods—Handbooks.]

Library of Congress Control Number: 2014940198

Developmental Editor: Betty Burns, CAE
Publishing Services Manager: Cyndi Scovel
Designer: Mary T. Burke
Medical Illustrations: Janice Cleary MS and Lobsang Studios

Printed in the United States of America.

10 9 8 7 6 5 4 3 2 1

Contributors

David J. Annibale, MD
Chief, Division of Neonatology
Program Director, Fellowship in Neonatal-Perinatal Medicine
Children's Hospital, Division of Neonatology
Medical University of South Carolina
Charleston, South Carolina

Robin L. Bissinger, PhD, APRN, NNP-BC, FAAN
Associate Dean of Academics
Neonatal Nurse Practitioner
College of Nursing
Medical University of South Carolina
Charleston, South Carolina

Carol Burke, MSN, APN/CNS, RNC-OB, C-EFM
Loyola University Chicago Perinatal Center
Chicago, Illinois

Fran Byrd, RN, NNP-BC, MPH
Director of Strategic Initiatives
The National Certification Corporation (NCC)
Chicago, Illinois

Cheryl A. Carlson PhD, APRN, NNP-BC
Neonatal Nurse Practitioner
Medical University of South Carolina
Charleston, South Carolina

Terri A. Cavaliere, DNP, RN, NNP-BC
Clinical Assistant Professor, School of Nursing
Stony Brook University
Stony Brook, New York;
Neonatal Nurse Practitioner
Cohen Children's Hospital at North Shore
Manhasset, New York

Margaret Conway-Orgel, MSN, APRN, NNP-BC
Neonatal Nurse Practitioner
Medical University of South Carolina
Charleston, South Carolina

Bresney Crowell, MSN, APRN, NNP-BC
Neonatal Nurse Practitioner
Medical University of South Carolina
Charleston, South Carolina

Ana Francisca Diallo, BSN, RN
Doctoral Student, School of Nursing
University of Connecticut
Storrs, Connecticut

James R. Kiger, MD
Assistant Professor
Children's Hospital, Pediatrics/Neonatology
Medical University of South Carolina
Charleston, South Carolina

Frances R. Koch, MD
Department of Pediatrics
Children's Hospital, Division of Neonatology
Medical University of South Carolina
Charleston, South Carolina

Jacqueline M. McGrath, PhD, RN, FNAP, FAAN
Associate Dean, Research and Scholarship
Professor, School of Nursing
University of Connecticut
Storrs, Connecticut;
Director of Nursing Research
Connecticut Children's Medical Center
Hartford, Connecticut

Rebecca J. Paquette, BS
School of Nursing
University of Connecticut
Storrs, Connecticut

Julie R. Ross, MD
Assistant Professor
Children's Hospital, Pediatrics/Neonatology
Medical University of South Carolina
Charleston, South Carolina

Haifa (Abou) Samra, PhD, RNC-NIC
Associate Professor, School of Nursing
South Dakota State University
Brookings, South Dakota

Jan Sherman, RN, NNP-BC, PhD
Associate Teaching Professor, Sinclair School of Nursing
Adjunct Associate Professor, Department of Child Health
School of Medicine
University of Missouri – Columbia
Columbia, Missouri

Gautham K. Suresh, MBBS, MD, MS
Associate Professor, Pediatrics and Community and Family Medicine
Dartmouth-Hitchcock Medical Center
The Dartmouth Institute for Health Policy and Clinical Practice
Lebanon, New Hampshire

Ellen Tappero, DNP, RN, NNP-BC
Coordinator, Neonatal Nurse Practitioner Program
NAL/MEDNAX
Phoenix, Arizona;
Clinical Faculty, Neonatal Nurse Practitioner Program
University of Missouri – Kansas City
Kansas City, Missouri

Catherine Theorell, RNC, APN, NNP-BC, PhD
Assistant Clinical Professor, College of Nursing
University of Illinois at Chicago
Chicago, Illinois

Lyn Vargo, PhD, RN, NNP-BC
Clinical Assistant Professor, Neonatal Nurse Practitioner Program
Stony Brook University
Stony Brook, New York;
Clinical Assistant Professor, Neonatal Nurse Practitioner Program
University of Missouri – Kansas City
Kansas City, Missouri

Introduction

The "Golden Hours" of care refers to the unique care of very low birth weight (VLBW) babies in the first few hours of life. VLBW babies (<1,500 g) comprise the majority of high-risk deliveries. Even when vigorous and crying, pink, and well-perfused, these infants are at risk and require a team of well-trained, experienced personnel.

Decisions made in the first hours of life can result in a smooth transition to extrauterine life or can hasten and worsen maladaptation. In addition, disease processes in these infants often require prompt intervention to lessen their severity and reduce the risk of lifelong complications.

Vulnerability in VLBW infants is especially high because of their premature development and the unique aspects of their physiology before, during, and after transition. These factors place multiple systems at risk.

Immature skin and high trans-epidermal water loss (TEWL) contribute to these infants' thermoregulatory needs and can result in electrolyte abnormalities and hypothermia. Limited skin barriers, with only 3–4 cell layers to their epidermis, contributes not only to TEWL, but also increases their risk of infection. They are born with surfactant-deficient lungs and diminished muscular strength that leads to respiratory distress that is progressive in nature if no intervention is provided.

Interventions — even lifesaving interventions — can impact their care.

Providing oxygen increases the risk of damage because of these infants' immature tissue. Anatomic and physiologic issues that impact cardiac output and perfusion may alter cardiac adaptation. Immature brain physiology increases the risk of disorders related, at least in part, to aberrations in perfusion associated with risks of intraventricular hemorrhage, periventricular white matter disease, and global cerebral hypoxia-ischemia that lead to poor neurodevelopment outcomes. A knowledgeable team skilled in the coordinated care of these infants is essential if outcomes are to be positive.

This book is an effort to assist health care providers to have real impact on the short- and long-term outcomes of VLBW infants during the Golden Hours of life. It is not just a guide to care, but a handbook with tools and resources to assist providers.

It is vital that health care providers understand the special needs of this very vulnerable group of infants. While all VLBW newborns require stabilization, approximately 10 percent also require resuscitation. The American Academy of Pediatrics (AAP) and the American Heart Association (AHA) have developed standards for neonatal resuscitation. Their guidelines are based on the International Liaison Committee on Resuscitation consensus and are used within the Neonatal Resuscitation Program (NRP) that is a national standard for all heath care providers who attend deliveries. These principles are stressed throughout this book.

Every VLBW infant deserves to have care from a dedicated and coordinated team that demonstrates a clear understanding of NRP guidelines through successful course completion and ongoing competency assessment.

It is imperative that you always follow your facility's protocols, guidelines, and dosage plans. We hope this book will be an additional, valuable resource to those who provide this vital care to these vulnerable infants. Our goal is to improve practice and outcomes.

We all want to make a difference in our work. Those of us who are fortunate enough to care for these infants in the Golden Hours of life know that we make huge differences in the lives of these infants and their families.

We would like to thank all of the authors who contributed their time, talents, and expertise. We would also like to thank NCC for publishing this book. We hope *Golden Hours: Care of the Very Low Birth Weight Infant* provides you, the practitioner, with another tool in your arsenal to bring about the best outcomes possible.

Robin L. Bissinger, PhD, APRN, NNP-BC, FAAN
David J. Annibale, MD

From the Publisher

Each year, NCC is faced with an imposing decision: How to allocate our resources for continuing-competency activities of our certified constituency. In the case of *Golden Hours: Care of the Very Low Birth Weight Infant*, the decision was simple. Robin Bissinger made us do it.

Robin approached us brimming with passion about the topic and how this book could help practitioners provide the best of care during the low birth weight neonate's first Golden Hours of life. We couldn't say no.

This is the first time that NCC has published a book. But we believe it could not be a better first effort. The book provides a general review of the critical aspects of care that are needed in these Golden Hours, as well as a list of resources and tools that practitioners can apply in real time.

We hope this resource will be valuable to those certified by NCC, and to the neonatal community at large. Here in a single reference are tools to help providers improve the outcomes for these special neonates and support their families during this challenging time.

Robin left the NCC presidency in 2013, but she has provided a great legacy with this effort. This valuable resource that she envisioned will help both practitioners and all those vulnerable neonates born too soon or too sick to make a normal transition.

Thank you to Robin and to all who made this book a reality.

Betty Burns, CAE
Executive Director
The National Certification Corporation (NCC)
Chicago, Illinois

Contents

1. **Fetal Assessment** 1
   *Carol Burke, MSN, APN/CNS, RNC-OB, C-EFM and
   Catherine Theorell, RNC, APN, NNP-BC, PhD*

2. **Maternal Risk Factors** 43
   Catherine Theorell, RNC, APN, NNP-BC, PhD

3. **Neonatal Assessment** 77
   Terri A. Cavaliere, DNP, RN, NNP-BC

4. **Transition at Birth and Umbilical Cord Blood Gas Analysis** 89
   Gautham K. Suresh, MBBS, MD, MS

5. **Basic Management of the Airway** 101
   Catherine Theorell, RNC, APN, NNP-BC, PhD

6. **Cardiac Support** 117
   Catherine Theorell, RNC, APN, NNP-BC, PhD

7. **Thermoregulation** 123
   Robin L. Bissinger, PhD, APRN, NNP-BC, FAAN

8. **Respiratory Diseases** 139
   Frances R. Koch, MD

9. **Pulmonary Emergencies** 159
   Cheryl A. Carlson, PhD, APRN, NNP-BC

10. **Cardiovascular Stability and Shock** 175
    Lyn Vargo, PhD, RN, NNP-BC

11. **Cardiac Emergencies** 185
    Julie R. Ross, MD

12. **Fluids, Electrolytes, and Nutrition** 209
    Jan Sherman, RN, NNP-BC, PhD

13. **Hypoglycemia** 221
    Jan Sherman, RN, NNP-BC, PhD

14. **Neonatal Sepsis** 231
    Jan Sherman, RN, NNP-BC, PhD

15. **Intraventricular Hemorrhage** 247
    *Bresney Crowell, MSN, APRN, NNP-BC
    and David J. Annibale, MD*

16 Hematologic Emergencies 265
James R. Kiger, MD

17 Surgical Emergencies: Abdominal Wall Defects 281
*Robin L. Bissinger, PhD, APRN, NNP-BC, FAAN
and Ellen Tappero, DNP, RN, NNP-BC*

18 Congenital Anomalies 289
Ellen Tappero, DNP, RN, NNP-BC

19 Developmentally Supportive and Family-Centered Care 315
*Jacqueline M. McGrath, PhD, RN, FNAP, FAAN;
Ana Francisca Diallo, BSN, RN; Rebecca J. Paquette, BS;
and Haifa (Abou) Samra, PhD, RNC-NIC*

20 Ethical Dilemmas 325
Margaret Conway-Orgel, MSN, APRN, NNP-BC

21 Teamwork and Communication 333
Margaret Conway-Orgel, MSN, APRN, NNP-BC

22 Neonatal Transport 343
Fran Byrd, RN, NNP-BC, MPH

23 Procedural Review 363
Cheryl A. Carlson, PhD, APRN, NNP-BC

Appendix A: Resource Toolbox 377

I. **Fetal Assessment** 378
   A. Fetal Lung Maturity 378
   B. Reference Values for Umbilical Cord Blood Gas Values 378
   C. Umbilical Sampling 378

II. **Respiratory System** 379
   A. Targeted Saturation Goal in the First 10 Min of Life 379
   B. Apgar Scoring at Birth 379
   C. Initial Positive-Pressure Ventilation (PPV) 380
   D. Intubation Guidelines 380

III. Thermoregulation 381
   A. Recommended Axillary Temperatures in Infants ≤1,500 Grams   381
   B. Recommended Stabilization Room Temperatures Based on Post-Menstrual Age and Birth Weight   381
   C. Example of Humidity Guidelines   382

IV. Cardiovascular System 383
   A. Treatment of Hypotension   383
   B. Recommended Volume Expanders in the Delivery Room   383

V. Fluids and Electrolytes 384
   A. Suggested Response to Blood Glucose ≤45 mg/dL or Symptomatic (Example of a Protocol)   384

VI. Neurological System 385
   A. Grading of Intraventricular Hemorrhage (IVH)   385

VII. Procedures 386
   A. Umbilical Line Measurements and Placement   386

VIII. Web Resources 387

Appendix B: Glossary of Acronyms   389

Index   395

Fetal Assessment

Carol Burke and Catherine Theorell

I. Pregnancy
A. Duration of pregnancy
1. Normal length of gestation is 280 days (40 weeks) from the first day of the woman's last normal menstrual period.
2. Because the actual date of conception is often unknown, the expected date of delivery or confinement (EDC) is a range of +/- 2 weeks to account for variations in ovulation timing. With assisted reproduction, timing is more accurate.
3. Pregnancy is divided into three trimesters:
   a. First trimester: 0–12 weeks
   b. Second trimester: 13–26 weeks
   c. Third trimester: 27 weeks until term
B. First trimester: Fertilization through 12 weeks gestation
1. Fertilization – zygote formation
   a. Occurs in the upper third of the fallopian tube
   b. Cell division continues into inner cell mass, giving rise to germ layers; and outer cell mass, giving rise to placental tissue
2. Multiple gestation
   a. Monozygotic — division of a single ovum after fertilization
      (1) Separation and duplication at 2–3 days after fertilization forms dichorionic-diamniotic gestation.
      (2) Separation and duplication of the inner cell mass 4–7 days after fertilization forms monochorionic-diamniotic gestation.
         (a) Most common for monozygotic formations
         (b) Twin-to-twin transfusion possible
      (3) Separation and duplication at day 7–13 forms monochorionic-monoamniotic gestation.
         (a) Higher rate of mortality due to cord entanglement
         (b) Twin-to-twin transfusion possible
      (4) Separation at 14 days and after is usually incomplete, resulting in conjoined twins.

b. Dizygotic — simultaneous fertilization of two ova (70% twins are dizygotic)
   (1) Strong maternal familial tendency
   (2) Increased incidence with increased parity, maternal age, maternal body mass index (BMI)
   (3) Always dichorionic-diamniotic, placentas may be fused or separated
3. Period of the embryo — 2 weeks after fertilization until end of 8 weeks of gestation
   a. Organogenesis completed
   b. All major systems established, greatest period of vulnerability and susceptibility to malformations
4. Period of the fetus — from 9 weeks gestation to delivery
   a. Rapid growth and gradual increase in functional ability
   b. Fetal organ growth not synchronous, systems have varying degrees of susceptibility to malformations due to environmental or maternal conditions
5. Ultrasound measurements
   a. To date, there is no proof that diagnostic ultrasound exposure has adverse effects on the developing human fetus.
   b. The gestational sac can be measured at 5–6 weeks
   c. A fetal pole with movement and cardiac activity can be measured by 7–8 weeks. This provides an estimated gestational age with +/- 9 days accuracy.
   d. Crown-rump length (CRL) has greatest accuracy, +/- 4.7 days.
6. Uterine growth — at 12 weeks, uterus fills pelvis and fundus is at symphysis pubis

C. Second trimester: 13–26 weeks gestation
1. Fetal growth
   a. From 20 weeks until term, further maturation of organ and body systems occurs, with a progressive increase in weight.
   b. Fetal anatomy may be evaluated and possible anomalies detected via ultrasound.
   c. By 24 weeks, 60% of the weight and 20% of the growth should be present.
   d. In the first half of pregnancy, the fetus grows by increasing the number of cells at a rapid rate (hyperplasia, or growth through increasing cell numbers).

2. Ultrasound measurements
   a. Fetal measurements, including biparietal diameter and femur length, may be used to estimate fetal age accurately.
   b. Biparietal diameter is a fairly accurate method of determining fetal age between 13 and 30 weeks of gestation, providing accuracy of +/- 10 days.
   c. An ultrasound in the mid-second trimester may be useful to evaluate fetal size and identify any size-date discrepancies.
3. Uterine growth provides a rough estimate of gestational age and is influenced by adiposity, variations in body shape, or presence of uterine fibroids.
   a. By 16 weeks, the uterine fundus is midway between the symphysis pubis and the umbilicus.
   b. At 20 weeks, the uterine fundus is expected at the umbilical level.
   c. Fundal height measurements, especially when confirmed by the onset of quickening and audible heart tones and an accurate menstrual history, can help to determine whether a size-date discrepancy exists.
   d. Maternal obesity, poor prenatal care, and uncertain menstrual history may confound assessment of fetal size-date measurements.
   e. Variations
      (1) Uterine size that is greater than expected may suggest multiple gestation, inaccurate dating, uterine anomalies, molar pregnancy, or polyhydramnios.
      (2) Uterine size that is less than expected may indicate inaccurate dating, intrauterine growth failure, or oligohydramnios, etc.
4. Fetal surveillance
   a. Goal is to prevent fetal death without false positive or false negative results that result in unexpected outcomes.
      (1) A false positive test implies that a condition exists when it actually does not exist.
      (2) A false negative test implies that a condition does not exist when it actually does exist.

b. Ultrasound may be used during the second half of pregnancy to assess blood flow changes in the fetal heart, aorta, cerebrum, and uterine and umbilical arteries.
  5. Viability
     a. The ability or capacity to survive outside the uterus
     b. Not defined by a worldwide, uniform, gestational age
D. Third trimester: 27–40 weeks gestation
  1. Fetal growth is governed by inherited genetic growth potential and can be influenced by maternal, placental, or uterine factors.
     a. Genetic determinants and environmental factors can play an important role in fetal development.
     b. Maternal nutrition, general maternal health, and exposure to legal and illicit drugs will influence fetal growth.
     c. Perfusion of the intervillous spaces and the availability of glucose, amino acids, and fats in maternal blood avail growth substrates to the fetus.
  2. Fetal growth continues through cellular hyperplasia, but the fetus primarily grows through cellular hypertrophy (growth through the enlargement of individual cells). Fetal growth increases linearly; as the infant reaches term, the rate of fetal growth slows.
     a. The fetus gains 85% of its body weight during the last half of pregnancy.
     b. Throughout gestation, there is a gradual decrease in total body water and in extracellular water; intracellular water increases as gestation progresses (**Fig. 1-1**).
     c. Rates of growth vary for specific organs and tissues.
     d. Based on the ratio of organ size to body size, the brain is the largest contributor to body mass, making up 13% in infants vs. 2% in adults.
     e. Infants' skin, kidneys, and liver are also twice as large in percentile as adults'.
  3. Gestational age definitions
     a. Early preterm: Birth at <34 weeks gestation
     b. Late preterm: Birth at 34 to 36-6/7 weeks gestation
     c. Early term: Birth at 37 to 38-6/7 weeks gestation
     d. Full term: Birth at 39 to 40-6/7 weeks gestation
     e. Late term: Birth at 41 completed weeks gestation
     f. Post term: Birth at ≥42 completed weeks gestation

4. Ultrasound measurements
    a. Ultrasounds are useful to detect other anomalies and to assess the volume of amniotic fluid (**Fig. 1-2**).
    b. Between 32 and 34 weeks, altered growth rates may be found in small for gestational age (SGA) and large for gestational age (LGA) fetuses.
    c. Growth curves are used in the third trimester.
        (1) SGA
            (a) Infants who are two standard deviations below the mean, or <10th percentile
            (b) Pathological or non-pathological factors may alter growth
        (2) Average for gestational age
        (3) LGA: ≥90th percentile
        (4) Intrauterine-growth restriction (IUGR)
            (a) Failure of a fetus to achieve its genetic growth potential *in utero.*
            (b) Occurs as a result of reduced growth potential or multiple maternal adverse effects, which places the fetus at increased risk for hypoxia.
            (c) Asymmetric growth restriction is usually due to extrinsic factors, such as maternal preeclampsia, placental insufficiency, and fetal malnutrition.

FIGURE 1-1
Changes in Body Water Throughout Gestation

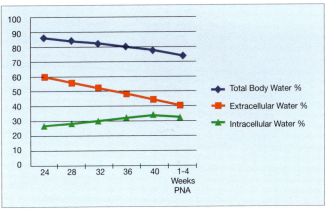

The fetus gains 85% of its body weight during the last half of pregnancy. Throughout gestation, there is a gradual decrease in total body water and in extracellular water; intracellular water increases as gestation progresses.

(d) The terms IUGR and SGA are not equivalent.
(e) Only 50% of these infants are identified prior to birth.
(f) The neonate is at risk for conditions such as perinatal asphyxia, meconium aspiration, hypoglycemia, cold stress, and polycythemia.

II. The placenta and placental physiology
A. Implantation
1. Mediated by coordinated actions between maternal and embryonic cells.
2. Implantation and placentation requires communication between the developing embryonic cells and maternal uterine receptivity, which includes increased vascularity, edema, increased secretory activity, and microvilli trophoblastic development.
3. The ideal window for implantation occurs ~6–10 days after ovulation.
4. The location for attachment is usually on the upper posterior wall of the uterus, but can occur on various other intrauterine and extrauterine sites.

FIGURE 1-2
Using Ultrasound to Measure Amniotic Fluid

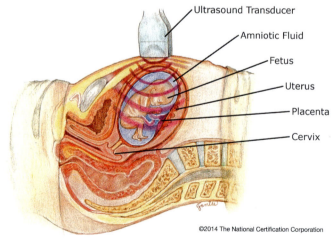

©2014 The National Certification Corporation

Ultrasounds are useful to detect anomalies and to assess the volume of amniotic fluid. Between 32 and 34 weeks, altered growth rates may be found in fetuses who are SGA or LGA.

5. Human chorionic gonadotropin (hCG) can be detected in maternal serum and urine 7–8 days after ovulation or around the time of implantation.
6. Slight bleeding may occur during implantation, which may be mistaken for a scanty, short menstrual period.
7. The endometrium following implantation is referred to as decidua. The decidua basalis forms the maternal portion of the placenta and is the site in which separation of the placenta occurs after delivery of the fetus.

B. Normal development
   1. The placenta is a fetal organ and the maternal-fetal interface.
   2. Development and function are directly related to the growth and well-being of the fetus; antenatal testing assesses the functionality.
   3. By 21–22 days, a primitive fetoplacental circulation is established between blood in the chorionic villi and embryonic vessels.
   4. The mature placenta is established at ~10–12 weeks of gestation, when maternal spiral arteries open and supply blood to the intervillous space.
   5. The intervillous space surrounds numerous chorionic villi within the placenta.
      a. The intervillous space is the site for simple (passive) diffusion, facilitated diffusion, active transport, bulk flow, and pinocytosis; which allow for the exchange of gases and nutrients and the removal of waste.
      b. Oxygen and carbon dioxide diffuse readily across the thin blood-blood barrier.
      c. Restriction of fetal oxygenation may result from acute or chronic conditions that reduce maternal blood entering the intervillous space.

C. Abnormalities of the chorionic villi may occur with the initial invasion of maternal spiral arteries and villi or the secondary destruction by infarction, thrombosis, hemorrhage, or infection.
   1. Hypoplasia may result in abortion or abruption and increase the risk of stillbirth, IUGR, and preterm delivery.
   2. Hyperplasia is possibly due to suboptimal oxygenation and has been observed in women with hypertension and prolonged pregnancy. Large placentas are seen with severe erythroblastosis, some class A–C diabetic pregnancies, and cigarette smokers.

3. Preeclampsia is thought to be associated with abnormal vascular invasion and remodeling at the level of the spiral arteries, which leads to abnormal perfusion of nutrients into the intervillous space.
D. Fetal/placental circulation
 1. Adequate blood flow to and through the placenta from both maternal and fetal circulation is essential for exchange of nutrients, gases, and waste products.
 2. Fetal circulation
    a. Umbilical vein
       (1) Carries blood from the placenta to the fetus.
    b. Ductous venosus
       (1) Connects the umbilical vein with the inferior vena cava.
       (2) Less than one-third enters the fetal ductus venosus, while the remainder enters the liver proper from the inferior border.
       (3) Blood travels via the inferior vena cava to the right atrium of the heart.
    c. Foramen ovale
       (1) Blood passes through an opening between the right and left atrium (the foramen ovale), bypassing pulmonary circulation.
       (2) Blood flow continues into the left ventricle and is pumped through the aorta, primarily to the head and into the body.
       (3) Blood returns from the head via the superior vena cava into the right atrium, enters the right ventricle, and is pumped into the pulmonary artery.
    d. Ductus arteriosus
       (1) A connection between the pulmonary artery and the aorta with the purpose of bypassing the lungs.
       (2) 90% of the blood flow passes through this ductus, while 10% enters the lungs.
       (3) From the ductus arteriosus, the blood moves from the aorta through the internal iliac arteries.
    e. Two umbilical arteries
       (1) A branch of the hypogastric arteries that return deoxygenated blood to the placenta, where carbon dioxide and other waste products from the fetus are taken up and enter the maternal circulation.

3. Changes at birth
   a. When the infant breathes for the first time, there is a decrease in the resistance in the pulmonary vasculature, which causes the pressure in the left atrium to increase relative to the pressure in the right atrium.
   b. An increase in left-sided pressure leads to the closure of the foramen ovale.
   c. The increase in the oxygen concentration in the blood leads to a decrease in prostaglandins, causing closure of the ductus arteriosus over 12–24 hours.
   d. These closures prevent blood from bypassing pulmonary circulation, allowing the neonate's blood to become oxygenated via the newly operational lungs.

E. Maternal circulation
   1. Blood flows to the uterus via the uterine arteries and reaches the placenta via the altered spiral arteries of the uterus.
   2. The intervillous space in the mature placenta contains ~150 mL of blood; the rate of flow increases during pregnancy, from 50 mL/min at 10 weeks to 500–600 mL/min by term.
   3. Uterine contractions limit the entry of blood into the intervillous space; oxygen transfer to the fetus may be decreased during a normal contraction.
   4. The blood flows around the chorionic villi, allowing exchange of materials between maternal and fetal circulation.
   5. Pressures within this system are low; increased blood flow is mediated by the low-resistance uteroplacental circuit, alteration in maternal cardiac output, system and peripheral vascular resistance, and hormonal/chemical influences.
   6. The spiral arteries underlying the placenta are almost completely dilated and become distended, flaccid, saclike structures with low resistance that are able to accommodate the blood needed to supply and provide reserve in the intervillous spaces. These arteries are no longer responsive to systemic circulatory pressor agents or influences of the autonomic nervous system.

F. Placental separation
   1. Separation occurs normally during the third stage of labor. Delivery causes sudden emptying of the uterus, leading to a decrease in the support base for the placenta and the shearing of the placenta from the decidua basalis.
      a. Gross examination for abruption, calcification, meconium staining, and infection of the placenta upon delivery is important and may yield the need for microscopic evaluation.
      b. Retained fragments of the placenta and membranes can lead to uterine atony, hemorrhage, or infection.

III. Antepartum fetal surveillance
   A. Initiation and frequency
      1. Testing is initiated when individual clinical circumstances warrant fetal monitoring. Initiating testing at 32–34 weeks of gestation is appropriate for most pregnancies with increased risk of stillbirth.
      2. A reactive test indicative of normal fetal acid-base balance should be repeated periodically (weekly or twice weekly) until delivery when a high-risk condition persists.
      3. More frequent testing intervals, with individualization based on the high-risk clinical setting or any significant deterioration in the clinical status (e.g. worsening preeclampsia, decreased fetal activity) requires fetal reevaluation, regardless of the amount of time elapsed since the last test.
   B. Maternal conditions that warrant antenatal testing
      1. Antiphospholipid syndrome
      2. Poorly controlled hyperthyroidism
      3. Diabetes mellitus
      4. Cyanotic heart disease
      5. Systemic lupus erythematosus
      6. Hypertensive disorders
      7. Chronic renal disease
      8. Hemoglobinopathies
      9. Substance/environmental exposures
      10. Decreased fetal movement
      11. Oligohydramnios
      12. Polyhydramnios
      13. IUGR
      14. Multiple gestation
      15. Post-term pregnancies

16. Previous fetal demise
17. Isoimmunization
18. Prolonged premature rupture of membranes
19. Unexplained third trimester bleeding

C. Fetal movement counting
1. Fetal movement is usually perceived at 18–20 weeks of gestation.
2. Several methods of fetal movement counting are in place; neither the ideal number of kicks nor the duration for counting has been determined.
3. There is not enough evidence to influence practice. In particular, no trials have compared fetal movement counting vs. no fetal movement counting to determine morbidity.
4. Decreased fetal movement may be affected by:
   a. Placental location
   b. Maternal smoking, opioid or steroid use, alcohol
   c. Maternal perception
   d. Decreased uterine space
   e. Adiposity
   f. Hypoglycemia or hyperglycemia
5. The fetus has periods of sleep when activity is lower and movement decreased.
6. Fetal heart rate (FHR) usually increases with movement.

D. Non-stress test (NST)
1. Definition
   a. Non-invasive test to evaluate the presence of accelerations in the FHR that are either spontaneous or in association with fetal movement
   b. Common method of fetal surveillance
2. Physiologic basis
   a. Fetal movement and accelerations require an intact central nervous system (CNS) reflective of adequate fetal oxygenation and autonomic function.
   b. The normal fetus moves at various intervals; the CNS and myocardium respond to movement with acceleration of the FHR.
   c. Since 1975, fetal movements and FHR accelerations have been recognized indicators of fetal well-being.
3. Procedure
   a. An external fetal monitor is applied, including both a tocodynamometer and an ultrasound transducer.
   b. A baseline FHR tracing is obtained.

c. The mother presses a button to indicate fetal movement.
d. The FHR tracing is evaluated for the presence of accelerations with fetal movement.
e. An acceleration is considered to be present if detected on the monitor, even if the mother does not perceive a fetal movement.

4. Interpretation of results
   a. Reactive NST ($\geq$32 weeks gestation)
      (1) Presence of two or more accelerations reaching a peak of $\geq$15 beats/min (bpm) above the baseline rate and lasting for $\geq$15 sec from onset to return in a 20-min period
      (2) An indicator of normal fetal acid-base balance
   b. Reactive NST (28 to 31-6/7 weeks gestation)
      (1) Presence of two accelerations $\geq$10 bpm lasting $\geq$10 sec over a 20-min interval
      (2) NST of non-compromised preterm fetus (24–28 weeks gestation) is frequently nonreactive
   c. Nonreactive NST
      (1) Defined as one that does not show such accelerations over a 40-min period

5. Considerations with nonreactive NST
   a. May be benign and temporary due to fetal immaturity, quiet fetal sleep, or maternal smoking
   b. May be a sign of fetal hypoxemia or acidosis and thus necessitate additional testing
   c. May be related to fetal neurological or cardiac anomalies, sepsis, or maternal ingestion of drugs with cardiac effects
   d. Use of vibroacoustic stimulation
      (1) Decreases testing time and may be used for the term infant
      (2) Applies a vibratory sound stimulus to the abdomen over the fetal head for 1–3 sec
      (3) May be repeated at 1-min intervals for a total of three stimuli
      (4) Will elicit an acceleration due to fetal startle reflex

6. Follow-up
   a. There is a <1% chance of fetal death within 1 week of a reactive NST.

- b. FHR decelerations during the NST, regardless of reactivity, warrant consideration of further testing or delivery.
- c. The nonreactive NST indicates a need for further testing and should be followed by a contraction stress test (CST) or biophysical profile (BPP).
- d. False negative/false positive
    - (1) False positive
        - (a) Results in a nonreactive NST when the fetus is normal.
        - (b) Between 28 and 32 weeks of gestation, 15% of normal fetuses have nonreactive NSTs.
        - (c) 90% of these fetuses have a negative CST.
    - (2) False negative
        - (a) Results in reactive FHR when a hypoxic condition actually exists.
        - (b) Rate is 6.8:1000.

E. CST
  1. Definition
     a. Antepartum observation assessing for evidence of transient fetal hypoxemia, demonstrated by late decelerations when the fetus is exposed to the stress of uterine contractions
     b. An infrequently used test to determine how the fetus responds to relative hypoxemia during a contraction
  2. Physiologic basis
     a. Fetal oxygenation will be transiently worsened by uterine contractions and, in the fetus with suboptimal oxygenation, the added stress will lead to late decelerations.
     b. Due to the state of hypoxemia with deteriorating reserves, the fetus may not withstand labor contractions without developing metabolic acidosis.
     c. Relative contraindications to the test include conditions that are associated with an increased risk of preterm labor and delivery, uterine rupture, or uterine bleeding. These include preterm labor, preterm premature rupture of the membranes (PPROM), history of extensive uterine surgery or prior classic cesarean birth, and known placenta previa.

3. Procedure
   a. May be performed by nipple stimulation or by administering an IV infusion with oxytocin. If at least three spontaneous contractions ≥40 sec are present in 10 min, no uterine stimulation is necessary.
   b. Nipple stimulation
      (1) With the mother in a semi-Fowlers position with a lateral tilt, apply external monitor and establish FHR baseline.
      (2) Assess maternal blood pressure every 15 min during the test.
      (3) Instruct the mother to brush the palmar surface of her fingers over the nipple of one breast through her clothes; continue 4 cycles of 2 min on and 2–5 minutes off; stop when contraction begins and re-stimulate when contraction ends. If not effective, she may brush both nipples simultaneously.
      (4) Discontinue nipple stimulation when three or more spontaneous contractions ≥40 sec occur in a 10-min period.
      (5) If nipple stimulation does not produce the desired uterine activity, an oxytocin-stimulated CST may be necessary.
   c. Oxytocin challenge
      (1) With the mother in a semi-Fowlers position with a lateral tilt, apply external monitors, establish FHR baseline, and begin mainline IV infusion.
      (2) Assess maternal blood pressure every 15 min during the test.
      (3) Piggyback oxytocin into the primary IV line in the port nearest the IV insertion site.
      (4) Begin oxytocin at 0.5–2.0 mU/min and increase the dosage by 0.5–1.0 mU/min at 15-min intervals until three contractions of ≥40 sec duration have occurred within 10 min.
      (5) Discontinue the oxytocin when three contractions have occurred within a 10-min period of interpretable data.
      (6) Discontinue the oxytocin with tachysystole, a prolonged deceleration, or recurrent late decelerations.
      (7) Terbutaline may be required for tocolysis.

                (8) Continue to monitor until uterine activity and
                    FHR return to baseline status.
        4. Interpretation of results
            a. Negative: No late decelerations
            b. Positive: Late decelerations with 50% or more of
               contractions
            c. Equivocal
                (1) Suspicious: Intermittent late decelerations are
                    present, but at a frequency of ≤50% of uterine
                    contractions.
                (2) Tachysystole: FHR decelerations occur in the
                    presence of contractions that occur more
                    frequently than every 2 min or with a duration of
                    ≥90 sec.
                (3) Unsatisfactory: Fewer than three contractions
                    occur in 10 min or a tracing that is not
                    interpretable.
        5. Follow-up
            a. Negative CST predicts continued fetal well-being for
               7 days and needs only to be repeated weekly, provided
               maternal well-being is the same.
            b. Equivocal CST should be followed with another form
               of fetal assessment (e.g. BPP).
            c. Positive CST should be followed by an assessment of
               variability to help determine the need for immediate
               delivery. A category-3 pattern requires an urgent
               management plan.
            d. False-positive rate is >50% and may be due to supine
               hypotension during the test (tachysystole, etc.). False
               negative is <1%.
F. BPP
    1. Definition
        a. Combines reactive NST with ultrasonography to
           evaluate fetal well-being over a 30-min observation
           period
    2. Physiologic basis
        a. Implies absence of significant CNS hypoxemia/
           acidemia at the time of testing
        b. Presence of five biophysical variables: FHR reactivity,
           fetal movement, tone, and breathing reflect acute
           fetal state; amniotic fluid volume serves as marker of
           chronic state of placental function

3. Procedure
   a. Ultrasound examination performed over a 30-min period to assess fetal tone, movement, breathing, fetal reactivity, and amniotic fluid
      (1) Gross body movements: Four or more discrete body or limb movements
      (2) Fetal muscle tone: One or more episodes of active extension with return to flexion of limb or trunk and/or opening and closing hand
      (3) Fetal breathing: Intermittent, multiple episodes of hiccups or rhythmic fetal breathing movements of $\geq$30-sec duration
      (4) Amniotic fluid index >5 cm total or at least one pocket >2 cm
      (5) Reactive FHR
4. Interpretation of results
   a. Each component is assigned a score of 2 if present, 0 if not, for a total of 10.
      (1) Score of 8–10 with normal amniotic fluid is normal and indicates a 0.8% chance of fetal death. Repeat test in 3-4 days.
      (2) Score of 6 is considered equivocal; the test should be repeated. A persistent score of 6 indicates delivery of a mature fetus. If the fetus is immature, repeat the test in 24 hours.
      (3) Score of $\leq$4 is abnormal. Unless extenuating circumstances exist, consider delivery by obstetrically appropriate method.
      (4) Score of 0–2 means immediate delivery is necessary and indicates a 40% chance of fetal death.
   b. Oligohydramnios (amniotic fluid index $\leq$5) constitutes an abnormal biophysical assessment, regardless of the overall score.
      (1) Increases risk of preterm delivery or low birth weight, lower Apgar scores, intrauterine fetal death, meconium-stained amniotic fluid, more admissions to NICU, and cesarean delivery.
      (2) Prolonged oligohydramnios may result in severe pulmonary hypoplasia, as seen in infants with renal aplasia.
   c. False negative rate is superior to that of the NST alone and compares with the CST 0.6/1000.

5. Factors affecting test results
   a. Administration of antenatal corticosteroids
      (1) Can be associated with transient FHR and behavioral changes that typically return to baseline by day 4 after treatment.
      (2) The most consistent FHR finding is a decrease in variability on days 2 and 3.
      (3) Fetal breathing and body movements are also commonly reduced, which may result in a lower BPP score or nonreactive NST.
   b. Onset of labor
      (1) Although fetal breathing and body movements decrease before the onset of spontaneous labor, other parameters that make up the BPP are present at early gestational ages and are useful in the evaluation of a very immature fetus.
   c. Sedation, stimulants, indomethacin, cigarette smoking
   d. Maternal hyperglycemia and hypoglycemia
G. Modified biophysical profile
   1. Definition
      a. An evaluation of fetal well-being
   2. Physiologic basis
      a. The NST is a short-term indicator of fetal hypoxemia.
      b. The amniotic fluid volume is an indicator of long-term placental function. Decrease in placental perfusion results in decreased blood flow and less oxygen to fetus, which diverts blood flow away from non-vital organs, including the kidneys. Decreased renal perfusion results in decreased fetal urine output, leading to decreased amniotic fluid.
   3. Procedure
      a. Combines the NST and ultrasonic evaluation of amniotic fluid volume (AFV)
      b. Performed once to twice weekly
   4. Interpretation of results
      a. Normal: Reactive NST, amniotic fluid volume >5 cm, and absence of variable or late decelerations
      b. Abnormal: Any of the following require complete BPP or CST
         (1) Nonreactive NST
         (2) Variable or late decelerations
         (3) AFV ≤ 5 cm

5. Follow-up
   a. Test is repeated twice weekly.
   b. False negative rate is 0.8/1000; false positive rate is 60%.
H. Umbilical Doppler velocimetry
   1. Definition
      a. A noninvasive method to assess the uteroplacental blood flow in the umbilical arteries.
      b. Umbilical artery, fetal aorta, and middle cerebral artery velocimetry is a relatively new antepartum fetal surveillance method used to assess placental function in women who may have fetal growth restriction.
   2. Physiologic basis
      a. Normally, the end-diastolic velocity in the umbilical arteries increases with advancing gestation secondary to decreased resistance in the placenta as more tertiary vessels develop.
      b. The velocity of blood flow through the umbilical artery can be detected with Doppler waveform analysis.
   3. Procedure
      a. Assist the mother into a supine position with a left tilt to facilitate adequate blood flow and reduce maternal positional side effects.
      b. A pulsed Doppler device is positioned over the fetus.
      c. The umbilical artery blood flow is distinguished from other blood flow by its characteristic waveform.
      d. The directed blood flow within the umbilical arteries is calculated using the difference between the systolic and the diastolic flow.
      e. Measurements are averaged from at least five waveforms.
   4. Interpretation of results
      a. Absent or reversed flow can occur when more of the vessels are abnormal.
         (1) Absent or end-flow velocity is an indication for preparation for delivery in consideration with other clinical factors.
         (2) Reversed end-flow velocity is an indication for immediate delivery.

b. Elevations of the systolic/diastolic ratio are seen in hypertensive disorders of pregnancy, fetal growth restriction, or other causes of uteroplacental insufficiency.
  c. Abnormal flow in the ductus venosus indicates serious compromise and increased morbidity and mortality.
5. Implications for management
  a. Abnormal Doppler flow precedes FHR abnormalities by 7 days.
  b. Doppler flow velocities of maternal and fetal circulation detect vascular resistance before onset of IUGR.
  c. Maternal uterine artery notching indicates preeclampsia and IUGR.
  d. Doppler flow velocity of the fetal middle cerebral artery has been used as a surrogate measure of fetal anemia; peak systolic velocity is inversely correlated to fetal hemoglobin.

IV. Intrapartum fetal monitoring

A. Overview
  1. Electronic heart rate monitoring has been used since the early 1970s; no decrease in intrapartum fetal deaths, morbidity, or cerebral palsy has been proven, despite several randomized controlled trials and retrospective studies.
  2. Labor is metabolically stressful to the fetus; a progressive decrease in fetal pH and oxygenation develops.
  3. Healthy fetuses tolerate and recover from labor.
  4. Continuous or intermittent monitoring is equally effective. The effect of electronic fetal monitoring on the perinatal death rate is unclear. Most obstetric units cannot provide the level of nursing care that intermittent auscultation requires.
  5. FHR monitoring is not a specific technique for identifying the compromised fetus. The high false positive rate (category 2 and 3) may induce clinicians to perform unnecessary interventions, with the intention of preventing of fetal neurologic injury.
  6. The NICHD convened a series of workshops to develop a standardized definition for FHR tracings to improve communication and allow evidence-based clinical management of intrapartum fetal compromise.

a. FHR patterns are produced by an external Doppler device detecting fetal cardiac motion or with a direct fetal electrode detecting the fetal EKG.
b. Patterns are categorized as baseline, periodic, or episodic.
    (1) Baseline patterns include baseline rate and variability.
    (2) Periodic and episodic patterns include FHR accelerations and decelerations.
        (a) Periodic patterns are those associated with uterine contractions.
        (b) Episodic patterns are those that occur spontaneously and are not associated with uterine contractions.
c. Abrupt shape is defined as the onset of the change in the FHR from the baseline to the nadir or peak in <30 sec (acceleration or variable deceleration).
d. Gradual shape applies to a deceleration that has a change in the FHR from the baseline to the nadir in ≥30 sec.
e. There are five basic components of a fetal heart rate tracing:
    (1) Uterine activity
    (2) Baseline rate
    (3) Baseline variability
    (4) Periodic or episodic changes (accelerations or decelerations)
    (5) Changes or trends over time (categories of FHR)

B. Uterine activity
  1. Definition
     a. The number of contractions present in a 10-min window, averaged over 30 min.
     b. Duration, intensity, and relaxation time between contractions are important in clinical practice.
  2. Terms
     a. Normal: Five contractions in 10 min, averaged over a 30-min window
     b. Tachysystole: More than five spontaneous or induced contractions in 10 min, averaged over a 30-min window
  3. Interpretation
     a. External (indirect) tocodynamometer
        (1) Determines contraction frequency and duration.

(2) Intensity requires palpation, which is described as mild, moderate, or strong, depending on the ability to indent the fundus with the fingertips.
(3) Resting tone should be palpated in between uterine activity.
  b. Internal (direct) intrauterine pressure catheter
    (1) Determines contraction frequency, duration and intensity
    (2) Intensity measured in mmHg for baseline tonus and peak intensity

C. Baseline FHR
  1. Definition
    a. The approximate mean FHR rounded to increments of 5 bpm during a 10-min segment (excluding periodic or episodic changes), periods of marked variability, and segments of baseline that differ by >25 bpm.
    b. A period of at least 10 min is required to determine baseline and at least 2 min of (not necessarily contiguous) information is required to establish a baseline.
    c. Baseline is reported as a single number, e.g., 145 bpm.
    d. The baseline is used as a reference point to determine variability and if accelerations or decelerations are present.
  2. Underlying physiology
    a. Regulated by the sinoatrial node, atrioventricular (AV) node, catecholamine release, and autonomic innervation (parasympathetic and sympathetic branches).
      (1) Sympathetic innervation and catecholamine release increases baseline FHR.
      (2) Parasympathetic innervation, carried by the vagus nerve, reduces the baseline rate.
    b. Chemoreceptors and baroreceptors located in the aortic arch and carotid arteries regulate the heart rate in response to changes in fetal partial pressure of oxygen (PO_2), partial pressure of carbon dioxide (PCO_2), and blood pressure.
  3. Rate
    a. Normal FHR baseline
      (1) Ranges from 110 to 160 bpm
      (2) Decreases with advancement of gestational age due to maturation of the parasympathetic pathway

b. Tachycardia – baseline >160 bpm
   (1) Any baseline FHR >160 bpm must be explained on some basis other than fetal prematurity.
   (2) Potential maternal conditions causing tachycardia:
      (a) Fever
      (b) Chorioamnionitis
      (c) Dehydration
      (d) Hyperthyroidism
      (e) Illicit substance use
      (f) β-sympathomimetic medications (terbutaline)
   (3) Potential fetal conditions causing tachycardia:
      (a) Anemia
      (b) Heart failure
      (c) Hypoxia
      (d) Infection or sepsis
      (e) Tachyarrhythmia
   (4) Implications
      (a) Increases myocardial oxygen demand, which utilizes fetal reserve.
   (5) Management
      (a) Base on the associated baseline FHR variability and the presence or absence of accelerations.
      (b) Maximize uteroplacental perfusion and identify if tachysystole exists.
      (c) Notify provider of fetal tachycardia.
c. Bradycardia – FHR <110 bpm
   (1) A sudden, profound bradycardia is a medical emergency.
   (2) Bradycardia that occurs during the second stage of labor following a previously normal FHR pattern may be due to increased vagal tone (head compression, rapid fetal descent) or, occasionally, umbilical cord occlusion.
   (3) Potential maternal conditions causing bradycardia:
      (a) Uterine rupture
      (b) Beta-blockers (propranolol [Inderal])
      (c) Hypoglycemia
      (d) Hypothermia
      (e) Urosepsis
      (f) Magnesium sulfate infusion
   (4) Potential fetal conditions causing bradycardia:
      (a) Dominance of AV node innervation with heart block arrhythmia

- (b) Chronic or acute hypoxemia
- (c) Prolapsed cord
- (5) Implications
  - (a) Bradycardia must be quickly distinguished from continuation of a prolonged deceleration.
  - (b) In the absence of a known cardiac condition, e.g., congenital heart block, bradycardia is a serious finding.
- (6) Management
  - (a) Differentiate maternal vs. fetal heart rate.
  - (b) Immediate delivery is usually required.

D. Baseline variability
  1. Definition
     a. Fluctuations in the baseline FHR of ≥ 2 cycles/min
     b. Fluctuations irregular in amplitude and frequency, quantitated in bpm, and measured from peak to trough in a single cycle
     c. Reflection of the interaction of the sympathetic and parasympathetic reflexes
  2. Categories
     a. Absent: Amplitude range undetectable
        (1) When associated with recurrent late or variable decelerations, it is most consistently associated with newborn acidosis and neonatal morbidity.
        (2) When present, it is an indication for obstetric evaluation and possible intervention.
     b. Minimal: Amplitude range detectable but ≤ 5 bpm
        (1) May be seen in states of fetal sleep, following administration of general anesthesia, and in response to maternal drugs (magnesium sulfate, opioids given for relief of labor pain, corticosteroids).
        (2) Minimal variability is a very nonspecific finding and must be interpreted in the context of other indicators of hypoxia; other causes of reduced variability must be considered.
        (3) Minimal variability without concomitant decelerations is almost always unrelated to fetal acidemia.
     c. Moderate: Amplitude range 6–25 bpm
        (1) Reliably indicates the absence of metabolic acidemia.

(2) Most important indicator of anatomic and functional integrity of pathways regulating cardiac function; reflects adequate cerebral oxygenation.
   d. Marked: Amplitude range >25 bpm
      (1) May occur with sympathetic stimulation in response to acute but temporary hypoxemia.
      (2) May also occur following administration of larger doses of ephedrine.
E. Periodic and episodic changes
   1. Accelerations (**Fig. 1-3**)
      a. Definition
         (1) Abrupt (onset to peak <30 sec) increase in FHR above baseline calculated from most recently determined portion of baseline
            (a) At ≥32 weeks of gestation, peak is ≥15 bpm above the baseline and entire event is ≥15 sec from onset to return to baseline.
            (b) At <32 weeks of gestation, peak is ≥10 bpm above the baseline and duration is ≥10 sec.
         (2) Prolonged if acceleration lasts 2–10 min in duration

FIGURE 1-3
Fetal Heart Monitor Strip Showing Accelerations

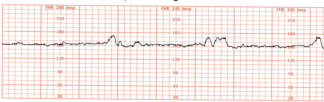
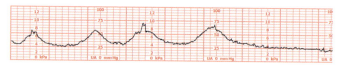

An abrupt (onset to peak <30 sec) increase in FHR above the baseline, calculated from the most recently determined portion of baseline, is thought to occur as a result of stimulation of peripheral proprioceptors, increased catecholamine release, and autonomic stimulation of the heart.

b. Physiologic mechanism
   (1) Thought to occur as a result of stimulation of peripheral proprioceptors, increased catecholamine release, and autonomic stimulation of the heart
c. Clinical significance
   (1) Indicator of normal fetal acid-base status when observed with fetal movements
   (2) Not required during active labor, but when present, denote a well-oxygenated fetus
d. Interventions
   (1) In the absence of spontaneous accelerations, fetal scalp stimulation or vibroacoustic stimulation performed when the fetus is at baseline can provoke fetal movement and FHR accelerations.

2. Early decelerations (**Fig. 1-4**)
   a. Definition
      (1) Gradual ($\geq$30 sec from onset to nadir) decrease in FHR from baseline and subsequent return to baseline associated with uterine contraction
      (2) Recurrent if occurring with $\geq$50% of uterine contractions in any 20-min segment
      (3) Decrease usually not >40 bpm
   b. Physiologic mechanism
      (1) Result of physiologic chain of events that begins with head compression during uterine contraction

FIGURE 1-4
Fetal Heart Monitor Strip Showing Early Decelerations

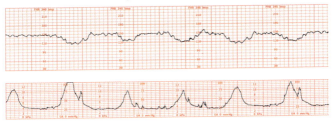

A gradual ($\geq$30 sec from onset to nadir) decrease in FHR from the baseline and subsequent return to the baseline is the result of a physiologic chain of events that begins with head compression during a uterine contraction. These are recurrent if they occur with $\geq$50% of uterine contractions in any 20-min segment.

(2) Caused by reduction in cerebral blood flow, hypoxemia, and hypercapnia
  (a) Hypercapnia results in hypertension that triggers a baroreceptor response mediated by the parasympathetic nervous system and a decrease in the FHR.
c. Clinical significance
  (1) Do not appear to be associated with poor outcome, therefore considered clinically benign.
  (2) May be included in the category-1 grouping.
d. Interventions
  (1) None required
3. Late decelerations (**Fig. 1-5**)
  a. Definition
    (1) Gradual ($\geq$30 sec from onset to nadir) decrease in FHR associated with uterine contractions
    (2) Deceleration begins after peak of contraction, gradual in shape
  b. Physiologic mechanism
    (1) Believed to reflect fetal response to transient or chronic disruption of oxygen transfer from the environment to the fetus, resulting in transient fetal hypoxemia
    (2) Interruption in uteroplacental blood flow sufficient to impair oxygen transfer to the fetus

FIGURE 1-5
Fetal Heart Monitor Strip Showing Late Decelerations

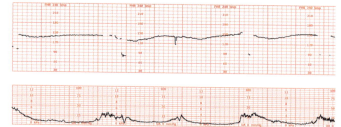

Late decelerations begin after the peak of the contraction and are gradual in shape. These are believed to reflect fetal response to transient or chronic disruption of oxygen transfer from the environment to the fetus, resulting in transient fetal hypoxemia.

(3) Reflex fetal response to transient hypoxemia during uterine contraction
   (a) Uterine contractions compress maternal blood vessels and disrupt maternal perfusion of the intervillous space.
   (b) Decreased oxygenation in the intervillous space can reduce the diffusion of oxygen into the fetal capillary blood, leading to a decline in fetal PO_2 below the normal range of 15–25 mmHg.
   (c) Chemoreceptors detect the change and initiate a protective reflex response of peripheral vasoconstriction, which redistributes perfusion to the brain, heart, and adrenal glands.
   (d) Vasoconstriction leads to an increase in fetal blood pressure, leading to a baroreceptor stimulation and gradual slowing of the FHR.
   (e) After the contraction, these reflexes subside.
(4) Risk to a fetus with decreased placental reserve
(5) Maternal factors potentially related to uteroplacental insufficiency:
   (a) Hypotension
   (b) Hypertension
   (c) Placental concerns: post-term, previa, abruption, or small or malformed placenta
   (d) Cardiopulmonary disease
   (e) Severe anemia
   (f) Tachysystole
   (g) Other high-risk conditions of pregnancy: preexisting chronic disease, maternal smoking, poor maternal nutrition, multiple gestation

c. Clinical significance
   (1) Baseline variability will determine if category 2 or 3.
   (2) Recurrent or sustained disruption may progress to metabolic acidemia.

d. Intervention
   (1) Must correlate with variability
      (a) If moderate variability occurs with late decelerations, it is believed to reflect a chemoreceptor-mediated response to a transient hypoxemic event.

(b) Late decelerations with absent variability occur when the amount of oxygen in blood coming from the placenta cannot support fetal myocardial function.
4. Variable decelerations (**Fig. 1-6**)
    a. Definition
        (1) Abrupt (onset to nadir <30 sec) decrease of ≥15 bpm below the baseline with a duration of ≥15 sec and <2 min
        (2) May occur with (recurrent) or without (episodic) uterine contractions and not necessarily associated with uterine contraction
        (3) Recurrent if occurring with >50% of uterine contractions in any 20-min segment
    b. Physiologic mechanism
        (1) Results from transient mechanical compression of umbilical blood vessels within the umbilical cord.
        (2) Results from baroreceptor detection of abrupt rise in blood pressure and signals abrupt decrease in heart rate.
        (3) Parasympathetic stimulation may result in AV rhythm that appears as relatively stable rate of 60–80 bpm at the base of a variable deceleration.
        (4) As cord is decompressed, this sequence of events occurs in reverse.

FIGURE 1-6
Fetal Heart Monitor Strip Showing Variable Decelerations

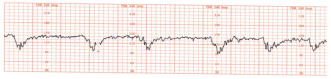
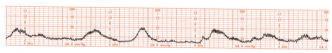

Variable decelerations are abrupt (onset to nadir <30 sec) decreases of ≥15 bpm below the baseline with a duration of ≥15 sec and <2 min. These may occur with (recurrent) or without (episodic) uterine contractions, but are not necessarily associated with uterine contractions.

c. Clinical significance
   (1) Recurrent variable decelerations can result in recurrent disruption of fetal oxygenation and lead to a cascade of changes; including hypoxemia, hypoxia, respiratory acidosis; and may progress to mixed acidosis.
   (2) This is a common type of deceleration that varies in depth, shape, and duration.
d. Intervention
   (1) Position change, fluid bolus
   (2) Category 2, may deteriorate to category 3 if accompanied by absent variability

5. Prolonged deceleration
   a. Definition
      (1) Abrupt or gradual deceleration of ≥15 bpm lasting 2–10 min
      (2) Characterized by duration of the event
   b. Physiologic mechanism
      (1) Prolonged interruption of oxygenation from cord compression, tachysystole, uterine tetany, etc.
   c. Clinical significance
      (1) If duration exceeds 10 min, it is a bradycardia.
      (2) The fetus may become academic, followed by myocardial depression.
   d. Intervention
      (1) Intrauterine resuscitation
      (2) Prepare for expeditious delivery if unresolved

6. Abnormal patterns
   a. Sinusoidal pattern (**Fig. 1-7**)
      (1) Visually apparent, smooth, sine wave-like undulating pattern above and below the baseline, with a cycle of ~2–5 times/min and an amplitude of 5–15 beats above and below the baseline that persists for >20 min
      (2) Actual baseline is indeterminate
      (3) Not a type of variability
      (4) Classically associated with fetal anemia due to Rh isoimmunization, massive fetomaternal hemorrhage, twin-to-twin transfusion syndrome, ruptured vasa previa, and fetal intracranial hemorrhage

(5) Other associated fetal conditions include fetal hypoxia or asphyxia, fetal infection, cardiac anomalies, gastroschisis
(6) Classified as category-3 tracing
(7) Will not resolve spontaneously and may become complicated by additional elements, such as late, variable, or prolonged decelerations

b. Arrhythmia
(1) Defined as any irregularity of the fetal cardiac rhythm
(2) Specific arrhythmias named according to anatomic site of aberrant impulse formation or conduction
(3) Usually not associated with uterine contractions, but characteristic of the baseline
(4) Rarely seen; may be detected during prenatal visit, NST, or labor
(5) Important to differentiate between arrhythmia and artifact
    (a) Arrhythmias may impair interpretation of intrapartum heart rate tracings. Direct fetal monitoring with a fetal scalp electrode will assist in determination of baseline.

FIGURE 1-7
Fetal Heart Monitor Strip Showing Sinusoidal Pattern

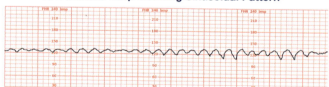
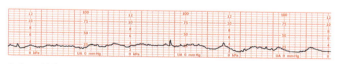

A sinusoidal pattern appears as a smooth, sine wave-like undulating pattern above and below the baseline, with a cycle of ~2–5 times/min and an amplitude of 5–15 beats above and below the baseline that persists for >20 min. It is classically associated with fetal anemia due to Rh isoimmunization, massive fetomaternal hemorrhage, twin-to-twin transfusion syndrome, ruptured vasa previa, and fetal intracranial hemorrhage.

(6) Significance
    (a) Arrhythmias usually disappear in the immediate neonatal period, although some are associated with structural cardiac defects.
    (b) Ultrasonic survey of fetal anatomy, as well as echocardiography, may be useful.
c. Supraventricular tachycardia (SVT)
    (1) Rate disorder that presents after 15 weeks of gestation and is most commonly seen at 30–32 weeks.
    (2) Atrial arrhythmia is sustained, rapid, and regular.
    (3) Rate may range upwards from 210 and increases workload on the fetal heart, resulting in decreased cardiac output.
    (4) May progress to hydrops, depending on the severity of hemodynamic compromise
    (5) Management ranges from observation to prenatal medication therapy, including digoxin.
d. Atrioventricular block
    (1) Thought to be due to a failure of union of the AV node and bundle of His in early fetal development; complete congenital heart block may also result from damage to the conducting system after it has been normally formed.
    (2) Categorized according to the severity of the block: first, second, and third (complete). Impulse conduction is through the AV node and is abnormally slow.
    (3) May be associated with maternal collagen vascular disease, fetal cardiac structural defects, fetal cytomegalovirus, antiphospholipid antibody syndrome, and maternal lupus.
e. Premature atrial contractions (PAC) and premature ventricular contractions (PVC)
    (1) Comprise more than half of the cases of fetal dysrhythmia.
    (2) Generally considered benign, but warrant observation.
    (3) With direct monitoring, vertical spikes above and below the baseline are characteristic.
    (4) Indirect (external) monitoring reveals irregular rhythm.

F. Categories of FHR
   1. Normal (category 1)
      a. Characteristics
         (1) Exhibit baseline rate of 110–160 and moderate variability with no late, variable, or prolonged decelerations
         (2) May or may not exhibit accelerations or early decelerations
      b. Significance
         (1) Almost always associated with non-acidotic fetus and vigorous newborn at delivery; high predictability of a normally oxygenated fetus
      c. Management
         (1) Routine measures to support labor progress, maternal coping, and fetal oxygenation
   2. Indeterminate (category 2)
      a. Characteristics
         (1) All FHR tracings that do not meet criteria for category 1 or 3
         (2) Includes tracings such as moderate or minimal variability and recurrent late or variable decelerations, tachycardia, prolonged decelerations, absent variability without decelerations
      b. Significance
         (1) Requires heightened surveillance and ongoing reevaluation
         (2) FHR patterns nonspecific; cannot reliably predict whether fetus will be well-oxygenated, depressed, or acidotic at birth
      c. Management
         (1) Supportive actions to promote maternal and fetal adaptation to labor
         (2) Intrauterine resuscitation measures (noted under category 3) may be used as appropriate
   3. Abnormal (category 3)
      a. Characteristics exhibit any of the following:
         (1) Absent variability with bradycardia
         (2) Absent variability with recurrent late or variable decelerations
         (3) Sinusoidal pattern

b. Significance
   (1) Abnormal FHR patterns may be associated with fetal acidemia.
   (2) The following conditions may indicate neurologic injury:
       (a) Profound acidemia (determined by umbilical artery pH of <7 and base deficit ≥12 mmol/L)
       (b) Five-minute Apgar scores of 0–3
       (c) Early onset of severe or moderate neonatal encephalopathy in infants born ≥34 weeks gestation
       (d) Multi-organ system involvement within 72 hours of birth
           i. The kidney is a very sensitive organ and renal damage may occur as a result of altered blood flow patterns adopted by the fetus when hypoxia is present.
       (e) Cerebral palsy of the spastic quadriplegic or dyskinetic type
   (3) Exclusion of other identifiable etiologies: trauma, coagulation disorders, infectious conditions, genetic disorders
c. Management
   (1) Initial assessment may include a cervical examination to rule out cord prolapse or imminent delivery.
   (2) One or more intrauterine resuscitation techniques should be used:
       (a) Maternal repositioning to a lateral position
       (b) Reduction of excessive uterine activity noted as hypertonus (basal tone >20–25 mmHg) or tachysystole
           i. Removal of pharmacologic agents used with cervical ripening
           ii. Decreasing or discontinuing oxytocin infusion
           iii. Lateral positioning
           iv. Administration of an IV fluid bolus of lactated Ringers solution
           v. Consideration of a subcutaneous dose of terbutaline (0.25 mg)

- (c) IV fluid bolus
  - i. Correction of maternal hypotension with bolus or ephedrine
  - ii. 500- to 1,000-mL lactated Ringer's solution
  - iii. Caution with repeated IV fluid boluses
    1) Caution with preeclampsia, preterm labor
    2) IV boluses of glucose-containing solutions should generally be avoided due to transfer of glucose to the fetus, which can cause fetal hyperglycemia and subsequent reactive hypoglycemia due to hyperinsulinism.
- (d) Oxygen administration
  - i. Provide 100% oxygen via a non-rebreather face mask at 10 L/min and discontinue as soon as possible, based on fetal response.
  - ii. Oxytocin should not be infused concurrently with maternal oxygen administration.
- (e) Amnioinfusion
  - i. Transcervical instillation of fluid into the amniotic cavity
  - ii. Used to resolve variable decelerations
- (f) Modification of maternal pushing efforts during second-stage labor
  - i. Continuation of coached pushing in the presence of category 2 and 3 patterns can lead to iatrogenic fetal stress.
  - ii. Shortening the active pushing phase, temporarily discontinuing pushing, and limiting pushing to every other or every third contraction can be effective methods to minimize risk of progression fetal oxygen desaturation.

V. Conditions affecting pregnancy that may impact fetal growth

A. Maternal nutrition
1. Maternal metabolic changes in pregnancy ensure that nutrients are continuously provided to the fetus.
   a. Substrates are delivered to the maternal side of the placenta for transport to the fetus.

b. If nutrient restriction occurs only during the first trimester, infant birth weights tend to be within normal limits. Restricted protein intake in early pregnancy has a detrimental effect on both fetal and placental development.
   c. Caloric restriction in third trimester may affect fetal weight.
2. Due to the release of human placental lactogen (hPL) and increase in maternal insulin resistance, providing glucose to the fetus causes the following to occur:
   a. Hypoinsulinemia reduces glucose uptake in insulin-dependent tissues, preserving glucose for fetal use.
   b. Alternative substrates, such as ketones, cross the placenta and can be utilized by the fetus for lipid or protein synthesis.
3. During maternal fasting, adaptive mechanisms preserve fetal growth.
   a. Fuel mobilization results in increased maternal ketones and free fatty acids.
   b. Mobilization of maternal adipose tissue stores is facilitated by a rapid decline in maternal insulin levels and enhanced secretion of human placental somatomammotropin.
   c. Somatomammotropin has lipolytic activity and directly diminishes maternal glucose utilization, allowing greater fetal glucose transport.
   d. Maternal glucose utilization decreases because free fatty acids and ketones replace glucose as a maternal energy source.
   e. Prolonged periods of starvation have adverse consequences on fetal outcome.

B. Insulin and fetal-growth hormone
  1. Maternal insulin does not cross the placenta; fetal insulin is from fetal pancreatic origin.
  2. Fetal insulin and insulin-like growth factors are critical to fetal health.
     a. Increase deposition of adipose tissue in fetus
     b. Increase fetal glycogen stores
     c. Stimulate fetal amino acid uptake and protein synthesis in the muscle
     d. Govern fetal growth

3. Fetal-growth hormone does not significantly influence growth; there are few fetal-growth hormone receptors in the liver.
    a. Infants with growth-hormone deficiency (panhypopituitarism) have birth weights that are similar to those of normal fetuses.
    b. In cases of IUGR, placental-derived growth hormone levels in maternal serum are low.
    c. Placental-derived growth hormone increases maternal nutrient provision to the fetus and enhances mobilization of maternal substrates for fetal growth.

C. Maternal conditions
   1. If the mother was small or large at her own birth, genetic factors may result in large or growth-restricted infants.
   2. Chronic maternal diseases may influence fetal growth.
      a. Hypertensive disorders
         (1) Gestational hypertension
         (2) Preeclampsia-eclampsia
         (3) Chronic hypertension
         (4) Chronic hypertension with superimposed preeclampsia
      b. Maternal hypoxemia from cyanotic heart disease or living at high altitude
      c. Diabetes mellitus, particularly if vascular complications are present
      d. Autoimmune diseases
      e. Sickle cell anemia
   3. Maternal ingestion of legal or illegal drugs
      a. Teratogens: isoretinoin, warfarin, toluene, methylmercury
      b. Pharmaceuticals: propranolol, prednisone
      c. Recreational: amphetamines, cocaine (may cause abruption from vasoconstriction), alcohol, heroin, phencyclidine
   4. Other factors
      a. Cigarette smoking and lower socioeconomic status have been linked to IUGR.
         (1) These conditions may actually be related to poor maternal nutrition or drug abuse.
      b. History of previous infant with either IUGR or SGA
      c. Low pre-pregnancy weight

D. Fetal conditions
   1. Chromosomal abnormalities, such as trisomy 8, 13, 18, and 21
   2. Deletion or addition syndromes
   3. Triplet sex-chromosome abnormalities
   4. Agenesis of the pancreas
   5. Other known syndromes
      a. Cornelia de Lange
      b. Potter syndrome
      c. Radial aplasia
      d. VACTERL syndrome
      e. Williams syndrome
      f. TORCH infectious syndromes
         (1) Toxoplasmosis
         (2) Other (syphilis, varicella)
         (3) Rubella
         (4) Cytomegalovirus
         (5) Herpes simplex

VI. Preterm labor and delivery
   A. Definition and incidence
      1. Defined by the World Health Organization as any delivery that occurs between 20 and 37 weeks of gestation
      2. Account for 60%–80% of infant deaths worldwide
      3. Rate of preterm delivery has not changed in last 40 years; may actually have increased in recent decades
      4. Rate in United States is 12%
   B. Risk factors
      1. Race
         a. Preterm delivery rate is 16%–18% for African Americans; 7%–9% for Caucasians.
      2. Socioeconomic factors
         a. Mother's age; <17 and >35 at higher risk
         b. Lower income
      3. Stress
      4. Previous preterm delivery most significant risk factor
         a. Risk ranges from 17% to 40%, depending on number of prior preterm deliveries
         b. Greater number and earlier time frame of prior preterm deliveries increases risk
         c. Spontaneous abortion prior to second trimester
      5. Uterine abnormalities and fibroid presence

6. Cervical incompetence (painless dilation at 12–20 weeks), may be associated with previous cervical biopsies or traumatic deliveries
7. Multiple fetus gestation
    a. One of the highest risk factors for preterm delivery and low birth weight
    b. 26% of infants with birth weight <2,500 g are twins
    c. 50% of twins and triplets are preterm
8. Placental factors: placenta previa or abruption

C. Management of preterm labor
  1. Determination of underlying cause, if possible
     a. PPROM
     b. Maternal underlying condition
     c. Fetal underlying condition
  2. Ultrasound to determine cervical length
     a. Dynamic changes of cervix over time
     b. Cervical funneling or wedging
  3. Goals of preterm labor management
     a. The initial goal of management is to delay delivery long enough using tocolytics to allow three adjunctive interventions that have been shown to reduce the neonatal morbidity and mortality related to prematurity.
        (1) Transfer of mother and fetus to a hospital equipped to care for a premature infant
        (2) Administration of glucocorticoids
        (3) Administration of antibiotic prophylaxis to decrease neonatal group B *Streptococcus* (GBS) infection
  4. Tests for lung maturity (**Table 1-1**)
     a. Overview
        (1) Tests of lung maturation are based on the premise that amniotic fluid accurately reflects the degree of differentiation of the type II cell population in the fetal lung.
        (2) Amniotic fluid phospholipids are far downstream in distance and time from the type II alveolar cell.
        (3) Surfactant secretion and the flow of fetal lung fluid are influenced by preterm labor and delivery.
     b. Ratio of lecithin (phosphatidylcholine) to sphingomyelin (L/S ratio)
        (1) Introduced by Gluck and associates in 1971.

(2) Standard against which all other tests are compared.
(3) Depends on sufficient flow of fetal lung fluid into amniotic fluid to change amniotic fluid phospholipid composition in a timely manner.
(4) Sphingomyelin is a membrane lipid, a nonspecific component of amniotic fluid not related to lung maturation.
(5) Sphingomyelin tends to decrease from ~32 weeks gestational age to term.
(6) Phosphatidylcholine, a large part of which is produced by the fetal lung, increases to a value of 2 by 35 weeks of gestation.
(7) In the normal fetus, values of 1.5–2 are considered immature; however, risk of respiratory distress syndrome (RDS) is low.
(8) If L/S ratio <1, incidence of RDS is high.
c. Phosphatidylglycerol (PG)
(1) Normally appears in amniotic fluid at the time of lung maturity, ~35 weeks gestation
(2) Absent from the amniotic fluid of tracheal aspirates of infants with RDS, appears as disease resolves
(3) Can be detected <30 weeks gestation in infants with early lung maturation
(4) Present in appreciable amounts only in lung tissue and surfactant
d. TDx-FLM II
(1) Measures relative concentrations of surfactant and albumin in the amniotic fluid

TABLE 1-1
Fetal Lung Maturity

Test	Normal	Abnormal
L/S ratio	>2: normal	1.5–2: immature, incidence of RDS low <1: incidence of RDS high
PG	Present	Absent
TDx-FML II	≥55 mg/g: likelihood of RDS small	40–54 mg/g: intermediate risk for RDS <39 mg/g: likelihood of RDS high

L/S ratio = ratio of lecithin to sphingomyelin; PG = phosphatidylglycerol;
RDS = respiratory distress syndrome

(2) Has several advantages over L/S ratio:
   (a) Less technical expertise required
   (b) Can be performed more easily
   (c) Results obtained faster
(3) Interpretation of results:
   (a) <39 mg/g: Risk for immature lungs, other conditions may weigh more heavily on decision to deliver early
   (b) 40-54 mg/g: Intermediate risk for development of RDS
   (c) ≥55 mg/g: Likelihood of RDS small
(4) Measures ratio of amniotic fluid surfactant to albumin
(5) Equivalent to L/S ratio for prediction of RDS
(6) Used less frequently today
   (a) Virtually all women at risk for preterm delivery are treated with antenatal corticosteroids.
   (b) The availability of postnatal surfactant administration has changed the nature of surfactant deficiency disease.

5. Glucocorticoid recommendations from the NICHD and the American College of Obstetricians and Gynecologists (ACOG)
   a. Antenatal steroids are recommended for mothers expected to deliver at <32 weeks of gestation to reduce mortality and the incidence of RDS and intraventricular hemorrhage, regardless of the status of the fetal membranes.
   b. At 32–34 weeks, both recommend antenatal steroid treatment for mothers with intact membranes who are likely to deliver within 7 days, but noted that the benefit for infants born to women with ruptured membranes after 32 weeks is still controversial.
   c. Corticosteroids have greatest effect if delivery occurs 24 hours after starting treatment or <7 days after the last dose. However, if delivery occurred <24 hours after administration, steroid administration provided benefits.
   d. Anticipate transient FHR changes that typically return to baseline by 4–7 days after treatment.
      (1) The most consistent FHR finding is a decrease in variability on days 2 and 3.

- (2) Fetal breathing and body movements are also commonly reduced, which may result in a lower BPP score or nonreactive NST.
- e. Corticosteroid treatment decreases the tendency of the preterm lung to develop pulmonary edema.
- f. Effects between corticosteroid and surfactant treatments are synergistic and additive. Because of increased lung volume, corticosteroid-treated fetuses have improved responses to postnatal surfactant.

D. Fetal neuroprotection
1. Pooling the results of the available clinical trials of magnesium sulfate for neuroprotection suggests that prenatal administration of magnesium sulfate reduces the occurrence of cerebral palsy when given with neuroprotective intent.
2. It is believed that magnesium sulfate not only reduces the risk of all levels of cerebral palsy (mild, moderate, severe), but also decreases the combined outcome of cerebral palsy on both fetal and infant death.
3. Use during 24–31 weeks of gestation, when risk of delivery is high.
    a. 6 g magnesium sulfate load followed by 2 g/hour up to 12 hours
    b. May be resumed when delivery is imminent

References

Association of Women's Health, Obstetric and Neonatal Nurses. *AWHONN's Fetal Heart Monitoring Principles and Practices*. 4th ed. Washington, DC: Association of Women's Health, Obstetric and Neonatal Nurses; 2009.

Berghella V, ed. *Maternal-Fetal Evidence Based Guidelines*. 2nd ed. New York, NY: Informa Healthcare; 2011.

Callen PW, ed. *Ultrasonography in Obstetrics and Gynecology*, 5th ed. Philadelphia, PA: Saunders Elsevier; 2008.

Chalak LF, Rouse DJ. Neuroprotective approaches: before and after delivery. *Clin Perinatol*. 2011;38(3):455-470.

Cloherty JP, Eichenwald EC, Hansen AR, Stark AR. *Manual of Neonatal Care*. 7th ed. Philadelphia, PA: Wolters Kluwer Health/ Lippincott Williams & Wilkins; 2012.

Gardner SL, Carter BS, Enzman-Hines M, Hernandez JA. *Merenstein and Gardner's Handbook of Neonatal Intensive Care*. 7th ed. St. Louis, MO: Mosby Elsevier; 2011.

Gilbert ES. *Manual of High Risk Pregnancy and Delivery*. 5th ed. St. Louis, MO: Mosby Elsevier; 2011.

Gomella TL, Cunningham MD, Eyal FG, eds. *Neonatology: Management, Procedures, On-Call Problems, Diseases, and Drugs*. 7th ed. New York, NY: McGraw Hill/Lange; 2013.

Jansson T, Powell TL. Placental nutrient transfer and fetal growth. *Nutrition*. 2000;16(7-8): 500-502.

Leveno KJ. *William's Manual of Pregnancy Complications*. 23rd ed. New York, NY: McGraw Hill Medical; 2013.

Martin RJ, Fanaroff AA, Walsh MC. *Fanaroff and Martin's Neonatal-Perinatal Medicine: Diseases of the Fetus and Infant*. 9th ed. St. Louis, MO: Mosby Elsevier; 2011.

Miller LA, Miller DA, Tucker SM. *Mosby's Pocket Guide to Fetal Monitoring: A Multidisciplinary Approach*. 7th ed. St. Louis, MO: Mosby Elsevier; 2013.

Monk D, Moore, GE. Intrauterine growth restriction: genetic causes and consequences. *Semin Fetal Neonatal Med*. 2004;9(5):371-378.

Signore C, Freeman RK, Spong CY. Antenatal testing: a reevaluation. *Obstet Gynecol*. 2009;113(3):687-701.

Simpson KR, Creehan PA, eds. *AWHONN's Perinatal Nursing*. 4th ed. Philadelphia, PA: Wolters Kluwer Heath/Lippincott Williams & Wilkins; 2014.

Wildschut H, Weiner CP, Peters TJ. *When to Screen in Obstetrics and Gynecology*. 2nd ed. Philadelphia, PA: Saunders Elsevier; 2006.

Maternal Risk Factors

Catherine Theorell

I. Introduction
A. In order to fully comprehend and manage critically ill newborns, one must explore the biological aspects of pregnancy and maternal physiology that impact neonatal development and outcome.

II. Maternal antenatal fetal screening
A. Overview
1. Currently, the American College of Obstetricians and Gynecologists (ACOG) recommends that all pregnant women be offered the option of early screening for the presence of fetal aneuploidy and neural tube defects.
2. Screening for such defects does not imply that parents are obligated to intervene in the pregnancy, but may present opportunities for intrauterine treatment, as well as for psychological preparation of the parents and family for the birth of a newborn with problems.

B. First trimester screening
1. Early ultrasound and evaluation of serum markers is performed between 10-4/7 weeks and 13-4/7 weeks of pregnancy.
2. Ultrasound is performed to date the pregnancy using crown-rump measurements and to evaluate the fetus for the presence of nuchal translucency.
3. The presence of nuchal translucency is a fetal marker that indicates a higher risk for the presence of aneuploidy and Down syndrome.
4. If the translucency is >3.5 mm, the fetus should undergo a targeted ultrasound and a fetal echocardiograph, which detect up to 70% of cases of Down syndrome.
5. If the presence of nuchal translucency is combined with the use of two maternal serum markers — pregnancy-associated plasma protein-A (PAPP-A) and human chorionic gonadotropin (hCG) — the antenatal detection rate for Down syndrome improves to 79%–90% of cases.

C. Second trimester screening
   1. Screening in the second trimester of pregnancy is performed between 15 and 20-6/7 weeks to detect trisomies and the presence of neural tube defects.
   2. An increase in maternal serum alpha-fetoprotein (AFP) may indicate the presence of an open neural-tube defect in the fetus.
   3. AFP is a specific molecule produced by the fetal yolk sac, gastrointestinal tract, and liver.
   4. Levels of AFP are lower in maternal serum than in fetal serum of liver tissue.
   5. Maternal serum AFP levels are drawn between 15 and 20 weeks of gestation; the results are reported as multiples of mean (MoM) and are based on gestational age of the fetus.
   6. AFP values greater than MoM are considered abnormal and should be repeated along with a targeted ultrasound assessment of the fetus.
   7. Accurate timing of fetal gestational age is key to appropriate interpretation of AFP levels.
   8. When maternal serum AFP levels are combined with hCG and unconjugated estriol levels, the testing array is called a "triple screen."
   9. The triple screen has an aneuploidy detection rate of 65%.
   10. The addition of the maternal serum marker ("quad screen") increases the aneuploidy detection rate to 80% of trisomies and neural-tube defects.
   11. The combination of nuchal translucency and the quad screen increases detection of trisomies and neural-tube defects to 90%.
   12. AFP and amniotic acetylcholinesterase are also used to detect open neural-tube defects, with a 96% accuracy rate and a low false positive rate of 0.14%, which occurs when the sample has become contaminated with blood.
   13. If a trisomy is suspected, the definitive diagnosis is a fetal karyotype obtained from fetal cells shed into the amniotic fluid.
   14. An elevated maternal serum AFP in the second trimester that cannot be explained by a structural anomaly or underlying maternal conditions is associated with increased risk of fetal demise, abruption, and preeclampsia.

III. Diabetes
  A. Overview
   1. Diabetes is one of the most frequent complications of pregnancy.
   2. 90% of all cases are caused by gestational diabetes.
   3. Each year, 135,000–200,000 women are diagnosed with gestational diabetes.
   4. Type 2 diabetes among women of childbearing age has increased 33%.
   5. Neonates born to women with gestational diabetes have a 3- to 5-fold increase in the incidence of metabolic syndrome, obesity, and diabetes during their lives.
   6. Diabetes, risk of obesity, and potential for adolescent obesity in offspring of diabetic women are major public health issues.
  B. Maternal pathophysiology and clinical correlates
   1. Severe hypoglycemia (serum glucose <60 mg/dL) and diabetic ketoacidosis are more common with type 1 diabetes.
   2. Insulin resistance is more common in type 2 diabetes.
  C. Type 1 insulin-dependent diabetes
   1. Autoimmune disease characterized by islet B-cell destruction.
   2. Islet cell autoantibodies, insulin autoantibodies, and other B-cell autoantibodies are present.
   3. Type 1 diabetes may result in systemic effects on the cardiovascular system and blood flow to the kidneys and pelvic vessels.
   4. Type 1 diabetics with pelvic vascular involvement may result in reduced uterine blood flow and, subsequently, fetal intrauterine growth restriction (IUGR).
   5. Viruses, dietary factors, and environmental exposure to chemicals have been investigated as causes of the disorder.
  D. Type 2 diabetes
   1. Characterized by hyperglycemia caused by an increased hepatic glucose production, abnormal insulin secretion, and increased insulin resistance.
   2. Decreased insulin action and increased glucagon secretion cause an increase in hepatic glucose production.
   3. Pathophysiology of type 2 diabetes and gestational diabetes is similar; some researchers have identified them as the same disease with different names.

E. Gestational diabetes
   1. Normal pregnancy is characterized by a state of hyperinsulinemia and insulin resistance caused by the diabetogenic effects on normal carbohydrate metabolism.
   2. Women who develop gestational diabetes have a higher insulin resistance before conception, often associated with obesity.
   3. Insulin resistance results in decreased glucose uptake by skeletal muscles, white adipose tissue, and liver, and in suppression of hepatic glucose production.
   4. Women who develop gestational diabetes are more likely to develop metabolic syndrome and/or overt diabetes later in life.
F. Fetal exposure to increased glucose
   1. Maternal glucose readily crosses the placenta; fetal glucose levels follow maternal levels.
   2. Maternal insulin does not cross the placenta in clinically significant amounts.
   3. High levels of fetal glucose stimulate increased secretion of fetal insulin.
   4. Fetal hyperinsulinemia causes:
      a. Increased cellular glucose use
      b. Increased hepatic glycogen deposits
      c. Decreased mobilization of lipids
      d. Increased protein production
      e. Increased amino acid uptake and protein synthesis
      f. Decreased protein catabolism
   5. In the last 12 weeks of gestation, infants of diabetic mothers (IDMs) deposit 50%–60% more fat than infants of non-diabetics.
   6. All organs of IDMs are larger, except the kidneys and brain.
   7. Growth abnormalities are a common risk in these infants.
      a. Macrosomia: In the United States, nearly 450,000 infants who are large for gestational age (LGA) are born each year.
         (1) Shoulder dystocia complicates ~50%–86% of LGA infants.
         (2) Infants whose birth weight is >4,000 g, and particularly those infants whose birth weight is >4,500 g, have higher mortality and morbidity than infants who are average for gestational age.

- (3) Since fetuses gain 95% of their weight in the last half of pregnancy, maternal glycemic control during that time may reduce the risks of these macrosomic infants.
  - b. Small for gestational age (SGA)
    - (1) 20% of IDMs will be SGA.
    - (2) Impaired fetal growth in these infants is secondary to maternal renovascular disease.
- G. Maternal hyperglycemia and resulting fetal hyperinsulinemia
  1. Neonatal complications of maternal diabetes include:
     - a. Fetal anomalies
     - b. Metabolic, hematologic, and respiratory issues
     - c. Increased NICU admissions and birth trauma
     - d. Increased fetal growth and stillbirth
  2. Congenital malformations account for 30%–50% of neonatal deaths, vs. 20%–30% for infants of non-diabetic mothers.
  3. Rate of congenital anomalies:
     - a. Similar for women with type 1 or type 2 diabetes
     - b. 3- to 5-fold higher than in infants of non-diabetic mothers
     - c. 4%–11% higher in fetuses of mothers with gestational diabetes
     - d. Most common anomalies include central nervous system (CNS) and cardiovascular malformations (see **Table 2-1**)
     - e. Most specific associated anomaly in IDMs is sacral agenesis
     - f. Sacral agenesis 300–400 times more common in diabetic pregnancies (most common associated risk factor for sacral agenesis is diabetes mellitus)
     - g. Other anomalies that develop as a result of embryologic disruption <8 weeks gestation (before completing organomegaly):
       - (1) Cardiac: Transposition of great vessels most common
       - (2) CNS: Neural tube defects and other anomalies
       - (3) Genitourinary defects
       - (4) Skeletal defects
       - (5) Early glycemic control a key factor in reducing perinatal morbidity and mortality

TABLE 2-1
Congenital Malformations and Lesions Found in Infants of Diabetic Mothers (IDMs)

\multicolumn{3}{c}{STRUCTURAL}		
Systems	**Defects**	**Specific**
Central Nervous	Neural tube defects	Meningocele, encephalocele, anencephaly
	Caudal regression syndrome (sacral agenesis)	300–400 times more common in diabetic pregnancies
	Holoprosencephaly	
Respiratory	RDS	
	Transient tachypnea of the newborn	
Cardiovascular	Transposition of the great vessels; truncus arteriosus	
	Ventricular and atrial septal defects	Tricuspid atresia
	Left-sided obstructive lesions	Hypoplastic left heart, aortic stenosis, coarctation of the aorta, ventricular septal hypertrophy
Genitourinary	Renal agenesis	
	Hydronephrosis	
	Ureteral duplication	
	Cystic kidneys	
Gastrointestinal	Intestinal atresias	Duodenal, anorectal
Musculoskeletal	Arthrogryposis	
	Hypoplastic femur	
FUNCTIONAL		
Cardiac	Intraventricular septal hypertrophy, cardiomyopathy (with ventricular hypertrophy), cardiac failure	
Intestinal	Small left colon syndrome, meconium plug syndrome	
OTHER		
Hematologic	Renal vein thrombosis, adrenal hemorrhage, polycythemia, thrombocytopenia	
Growth Anomalies	Macrosomia (LGA) when hyperglycemic states are predominant; SGA when pelvic vascular disease has developed.	
Metabolic and Electrolyte	Hypoglycemia, hypocalcemia, hypomagnesemia, iron abnormalities	
Increased Risks	Asphyxia, hyperbilirubinemia, birth trauma, palsies (brachial plexus, Erbs, Klumpke)	

H. Diagnosis
  1. Type 1 or type 2 diabetes should be identified and treated by the first prenatal visit.
  2. Gestational diabetes is identified when a women with normal glucose control develops abnormal glucose while pregnant.
  3. Approximately 2%–10% of diabetes classified as gestational are actually type 2 diabetes first identified during pregnancy.
  4. Since diabetes carries long-term chronic disease implications, pregnancy remains an important screening period.
  5. Because of the frequency of type 1 diabetes, type 2 diabetes, and obesity in childbearing women, all pregnant women should be screened with a 100-g glucose load and a 3-hour glucose tolerance test.
  6. A single abnormal value probably indicates gestational diabetes and resultant risk for excessive fetal growth.
  7. The National Diabetes Data Group, which is endorsed by ACOG and the American Diabetes Association, defines normal glucose levels (fasting) as shown in **Table 2-2**.
  8. Women at risk for developing gestational diabetes mellitus present with:
     a. Abnormal fasting glucose
     b. Previous diagnosis of gestational diabetes before 20 weeks
     c. Previous infant of diabetic mother
     d. Obesity
I. Management during pregnancy
  1. Goals
     a. Establish glycemic control **prior** to conception.
     b. Diminish rate of hyperglycemia and ketosis.

TABLE 2-2
Normal Fasting Glucose Levels in Pregnancy

Time	Range (mg/dL)
Fasting	95–105
1 hour	180–190
2 hours	155–165
3 hours	140–145

- c. Achieving glycemic control (not the type of pharmacologic therapy) is key to improving perinatal outcomes in gestational diabetes.
 2. Interventions
    a. Diet
    b. Exercise
    c. Medications
       (1) Oral anti-hyperglycemic agents
       (2) Insulin
J. Management during pregnancy that impacts fetal/neonatal well-being
 1. Establish best timing to begin fetal testing to prevent stillbirth and reduce fetal compromise.
 2. Establish timing of lung maturity to prevent respiratory distress syndrome (RDS).
    a. Use biochemical indices to determine lung maturation; do not rely on gestational age or fetal size.
    b. Test at 24–26 weeks, when fetus is viable to assist in timing of delivery.
    c. To prevent RDS in infants of diabetic women, determine lung maturation prior to delivery.
    d. Poor maternal glycemic control results in delayed lung maturation of phospholipid synthesis in the fetal lung by 1–2 weeks vs. non-diabetic pregnancies.
    e. Clinician must evaluate risks and benefits of delivering a fetus with immature lungs vs. continuing pregnancy of noncompliant or poorly controlled diabetes.
 3. Determine time and method of delivery, particularly if the fetus is macrosomic.
 4. Delivery should be term or earlier if macrosomia is present, if there is a history of previous stillbirth, or if there is poor compliance with testing or poor glycemic control.
K. Issues for fetus
 1. Poor glycemic control during pregnancy is associated with a higher incidence of early spontaneous abortion and fetal demise and late-gestation stillbirth.
 2. Maternal glucose crosses placenta; maternal insulin does not.
 3. Fetal glucose levels mirror those found in the mother.
 4. Fetal glucose levels stimulate beta cells of the fetal pancreas to secrete insulin.

5. Since insulin is one of the main fetal growth hormones, the infant undergoes increased protein synthesis and fat deposition and develops macrosomia.
6. Due to fetal beta cell hyperplasia and hyperinsulinemic state, loss of continual glucose infusion across the placenta may cause fetal hypoglycemia within a few hours of delivery.
    a. Hypoglycemia may be asymptomatic or may include jitteriness, cyanosis, irritability, seizures, and apnea.
    b. Monitor serum glucose levels frequently; early feedings and/or parenteral dextrose infusions may be necessary to maintain normal infant glucose levels.
7. Infants born to mothers with type 1 diabetes are at risk for developing:
    a. Hypoglycemia
    b. Asphyxia
    c. RDS
    d. Hyperbilirubinemia
    e. Electrolyte disturbances (hypocalcaemia, hypomagnesemia)
    f. IUGR
8. In addition, infants born to mothers with type 2 or gestational diabetes have an increased incidence of:
    a. Adolescent obesity
    b. Metabolic syndrome
    c. Type 2 diabetes later in life
9. Although breast-feeding is best for all infants, it has even greater importance in infants of diabetic mothers; reducing long-term risks of obesity, type 2 diabetes, hypertension, and cardiovascular disease; even if breast-fed for only 2 months.
10. Due to their hyperinsulinemic condition, all infants born to diabetic mothers must be carefully screened and evaluated for hypoglycemia in the first few days of life, particularly if breast feeding.

L. Issues for very low birth weight (VLBW) infants
1. Fetal growth abnormalities
    a. Macrosomia
        (1) Characteristic appearance includes generous adipose tissue deposits, organomegaly, a full round face, and plethora.

- (2) Kidneys and brain size are not enlarged in IDMs.
- (3) Frequently, infants have abundant vernix; placenta and umbilical cord are also large.
- (4) Even in low birth weight infants, can experience greater than expected growth in response to maternal hyperglycemia and fetal hyperinsulinemia.
- (5) VLBW infants may appear larger than expected for gestational age; since gestation was shortened, they have not been exposed to maternal hyperglycemia for as long and they do not exhibit typical facial or body morphological appearance of IDMs.
- (6) Larger size does not indicate greater maturity; evaluate based on gestational age.
  b. Fetal growth restriction
  - (1) Up to 3-fold more common in infants born to insulin-dependent diabetic mothers vs. non-diabetic population.
  - (2) May be related to abnormalities in fetal cell replication and reduction in number of cells, resulting in an impaired pattern of fetal growth that is early in onset and symmetrical in distribution.
  - (3) Early-onset growth restriction may be related to fetal malformations.
  - (4) Low maternal glucose levels and vasculopathy of pelvic vessels result in fetal growth restriction.
  - (5) IUGR infants have higher risk of asphyxia, immune deficiency, polycythemia/hyperviscosity, pulmonary hemorrhage, meconium staining, and intrauterine fetal death.
  - (6) Developmental outcome and postnatal growth are dependent upon the degree and cause of IUGR.
  - (7) Temperature instability is common.
2. Congenital anomalies: Cause 50% of perinatal mortality for IDMs
   a. Increased 2- to 3-fold in insulin-dependent diabetics; also increased anomalies in gestational diabetics, but not in diabetic fathers.
   b. Frequency is increased if there has been poor diabetic control and elevated hemoglobin A1C in early gestation.

- c. The most common anomalies involve the cardiac, musculoskeletal, and central nervous systems (see **Table 2-1**).
- d. Congenital anomalies are thought to result from maternal hyperglycemia during the first seven weeks of pregnancy.
- e. The incidence of congenital heart disease (most commonly transposition of the great arteries, septal defects, and coarctation of the aorta) is 3–5 times higher than in the general population.
- f. Skeletal anomalies include delayed ossification and osseous defects; caudal regression syndrome (sacral agenesis) and hypoplasia of the femur are much more common in IDMs.
- g. CNS anomalies include hydrocephalus, neural tube defects, and anencephaly. Small left colon is a rare functional, rather than structural, disorder that results in partial intestinal obstruction and delayed passage of meconium. Usually resolves over the first few days of life without need for surgical intervention.

3. Hypoglycemia
   a. The American Academy of Pediatrics (AAP) target glucose screen is ≥ 45 mg/dL for SGA infants, IDMs, and late preterm infants.
   b. Nadir of hypoglycemia occurs at 30–90 min of age. Most infants are asymptomatic but should be corrected with parenteral glucose solution.
   c. Mini bolus of 2mL/kg of D10W can be given to hypoglycemic infants, followed by a constant glucose infusion rate of 5–8 mg/kg/min of dextrose to maintain glucose between 40 and 50 mg/dL.
   d. Since most VLBW infants are started on parenteral glucose infusions after delivery and have their serum glucose levels monitored closely, this complication is not seen as frequently as in infants born at later gestational ages.
   e. Shortened gestation period in preterm infants results in decreased level of pancreatic beta cell hyperplasia from fetal hyperglycemia.
   f. Carefully monitor glucose infusion rate and serum glucose, particularly as feedings are being initiated and advanced.

4. RDS
   a. Maternal hyperglycemia and resulting fetal hyperinsulinemia inhibit production of phospholipids and decrease the synthesis of pulmonary surfactant, resulting in RDS.
   b. There is usually a 2-week delay in pulmonary maturation for IDMs.
   c. Fortunately, due to improved antenatal testing, administration of antenatal steroids, and the wide availability of surfactants, this complication of maternal diabetes is not as problematic today.
5. Hypocalcemia and hypomagnesemia
   a. Frequently seen in infants of insulin-dependent diabetic mothers.
   b. Symptoms resemble hypoglycemia; these parameters must be followed closely.
   c. Hypocalcemia (<7 mg/dL) develops in the first 72 hours after birth in infants born to insulin-dependent diabetics; may be due to diminished parathyroid response, persistently elevated levels of calcitonin, and, possibly, alterations in vitamin D metabolism.
   d. Neonatal hypomagnesemia (<1.5 mg/dL) is usually transient, with uncertain physiologic significance.
   e. Since VLBW infants are started on total parenteral nutrition within an hour after birth, these electrolytes may need to be adjusted or added to standard mixtures.
6. Polycythemia and renal vein thrombosis
   a. Seen frequently in IDMs; thought to be due to relative chronic hypoxic state in the fetus, which stimulates red blood cell production.
   b. Symptoms include jitteriness, tachypnea, cyanosis, and priapism; oliguria in larger infants.
   c. In VLBW infants, stimulation of red blood cell synthesis is interrupted by shortened gestation time; polycythemia is much less common.
   d. Treatment of a partial reduction exchange transfusion may be needed; rarely needed in VLBW infants.
   e. When present, however, polycythemia may lead to hyperviscosity and intravascular thrombosis, including renal vein thrombosis.
      (1) Symptoms of renal vein thrombosis include hematuria and a palpable renal mass.

(2) Medical treatment may be necessary to dissolve the thrombus; nephrectomy may be required, but is rare.
7. Myocardial dysfunction in IDMs
   a. Myocardial dysfunction and neonatal heart failure is related to fetal ventricular septal hypertrophy and left ventricular outflow obstruction.
   b. Even in asymptomatic infants, diastolic function is altered, along with decreased passive compliance of the ventricle.
   c. The infant presents with delayed peripheral capillary refill time, diminished perfusion, and decreased pulses.
   d. Placing the infant on inotropes increases the outflow obstruction; cardiac function deteriorates as the inotropes cause the ventricular wall to press into the hypertrophied septum below the aortic valve, further obstructing outflow.
   e. Stopping the inotropes and beginning an infusion of isoproterenol mediates this condition.
   f. This condition, now rare, usually occurs in infants whose mothers had very poor glycemic control.
   g. The condition is transient and disappears spontaneously within 6 months after birth.
8. Hyperbilirubinemia
   a. Unconjugated bilirubin may be increased because of increased red blood cell mass, diminished activity of the hepatic glucuronidase enzymes, withholding of early enteral feedings, and delayed passage of meconium from small left colon syndrome.
   b. Peak bilirubin is increased and hyperbilirubinemia is prolonged for IDMs.

IV. Maternal thyroid disease
A. Overview
   1. Maternal and fetal thyroid disorders are closely tied.
   2. Drugs used to treat maternal thyroid disease also affect the fetal thyroid gland.
   3. Maternal thyroid autoimmune disorders have been associated with increased early spontaneous abortions and uncontrolled thyrotoxicosis.
   4. Undertreated hypothyroidism can result in adverse pregnancy outcomes.

5. Fetal thyrotropin-releasing hormone (TRH) is detectable in mid-pregnancy and the level remains stable throughout gestation.
6. Maternal thyroid-stimulating hormone (TSH) does not cross the placenta; thyroxine (T4) does.
7. Throughout pregnancy, maternal T4 is used for normal fetal brain development, especially prior to the development of the fetal thyroid gland.
8. Despite fetal thyroid function beginning as early as 12 weeks, transfer of maternal T4 accounts for 30% of T4 in fetal serum at term.
9. The major maternal thyroid disorders include hyperthyroidism and hypothyroidism.
10. Most maternal thyroid disorders are linked to the presence of autoimmune antibodies, which may stimulate thyroid function, block thyroid function, or result in thyroid inflammation, leading to thyroid follicular cell destruction.
11. Thyroid-stimulating autoimmune antibodies bind to TSH receptors and activate the cells, resulting in thyroid hyperactivity and growth.
12. Thyroid-stimulating autoimmune antibodies are found in most patients with Graves' disease (hyperthyroid); thyroid-blocking autoimmune antibodies are found in women with Hashimoto's thyroiditis (hypothyroid).
13. The presence of thyroid-peroxidase autoimmune antibodies is associated with early pregnancy loss and postpartum thyroid dysfunction.

B. Hyperthyroidism (Graves' disease)
   1. Overview
      a. Pregnancy outcomes depend upon whether metabolic control and a euthyroid state can be achieved.
      b. Women with excessive T4 levels have greater early pregnancy loss and a higher incidence of preeclampsia, heart failure, and adverse perinatal outcomes.
      c. Systemic hyperthyroidism or thyrotoxicosis develops in 1 in 1,000 to 1 in 2,000 pregnancies; causes are Graves' disease or Hashimoto's thyroiditis.
      d. Mild thyrotoxicosis may be difficult to assess due to the natural changes in levels of TSH and T4 during pregnancy; they mimic the clinical findings of hyperthyroidism.
   2. Thyroid storm: An acute, life-threatening hypermetabolic state, rare in pregnancy

a. Excessive levels of T4 cause pregnant women to develop pulmonary hypertension and heart failure from cardiomyopathy.
  b. A pregnant woman with thyrotoxicosis has minimal cardiac reserve and decompensates if preeclampsia, anemia, and/or sepsis develop.
  c. Gestational thyrotoxicosis, a transient condition, develops when the normal pregnancy levels of hCG stimulate maternal TSH receptors to secrete massive amounts of T4, which causes suppression of endogenous TSH secretion and hyperemesis gravidarum.
3. Issues for the fetus
  a. Abnormalities of maternal thyroid function and treatment may affect the neonate.
  b. TSH receptor antibodies cross the placenta, stimulate the fetal thyroid gland, and cause a fetal goiter; maternal administration of thionamides may be therapeutic for the fetus.
  c. Although thionamides have the potential to cause fetal complications, these are uncommon.
  d. After pre-pregnancy maternal radioiodine thyroid ablation, fetal thyrotoxicosis may still develop as a result of transplacental passage of long-lived thyroid-stimulating antibodies.
  e. In most cases, the neonate is euthyroid; however, hyper- or hypothyroidism can develop, with or without a goiter.
  f. Approximately 1% of neonates born to mothers with Graves' disease develop fetal hyperthyroidism from the transplacental passage of thyroid-stimulating antibodies.
  g. Placental transfer of autoimmune antibodies may result in fetal goiter and thyrotoxicosis, which may progress to nonimmune hydrops and fetal demise. Fetal sonogram evaluation of thyroid volume can be performed antenatally.
  h. The lowest level of fetal risk for thyroid dysfunction is associated when no maternal antithyroid medications are required, the mother is euthyroid, and there is an absence of anti-thyroid autoimmune antibodies in the third trimester.

    i. Women who require anti-thyroid medications and have thyroid receptor antibodies present have a higher incidence of a fetus with goiters and either hyper- or hypothyroidism.
4. Issues for the VLBW infant
    a. Infants who are hyperthyroid at delivery may have tachycardia, cardiac failure, and an increased metabolic rate.
    b. Increased metabolic rate places the VLBW infant at greater risk for intolerance to labor, perinatal asphyxia, intrauterine and postnatal growth failure, and hypoglycemia.
    c. After delivery, neonatal thyrotoxicosis may require short-term anti-thyroid therapy.
        (1) Symptoms of neonatal thyrotoxicosis include poor weight gain or excessive weight loss, goiter, irritability, tachycardia, flushing, and exophthalmos.
        (2) Many infants are SGA.
        (3) May have elevated or high-normal T4 and suppressed TSH levels.
        (4) Large goiters may cause tracheal obstruction; cardiac failure may need to be treated with propranolol.
        (5) Onset of thyrotoxicosis develops within the first week of life but may be delayed until the second week of life.
        (6) Dysrrhythmias, such as paroxysmal atrial tachycardia and cardiac failure, and death may occur if thyrotoxicity is severe.
        (7) Prognosis is good as thyrotoxic state is transient; most resolve by 9 months of age.
        (8) May have rapid advance in skeletal maturation and advanced bone age, premature closure of cranial sutures.
C. Hypothyroidism (Hashimoto's thyroiditis)
    1. Overview
        a. The most common cause of hypothyroidism in pregnancy is Hashimoto's thyroiditis, caused by glandular destruction of the thyroid by autoimmune antibodies, particularly anti-thyroid peroxidase antibodies.

b. This disorder complicates from 2 in 1,000 to 3 in 1,000 pregnancies.
c. Overt maternal hypothyroidism or inadequate treatment results in a greater frequency of adverse perinatal outcomes; adequate T4 replacement therapy during pregnancy minimizes the risk of adverse outcomes.
d. Transplacental passage of maternal TSH receptor-blocking antibodies may cause fetal hypothyroidism without the development of goiter.
e. Fetal thyroid begins to produce T4 at 14 weeks of gestation; prior to that time, normal maternal thyroid hormone production is important for fetal neurologic development.

2. Congenital hypothyroidism
   a. May be caused by thyroid agenesis, errors of T4 synthesis, genetic factors, and drug-induced environmental factors.
   b. Universal newborn screening mandates testing of all newborns for hypothyroidism.
   c. In the United States, 1 in 2,500 newborns annually are diagnosed with this condition, 80%–90% resulting from thyroid agenesis or hypoplasia.
   d. Early and aggressive T4-replacement therapy is critical for these infants.
   e. Severity of the hypothyroidism, not timing of replacement therapy, is an important factor in long-term cognitive outcomes.

3. Issues for the fetus
   a. Maternal and fetal thyroid abnormalities are inescapably related.
   b. Both require adequate iodide intake; deficiency early in pregnancy results in both maternal and fetal hypothyroidism.
   c. Transplacental passage of maternal TSH receptor-blocking antibodies results in destruction of the fetal thyroid gland and hypothyroidism.
   d. Anti-thyroid peroxidase and anti-thyroglobulin antibodies seem to have little to no effect on fetal thyroid function, despite their transplacental passage.
   e. Women with Hashimoto's thyroiditis typically have fetuses with normal thyroid function.

f. Any fetus inadvertently exposed to radioactive iodine should be carefully evaluated for hypothyroidism after birth; potential for fetal hypothyroidism depends on the size and timing of the dose and the gestational age of the fetus.
4. Issues for the VLBW infant
   a. Infants with decreased thyroid function are at greatest risk for cognitive delays, which are related to the severity of hypothyroidism, rather than simply the timing of replacement therapy.
   b. Hypothyroidism during the critical first weeks of embryologic neurologic development results in neuro-developmental delay, even with early replacement therapy.
   c. Results of universal newborn screening tests for congenital hypothyroidism should be readily available with treatment prior to one month of age.
   d. After diagnosis of hypothyroidism, thyroid hormone (L-thyroxine) should be provided in sufficient doses to achieve a high euthyroid state within 2 weeks of starting therapy.
   e. After starting thyroxine therapy, T4 levels are monitored early in therapy (first 4–6 weeks).
   f. After 4–6 weeks of therapy, the TSH level is the best indicator of adequate treatment.
   g. If the TSH level remains elevated, then the dose of thyroxine needs to be increased.

V. Preeclampsia and HELLP syndrome
A. Overview
   1. This can be fatal to both the mother and the fetus.
   2. The term "pregnancy-induced hypertension" is misleading; does not address the underlying cause of hypertension.
   3. The NIH work group defined four categories of hypertension seen during pregnancy:
      a. Preeclampsia/eclampsia
      b. Gestational hypertension
      c. Chronic hypertension
      d. Preeclampsia/eclampsia superimposed on chronic hypertension
B. Pathophysiology
   1. The fundamental abnormality that underlies preeclampsia/eclampsia is uteroplacental ischemia.

2. Reduced uteroplacental perfusion is demonstrated by ischemic lesions and atherosis of the vascular bed of the placenta, restricted fetal growth secondary to decreased uteroplacental blood flow, and radionucleotide studies.

C. Diagnosis of preeclampsia
   1. Symptoms include new-onset hypertension with proteinuria and with or without edema.
   2. Proteinuria >30 mg in a random specimen or >300 mg in a 24-hour collection is abnormal.
   3. Pathologic edema consists of rapid weight gain (>2.25 kg/week), edema in nondependent sites, or persistent facial edema after patient is upright for a few hours.
   4. The classic definition of hypertension is blood pressure (BP) >140/90 or mean of 105.
   5. BP in the first half of pregnancy is generally lower than the patient's baseline; an increase in systolic BP of 30 and/or an increase in diastolic pressure of 15 do not reliably identify preeclampsia.
   6. Women who later develop preeclampsia have greater decreases in BP in the first half of pregnancy.
   7. Eclampsia presents with seizures, coma, or both, in the setting of preeclampsia.
   8. Severe preeclampsia occurs when a woman with a BP ≥160/110 who meets the basic criteria for a diagnosis of preeclampsia develops other complications, such as a platelet count <100,000, impaired liver function, renal insufficiency, pulmonary edema, visual disturbances (particularly black spots or flashes), epigastric pain, cerebral symptoms (persistent frontal headache), or cyanosis.

D. Assessment and screening during pregnancy
   1. Screening for hypertension and proteinuria is an essential component of standard prenatal care.
   2. Monitoring the progression of hypertension and proteinuria help to distinguish preeclampsia from gestational hypertension (with onset after the 20th week of pregnancy) and chronic hypertension (diagnosed before pregnancy or before the 20th week of gestation).
   3. Preeclampsia is a progressive disease with increasing severity; chronic hypertensive disorders are stable. Both diseases may coexist.
   4. The management goal for preeclampsia is to maximize perinatal outcome within the bounds of maternal and fetal safety.

5. Preeclampsia is more common in first pregnancies and occurs more commonly at the extreme ages of childbearing.
6. Higher levels of proteinuria are more common among African Americans.
7. Preeclampsia may occur more frequently in daughters and sisters of preeclamptic women.
8. The incidence of preeclampsia is higher in lower socioeconomic strata, in twin pregnancies, and diabetic pregnancies.

E. Management during pregnancy
1. Severe hypertension results in serious cerebrovascular events, including parenchymal ischemia and hemorrhage.
2. Antihypertensive therapy includes sublingual nifedipine and intravenous boluses of hydralazine or labetalol.
3. Caution should be taken when using nifedipine; it may cause inadvertent precipitation of angina and myocardial infarction.
4. Corticosteroids are used safely in patients with preeclampsia to accelerate fetal lung maturity and improve neonatal outcomes.
5. Magnesium sulfate infusion is the agent of choice to prevent maternal seizures and can be used in conjunction with nifedipine.
6. Infuse magnesium as a bolus of 2–4 g over 5–30 min, followed by a continuous infusion starting at 1 g/hour and increasing the dose to maintain therapeutic levels of 4–6 mEq/L.
7. Monitor maternal deep-tendon reflexes and urine output in preeclamptic women.

F. Issues for the fetus
1. Greatest risks are due to chronic uteroplacental insufficiency, restricted fetal growth, and fetal hypoxia.
2. These infants have little to no placental reserve and are often intolerant of labor.
3. Interventional preterm delivery, a complication in maternal preeclampsia, is a major cause of perinatal morbidity.
4. The highest fetal death rates occur in women with the greatest increases in hypertension, proteinuria, and uric acid levels.
5. Fetal growth restriction increases the risk of postnatal hypoglycemia and maladaptation to extrauterine life.

6. Chronic fetal hypoxia may result in perinatal asphyxia, abruption, placental insufficiency from placental infarcts, polycythemia, hyperviscosity, neurologic impairment, and fetal death.

G. Issues for VLBW infants
1. Interventional prematurity is the major complication for VLBW infants, due to deteriorating maternal condition, and may result in hypoglycemia, growth abnormalities, increased risks of intraventricular hemorrhage, RDS, patent ductus arteriosus, necrotizing enterocolitis, and an increased risk of infection.
2. Women may present with rapidly progressive, severe preeclampsia and a fetus with a poor biophysical profile, necessitating delivery prior to corticosteroid therapy for fetal lung maturation.
3. If the mother was treated with magnesium sulfate, the fetal serum level is very similar to the maternal level and may result in hypotonia, respiratory depression, hypocalcemia, and poor feeding.
4. Although Apgar scores do not closely correlate to maternal magnesium levels, fetuses exposed to magnesium *in utero* have a higher frequency of hypotonia for their age, as well as decreased intestinal motility and decreased diaphragmatic strength until the magnesium is cleared from their system by renal excretion.
5. Intrauterine growth is frequently impaired in a fetus born to a preeclamptic mother and these infants must be screened for hypoglycemia.
6. Infants born to preeclamptic mothers frequently have a reduced total white blood cell count, neutropenia, and thrombocytopenia.
7. Alterations in white blood cell counts may result in increased susceptibility to infections and bleeding.
8. Impaired placental perfusion seen in this condition may negatively affect transplacental passage of maternal antibodies and reduce passive immunity.

VI. Human immunodeficiency virus (HIV)
A. Overview
1. In the last several years, women represent the greatest number of new HIV cases; more than 50% are among African-American women.

2. Current estimates indicate 110,000–150,000 asymptomatic HIV carriers in the United States.
3. With appropriate recognition and treatment of HIV in pregnancy, the risk of transmission to the newborn, which was once certain, is now <2%.
4. Universal HIV screening in pregnancy is recommended by ACOG and is mandatory in many states.

B. Pathophysiology
1. HIV infection leads to a progressive incompetence of the immune system, leading to opportunistic infections and unusual neoplasms.
2. Diseases may present as AIDS, the condition of an HIV infection, along with opportunistic infections, neoplasia, dementia encephalopathy (wasting syndrome), CD4 counts <200, cervical cancer, pulmonary tuberculosis, and/or recurrent pneumonia.
3. Pregnancy does not alter the progression of HIV disease.
4. Diagnosis is made by rapid testing using enzyme-linked immunoabsorbant assay and is confirmed by a Western blot.

C. Treatment of HIV-positive mothers during pregnancy
1. Treatment during pregnancy involves multiple, potent antiviral medications (nucleoside reverse transcriptase inhibitors, non-nucleoside reverse transcriptase inhibitors, and protease inhibitors), which provide the best long-term control over viral replication.
2. The goal of treatment in pregnancy is to control maternal disease and prevent vertical transmission.
3. All pregnant women who are HIV positive should be treated with antiviral agents (even if they do not meet criteria for non-pregnant women), based on the reduction of vertical transmission to the newborn.
4. Antiviral therapy should drive the viral load below limits of detection.

D. Risks to the fetus
1. Transplacental transmission of HIV has been documented; the virus has been isolated from early trophoblastic tissue, amniotic fluid, membranes, placenta, and breast milk.
2. HIV-positive women in the United States, where formula is readily available, should not breast feed.
3. Intrapartum infections account for 70%–80% of vertical transmission; without treatment, 25%–30% of these infants develop HIV infections.

4. Considerations to reduce vertical transmission include:
    a. Decrease instrumentation.
    b. Reduce length of time membranes are ruptured prior to delivery.
    c. Reduce episiotomies.
    d. Perform operative deliveries before the onset of labor, rupture of membranes, or if viral load is >1,000 copies /mL.
    e. The risk of vertical transmission is correlated to viral load; there is a 1% risk of transmission with viral loads <50 copies/mL.

E. Treatment of HIV-positive mothers during labor
    1. To reduce fetal transmission, intrapartum intravenous zidovudine is recommended for all HIV-infected pregnant women, regardless of their antepartum regimen.
    2. For HIV-positive women in labor who have not received any antepartum antiretroviral therapy, intravenous zidovudine is recommended.
    3. Infants born to HIV-infected women who have not received antepartum antiretroviral drugs should receive prophylactic treatment of a combination antiretroviral drug regimen; begin as soon as possible after birth and continue for 6 weeks.
        a. For the most current NIH guidelines for reduction in the perinatal transmission of HIV, refer to http://aidsinfo.nih.gov/guidelines/html/3/perinatal-guidelines/0.
        b. For up-to-date parental and teaching information, refer to http://aidsinfo.nih.gov/contentfiles/Perinatal_FS_en.pdf.
    4. A randomized, controlled trial has shown that a 2-drug regimen of zidovudine given for 6 weeks, combined with 3 doses of nevirapine in the first week of life (at birth, 48 hours after the first dose, and 96 hours after the second dose), is as effective as, but less toxic than, a 3-drug regimen.
    5. The 3-dose regimen for nevirapine antiretroviral therapy in the first week of life is:
        a. Infants with birth weights of 1.5–2 kg:
            8 mg/dose x 3 doses
        b. Infants with birth weights of >2 kg:
            12 mg/dose x 3 doses

6. Neonatal antiretroviral prophylaxis includes 6 weeks of zidovudine for all HIV-exposed neonates to reduce perinatal transmission of HIV.
7. Zidovudine should be initiated as close to the time of birth as possible, preferably within 6–12 hours of delivery.
8. The 6-week course of zidovudine prophylaxis is recommended at age-appropriate doses.
9. The dosing schedule for zidovudine should be given either intravenously or orally (not both). See **Table 2-3**.

F. Testing
1. If an infant is born to a mother with unknown HIV status, rapid HIV testing of the mother and/or infant should occur as soon as possible after birth; immediately start antiretroviral treatment for the newborn if the rapid test is positive.
2. If the rapid test is positive, confirm with Western blot. Do not wait for the results of the Western blot before initiating antiviral prophylaxis.
3. If the Western blot is positive, perform an HIV DNA polymerase chain reaction (PCR) test on the infant.
4. If the HIV DNA PCR is positive, discontinue the antiretroviral therapy; immediately refer the infant to a pediatric infectious disease specialist for diagnostic confirmation and management.

TABLE 2-3
Dosing Schedule for Zidovudine

Gestational Age	IV Dose/Interval	PO Dose/Interval	Length of Therapy
≥35 weeks	3.0 mg/kg/dose Q 12 hours	4 mg/kg/dose Q 12 hours	6 weeks
≥30–<35 weeks	1.5 mg/kg/dose Q 12 hours for the first 2 weeks of life, then increase to 2.3 mg Q 12 hours for the next 4 weeks	2 mg/kg/dose Q 12 hours for first 2 weeks of life, then increase to 3 mg Q 12 hours for next 4 weeks	6 weeks
<30 weeks	1.5 mg/kg/dose Q 12 hours for the first 4 weeks of life, then increase to 2.3 mg Q 8 hours for the next 2 weeks	2 mg/kg/dose Q 12 hours for the first 4 weeks of life, then increase to 3 mg Q 8 hours for the next 2 weeks	6 weeks

Note: Verify all dosages with your institution's guidelines and current practice.

VII. Herpes simplex virus (HSV)

A. Overview
 1. HSV is a double-stranded-DNA virus that only infects humans.
 2. There are two serotypes: HSV-1 and HSV-2.
 3. HSV is one of the most common sexually transmitted infections worldwide and responsible for 70%–80% of genital ulcers.
 4. There are more than 600,000 new cases annually in the United States; 50 million people in the United States have been exposed to HSV.
 5. There are three types of HSV genital infections:
    a. A primary infection can result from exposure to HSV-1 or HSV-2, without prior exposure to either serotype.
    b. A non-primary first episode can occur when the first clinical episode with HSV-1 or HSV-2 is in an individual with prior exposure to the other serotype.
    c. A recurrent infection is reactivation of a latent virus.
 6. Primary infections are associated with multiple, painful genital lesions with pelvic lymphadenopathy; systemic symptoms include malaise and fever.
 7. Manifestations of non-primary and recurrent infections are not as severe and tend to resolve more quickly.
 8. Recurrences are common; 80%–85% of women with primary HSV-1 have at least one recurrence in their lifetimes.
 9. Of the women who are seropositive for HSV, 20%–30% have never been symptomatic.
 10. Asymptomatic viral shedding occurs in 3%–16% of pregnant women and may be as high as 33% in women who are infected during pregnancy.
 11. Viral shedding is more common in the following cases:
    a. After infection with HSV-2 (rather than HSV-1)
    b. When a second infection occurs soon after the primary outbreak resolves
    c. In a patient who is subject to frequent recurrences

B. Diagnosis and treatment
 1. Perform viral cultures of skin (eye, rectal, conjunctiva, nasopharyngeal) and obtain blood and cerebral spinal fluid for HSV DNA detection using PCR techniques with HSV type-specific serology.

2. There are three viral agents used to treat HSV:
   a. Acyclovir
   b. Valacyclovir
   c. Famciclovir
3. Acyclovir has been used in pregnancy extensively and reduces viral shedding by 90%.
4. An estimated 2% of pregnant women develop a primary HSV infection during pregnancy; the fetus is infected by vertical transmission.

C. Risk to the fetus
   1. If the primary infection develops in the first trimester, there is an increased incidence of early spontaneous abortion, stillbirth, and prematurity.
   2. Infants infected during the first trimester may be born with hallmark skin vesicles or scarring (10%–15%), chorioretinitis (40%–50%), microcephaly (60%), and microphthalmia (25%). Intracranial calcifications (15%), seizures (30%), or evidence of hydranencephaly may be present.
   3. Infants may be born with symptoms or develop them in the first day of life; ~66% of infants are ill by the end of the first week of life, but can develop symptoms of skin, eyes, and mouth (SEM) disease at 10–11 days of life.
   4. Congenital HSV infection occurs in 4% of infected infants; 40% have disease confined to skin, eyes, or mouth; 34% have disease confined to the CNS; 22% of infected infants have the disseminated infection.
   5. Mortality rate is 40%–80%, depending upon organ system involvement, despite treatment with acyclovir; one-half of survivors are expected to have significant long-term residual problems, including psychomotor delay, seizure disorder, spasticity, blindness, and deafness.
   6. The major risk of infection for the fetus is intrapartum exposure to an infected birth canal. The risks are increased when the maternal infection is primary, when multiple lesions are present on the cervix, when the infant is premature, when there is prolonged rupture of membranes, and if fetal scalp electrodes/invasive instrumentation are used.
   7. Vaginal deliveries in women with asymptomatic primary infections infect 30%–50% of neonates.

8. About 60%–80% of infants with HSV infection are born to mothers who are asymptomatic at time of delivery or in whom there is no history of HSV infection.
9. If lesions are from recurrent disease, the risk of transmission is reduced to 3%–5% and further reduced to 0.004% in the presence of asymptomatic viral shedding.
10. Neonatal manifestations involve SEM disease, SEM disease plus CNS involvement, or disseminated disease.
11. Although most infected infants are born with SEM disease, 60%–70% progress to SEM plus CNS or disseminated disease.
12. Most infants with herpes infections are born to mothers who have no history of HSV and have never had symptoms, making the neonatal diagnosis more challenging.
13. Prevention of vertical transmission can be accomplished by performing a cesarean section before or shortly after rupture of membranes, when active lesions are present.
14. Prophylactic acyclovir from 36 weeks onward reduces the recurrence of genital lesions and positive cultures at the time of labor; fewer cesarean sections are required.

VIII. Hepatitis viruses
A. Overview
  1. Hepatitis infections are common and highly contagious.
  2. Hepatitis B and hepatitis C can be sexually transmitted; the fetus can be infected by vertical transmission.
B. Hepatitis B (HB)
  1. Overview
     a. There are three major structural antigens:
        (1) HBsAG
        (2) HBcAG
        (3) HBeAG
     b. HB virus (HBV) is responsible for 40%–50% of acute hepatitis cases in the United States.
     c. 300,000 new cases occur annually.
     d. 12,000–20,000 of those infected develop a chronic-carrier state.
     e. The incubation period lasts from 2 to 4 months.
     f. It manifests with nausea, vomiting, malaise, weakness, abdominal pain, jaundice, hepatic tenderness, and weight loss.

g. The acute course lasts 3–4 weeks, but may persist for months.
h. After infection, 80%–85% have complete resolution with development of protective anti-HBs antibodies.
i. 10%–15% become chronic carriers.
   (1) HBsAG persists in the serum.
   (2) HBeAG may persist for years, followed by a gradual seroconversion to HBeAG antibodies.
j. Asymptomatic carriers have normal liver function tests and HBsAG and anti-HBcAG.
k. Fulminant hepatitis occurs in <1% with acute hepatic failure, encephalopathy, coma, and death.

2. Diagnosis
   a. After exposure to HBV, HBsAG develops and is present for 2–4 weeks before the onset of clinical symptoms and acute infection.
   b. HBeAG develops at this time and the antigen disappears before the symptoms resolve.
   c. Anti-HBeAG develops.
   d. During the convalescent period, anti-HBsAG develops and is evidence of immunity.

3. HB infection in pregnancy
   a. Complicates 1 in 1,000 to 2 in 1,000 pregnancies; chronic-carrier states complicate from 5 in 1,000 to 15 in 1,000 pregnancies.
   b. If maternal infection develops during the first or second trimester, the infection is rarely transmitted to the fetus.
   c. If maternal infection develops during the third trimester, there is an 80%–90% risk of neonatal infection.
   d. Most infants are infected by genital tract secretions or mixing of maternal blood.
   e. The best predictor of neonatal infection is the presence of HBeAG in maternal blood or secretions.
   f. If the mother is a chronic HB carrier and anti-HBeAG positive, the risk of fetal transmission is reduced to 10%–20%.
   g. Most infants who are infected at birth and untreated become chronic carriers and can develop cirrhosis, chronic active hepatitis, or hepatocellular carcinoma.

4. Recommendations in pregnancy and perinatal period
   a. All pregnant women should be screened for HBsAG during pregnancy; repeat for high-risk patients.
   b. Infants who are exposed to HBV or born to mothers with unknown HB status should receive prompt administration of HB immune globulin (HBIG) and HB vaccine.
   c. HBIG reduces the infection rate from 94% to 75% and reduces the carrier state from 91% to 22%.
   d. HBIG should be given within 12 hours of delivery.
   e. HB vaccine further reduces chronic carrier state from 14% to 9%.
   f. HB vaccine should be given within the first week of life.
   g. All newborns should receive HB vaccine after birth, even if the mother is HB negative.
   h. Breast-feeding is not contraindicated.
C. Hepatitis C (HC)
   1. Overview
      a. HC is sometimes called non-A, non-B hepatitis.
      b. The major source of infection occurs by parenteral route, with only a minor percentage as result of sexual transmission.
      c. It is the most common blood-borne infection, responsible for 20%–40% of acute hepatitis cases.
      d. The incubation period is 30–60 days; the disease is asymptomatic in 75% of cases.
      e. Symptoms, when they occur, are milder than HB.
      f. Seroconversion begins by 8–9 weeks; 97% of patients have seroconversion by 6 months.
      g. Fulminant hepatitis is rare; most patients develop chronic liver disease demonstrated by persistence of the HC virus (HCV), RNA, and abnormal liver function tests.
      h. The disease progression is slow and insidious, sometimes taking 20 years.
      i. There is no effective treatment and no vaccine presently available.
      j. HCV occurs in 1%–3% of pregnancies.
      k. Risk factors include IV-drug use, multiple sexual partners, the presence of other infections such as HIV or HBV, and absence of prenatal care.

l. 30%–60% have no identifiable risk factor.
m. The risk of vertical transmission is 5%; if the mother also has HIV disease, incidence of vertical transmission is increased to 23%.
n. Most infected neonates develop a chronic-carrier state and chronic hepatitis.
o. There is no treatment available and immunoprophylaxis is not effective.
p. The mode of delivery does not affect transmission rates.
q. Breast-feeding is not contraindicated, particularly if viral load is low.

IX. Gonorrhea

A. Overview
1. Gonorrhea remains one of the most common sexually transmitted communicable diseases in the United States.
2. More than 300,000 new cases are reported each year; more than 80% occur in 15- to 29-year-olds.
3. The Gram-negative *diplococcus* is found in the genitourinary tract, pharynx, and conjunctiva, and may cause sepsis and arthritis in infected individuals.
4. Gonorrhea infections during pregnancy tend to be asymptomatic, with only some vaginal discharge and dysuria.
5. Screening is done on the first prenatal visit by culturing the cervix; repeat cultures may be indicated for high-risk women.
6. Untreated gonorrhea infection during pregnancy may result in endometritis, premature rupture of membranes, chorioamnionitis, IUGR, or neonatal sepsis.
7. Treatment of maternal gonorrhea during pregnancy incorporates the use of cephalosporins; strains of gonorrhea in the United States are becoming penicillinase-producing and thus, resistant to penicillin.

B. Treatment of the fetus
1. Newborns born to untreated gonorrhea-positive mothers should be given a single dose of ceftriaxone.
2. Newborn eyes should be treated with erythromycin ointment or tetracycline ointment, which reduces the incidence of neonatal gonorrhea ophthalmitis from 10% to <0.5%.

3. Gonorrhea ophthalmitis develops within 4 days with frank, purulent discharge from both eyes. If left untreated, corneal ulceration develops, which leads to corneal scarring and blindness.

X. Syphilis
A. Overview
1. Syphilis is a serious, highly contagious, sexually transmitted disease caused by the organism *Treponema pallidum*.
2. Rates of syphilis vary widely across the country, with higher rates seen in women who are prostitutes, have multiple random partners, and who have little to no prenatal care.
3. The incubation period is 10–90 days after exposure to the organism.
4. The hallmark lesion of primary syphilis infection — a painless chancre, which is indurated with raised borders — develops at the site of exposure, usually the penis or cervix.
5. Primary syphilis is a local infection.
6. If primary syphilis is not treated, secondary syphilis develops 4–10 weeks later and is a systemic infection, which is disseminated throughout the body by the bloodstream.
7. Symptoms of secondary syphilis include fever, lymphadenopathy, condyloma lata, and a generalized maculopapular rash on the trunk, limbs, palms and soles.
8. After the rash fades, a latent period begins which may last for years.
9. If untreated, one-third of those infected develop tertiary syphilis, with involvement of the CNS and cardiovascular system, and gumma formation within 10–30 years.

B. Diagnosis
1. Non-treponema antigen screening tests include rapid plasma reagin (RPR) and the Venereal Disease Research Laboratory (VDRL).
2. False positives occur in 1%–2% due to subclinical autoimmune disease, recent fever, and laboratory error.
3. Confirm all positive results from either the RPR or VDRL with a specific antibody test using microhemagglutination assay or fluorescent treponemal antibody absorption test to detect antibodies to *T pallidum*.

C. Management and treatment
1. Prenatal care identifies women who have been exposed and infected with syphilis.
2. Individuals with syphilis require treatment with penicillin.
3. The number of doses depends upon the stage of the disease at the time of treatment.
4. Penicillin is safe to use in pregnancy; test of cure should be done to assure adequate treatment.
5. Erythromycin does not cross the placenta and does not treat the fetus; tetracycline causes fetal dental darkening; both drugs should be avoided.
6. The mother should be monitored monthly with either RPR or VDRL screening to detect an increase in titers or a lack of a 4-fold increase in titers over 3 months, which indicates a need for re-treatment.
7. Women who test positive for syphilis should also be screened for HIV, a known comorbidity.

XI. Congenital syphilis
A. Overview
1. Infants can be infected during the transplacental passage of the organism to the fetus during pregnancy or from fetal contact with active genital lesions during labor and delivery.
2. Up to 40–50% of congenital syphilis cases are fatal.
3. Early fetal infection may result in spontaneous abortion due to overwhelming infection of the placenta and the development of non-immune hydrops.
4. While nearly all infants born to mothers with primary or secondary syphilis have treponemes transmitted to them, only 50% of the infants are symptomatic.
5. If the infant is born in the early latent stage, there is a 40% chance of organism transmission, whereas if the infant is born during the late latent stage, the risk of transmission is 6%–14%.
6. Even with treatment, 11% of fetuses have CNS involvement.
B. Symptoms of untreated congenital syphilis include:
1. Non-immune hydrops
2. IUGR
3. Hemolytic anemia
4. Hepatosplenomegaly
5. Jaundice rhinitis

6. Maculopapular rash
7. Condyloma lata
8. Bone abnormalities, such as periostitis and osteochondritis
9. CNS involvement
C. Infections that occur late in pregnancy or are undertreated result in neurologic involvement, hearing loss from damage to the eighth cranial nerve, hydrocephalus, dental abnormalities (Hutchinson's teeth, mulberry molars), rhagades, saddle nose, saber shins, and clutton joints.

XII. *Chlamydia trachomatis*
A. Overview
1. More than 4 million infections occur annually.
2. *C. trachomatis* is an obligate intracellular bacterium that depends upon the invaded cell for its energy supply and destroys that cell with its replication.
3. Serotypes D–K cause inclusion conjunctivitis, newborn pneumonia, urethritis, cervicitis, salpingitis, acute urethral syndrome, and perinatal infections.
4. High-risk groups include inner-city women, particularly African Americans.
5. 40%–60% of women with positive gonorrhea cultures are also positive for chlamydia.
6. The cervix is the primary site of infection.
7. The woman may be asymptomatic or the infection may cause hypertrophic cervical erosion and copious mucopurulent discharge.
8. Chlamydial infections are a common cause of tubal infertility.
B. Diagnosis and treatment
1. Diagnosed with nucleic acid amplification tests.
2. Treatment of choice in pregnancy is azithromycin; erythromycin and amoxicillin are alternatives.
C. Risks to the fetus
1. Untreated chlamydia may cause a higher incidence of premature rupture of membranes, birth weight <2,500 g, and lower incidence of neonatal survival.
2. Newborns delivered to mothers with active chlamydial cervical infections have a 25%–60% chance of becoming infected.
3. The clinical presentation of chlamydial infection include conjunctivitis, which develops in 18%–45% of infants; and neonatal pneumonia, which develops in 20%.

4. Conjunctivitis is treated with erythromycin ointment.
5. Neonatal chlamydial pneumonia develops 4–11 weeks after birth and manifests with signs of congestion and obstruction, little nasal discharge, minimal fever, tachypnea, and a prominent staccato cough.
6. Bilateral infiltrates and lung hyperexpansion are found on chest radiograph.
7. Blood gases demonstrate mild to moderate hypoxemia.
8. Approximately 50% of these infants had conjunctivitis after delivery.
9. Most infants recover quickly with erythromycin treatment.

References

American College of Obstetricians and Gynecologists Task Force on Hypertension in Pregnancy. *Hypertension in Pregnancy*. Washington, DC: American College of Obstetricians and Gynecologists; 2013.

Berghella V, ed. Maternal-Fetal Evidence Based Guidelines. 2nd ed. New York, NY: Informa Healthcare; 2011.

Cloherty JP, Eichenwald EC, Hansen AR, Stark AR. *Manual of Neonatal Care*. 7th ed. Philadelphia, PA: Wolters Kluwer Health/Lippincott Williams & Wilkins; 2011.

Gardner SL, Carter BS, Enzman-Hines M, Hernandez JA. *Merenstein and Gardner's Handbook of Neonatal Intensive Care*. 7th ed. St. Louis, MO: Mosby Elsevier; 2011.

Gomella TL, Cunningham MD, Eyal FG, eds. *Neonatology: Management, Procedures, On-Call Problems, Diseases, and Drugs*. 7th ed. New York, NY: McGraw Hill/Lange; 2013.

Leveno KJ. *William's Manual of Pregnancy Complications*. 23rd ed. New York, NY: McGraw Hill Medical; 2013.

Martin RJ, Fanaroff AA, Walsh MC. *Fanaroff and Martin's Neonatal-Perinatal Medicine: Diseases of the Fetus and Infant*. 9th ed. St. Louis, MO: Mosby Elsevier; 2011.

Wildschut H, Weiner CP, Peters TJ. *When to Screen in Obstetrics and Gynecology*. 2nd ed. Philadelphia, PA: Saunders Elsevier; 2006.

Neonatal Assessment

Terri A. Cavaliere

I. Introduction
A. The use of an organized, structured approach is critical when caring for a very low birth weight (VLBW) neonate during the Golden Hours.
B. Basic to this systemic method is a comprehensive assessment, which, depending on the clinical condition of the neonate, may take place in the delivery room, the stabilization area, or the NICU.
C. It may be possible to perform an entire assessment at one time or it may be necessary to complete the examination in stages, depending on the stability and tolerance of the patient.
D. The assessment should be performed as a team activity to protect the infant from multiple examinations during a very vulnerable time period.

II. Neonatal Resuscitation Program (NRP) and Apgar score
A. Assessment of the neonate begins in the delivery room.
B. Immediately upon delivery, emphasis is placed on cardiorespiratory stabilization, which is guided by the principles of the NRP.
C. Assignment of the Apgar score represents another component of the initial newborn assessment.

III. Assessment: A continuous process
A. Overview
  1. Once initial cardiorespiratory stabilization is achieved, consideration must be given to other aspects of care, including:
     a. Risk and prevention of thermal challenges and injury to the central nervous system
     b. Predisposition to sepsis and bleeding
     c. Fluid requirements
  2. Interventions are guided by the ongoing assessment of the neonate's response to resuscitation and clinical condition.
  3. According to the American Academy of Pediatrics (AAP) and the American Heart Association (AHA), rapid systematic intervention for critically ill infants is key to preventing progression to more serious conditions, such as cardiorespiratory arrest.

4. Employing an organized approach to neonatal assessment enables the provider to rapidly identify cardiorespiratory instability (respiratory distress or hypotension), facilitating immediate interventions.
5. Clinical compromise and deterioration (respiratory arrest, shock) can result from failure to provide expeditious treatment.

B. Approach
1. Assessment is an important aspect of the Golden Hours bundle.
2. This bundle incorporates and expands on NRP guidelines to ensure that the unique needs of the VLBW population are addressed.
3. A systematic approach to assessment is not ideally suited for the needs of the neonate <1,500 g, however, it can be modified and used as a framework for neonatal assessment during the Golden Hours.

C. Evaluation
1. A structured yet flexible process is suggested, which coordinates evaluation with intervention.
2. This facilitates emergent intervention but also allows treatment to be delayed, if appropriate, until the assessment is complete.
3. The cyclic nature of the assessment process, in which each step flows into the next, is illustrated in **Fig. 3-1**.
4. Evaluation, identification, and management should continue:
    a. Until stabilization is achieved
    b. After any intervention
    c. When the patient's condition changes
5. An essential skill for neonatal care providers is the ability to identify and differentiate between life-threatening and non-life-threatening problems.
6. In addition to cardiac arrest, advanced management or emergency responses should be activated per NRP or unit protocol for life-threatening problems, such as:
    a. Airway obstruction
    b. Apnea/bradypnea that is unresponsive to simple interventions (suctioning, repositioning)
    c. Significantly increased work of breathing
    d. Pneumothorax
    e. Absence of palpable pulses
    f. Poor perfusion

g. Bradycardia accompanied by other signs of cardiovascular instability
h. Hypotension
i. Severe hypothermia
j. Bleeding
7. Once the infant is clinically stable, secondary assessment can begin.
8. Physical evaluation can continue in the face of non-life-threatening problems.
9. Examples of life-threatening conditions are listed in **Box 3-1**.

FIGURE 3-1
Suggested Approach to Neonatal Evaluation During the Golden Hours

ANTENATAL PERIOD
Obtain Comprehensive History (if time permits)

DELIVERY
NRP Stabilization
APGAR Score

EVALUATION
Primary
Secondary

IDENTIFICATION OF PROBLEMS/DIAGNOSIS

INTERVENTION

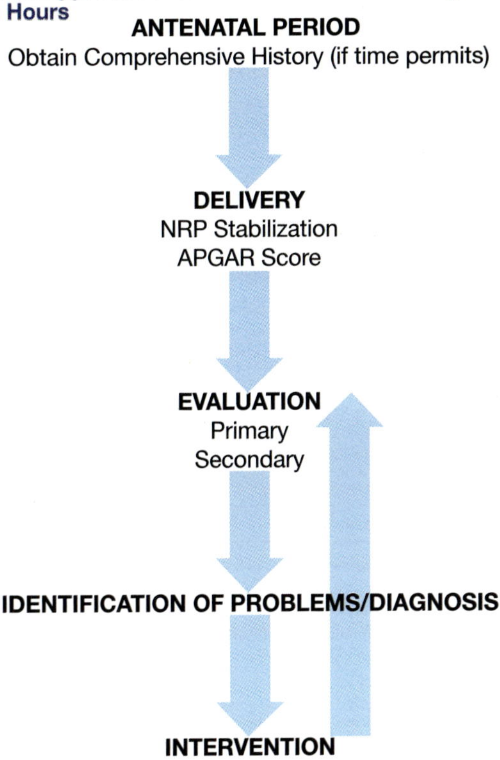

A structured yet flexible process is suggested to evaluate the neonate during the Golden Hours to facilitate emergent management while allowing treatment to be delayed, if appropriate, until assessment is complete. Evaluation, identification, and management should continue until stabilization is achieved, after any intervention, and when the patient's condition changes.

IV. Primary evaluation of ABCO (airway, breathing, circulation, and other) (Fig. 3-2)

A. Upper airway patency
   1. Observe chest and abdominal movement.
   2. Auscultate air movement and breath sounds.
   3. Suspect obstruction if there is increased work of breathing, retractions, adventitious inspiratory sounds (stridor, snorting), apparent respiratory efforts without breath sounds, difficulty passing catheter through one or both nares, and copious oral or nasal secretions.
      a. If there is concern regarding obstructed nares, a suction catheter may be gently inserted through one or both nares.
      b. Routine passage of suction catheters in an asymptomatic neonate is not recommended, as it could result in swelling and edema that leads to an obstruction that was not originally present.

BOX 3-1
Life-Threatening Conditions

REQUIRE IMMEDIATE INTERVENTION
Any condition or abnormality that causes cardiorespiratory instability
Obstructed airway not restored by simple measures (positioning/suctioning)
Cardiorespiratory arrest
Agonal breathing, gasping
Absent breath sounds (unilateral, bilateral)
Bilateral choanal atresia
Cyanosis, grunting, retracting, nasal flaring
Sustained bradycardia, tachycardia
Hypotension, shock, hypoperfusion, pallor, absent pulses
Bleeding
Scaphoid abdomen with barrel chest (diaphragmatic hernia)
Severe hypothermia
Symptomatic hypoglycemia
Seizures
Abdominal wall defects (gastroschisis, omphalocele, bladder exstrophy)
Dermatological problems (epidermolysis bullosa, ichthyosis)

B. Breathing/respiratory rate
   1. The normal rate is 30–60 breaths/min, with wide variations.
      a. Abnormalities include tachypnea, bradypnea, apnea, or gasping.
      b. A sustained increase or decrease from the infant's baseline respiratory rate can be suggestive of problems.
      c. Increased respiratory effort can be caused by increased resistance to airflow or by non-compliant lungs.
      d. Nasal flaring and retractions are signs of respiratory distress.
   2. Evaluate chest expansion, air movement, and lung/airway sounds.
      a. Expansion should be bilaterally symmetric and readily visible during inspiration.
      b. Evaluate the intensity of breath sounds and the quality of air movement; diminished distal air entry suggests airflow obstruction or lung disease.

FIGURE 3-2
Aspects of Primary Evaluation (ABCO)

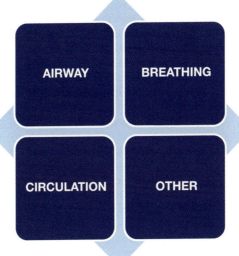

Primary evaluation of ABCO includes: upper airway patency; breathing/respiratory rate; chest expansion, air movement, and lung/airway sounds; circulation; and other considerations, such as skin color, hypothermia, glucose levels, and birth defects.

c. Stridor can indicate upper airway obstruction or congenital airway abnormalities.
d. Grunting is a compensatory mechanism that may signal lung disease or pulmonary edema; the cause should be identified and treated rapidly.
e. Gurgling signals upper airway obstruction due to secretions.
f. Crackles can be caused by fluid accumulation and are most generally associated with lung disease or atelectasis.
g. Rhonchi are caused by secretions or aspirated matter in large airways.
h. Diminished or unilateral breath sounds can be noted in pneumothorax or misplaced endotracheal tubes.
i. A barrel-shaped chest is the result of air trapping in pleural spaces (pneumomediastinum), space-occupying lesions (diaphragmatic hernia), or over-distention from mechanical ventilation.

C. Circulation
1. Heart rate typically ranges from 120–160 beats/min (bpm), depending on the infant's state and gestational age.
2. Resting heart rate is most representative; premature babies have higher resting heart rates; rhythm should be regular.
3. Sustained bradycardia, tachycardia, or asystole may be due to shock, asphyxia, or conduction defects.
4. Brief asymptomatic irregularities in rate and rhythm are not unusual. Sinus bradycardia and tachycardia and premature atrial or ventricular contractions are commonly benign.
5. Blood pressure (BP) varies according to chronologic and gestational age.
   a. Hypotension is defined as mean arterial pressure (MAP) <10th percentile for gestational age, weight, and postnatal age **or** MAP <gestational age in weeks during the Golden Hours.
   b. BP alone should not be the sole parameter prompting treatment for hypotension; consideration should be given to signs of cardiac instability before volume expanders or inotropic agents are employed:
      (1) Heart rate
      (2) Perfusion
      (3) Capillary refill time (CRT)
      (4) Pulses

(5) Oxygenation
(6) pH
(7) Hypothermia
6. If hypotension exists, management is needed to prevent development of shock and end organ damage or irreversible shock and death.
7. Pulses reflect perfusion status.
    a. Palpate central (femoral) and peripheral (radial, brachial) pulses.
    b. Central pulses are generally stronger than peripheral; differences in quality can occur in shock.
    c. Peripheral pulses can be diminished in a cool environment.
    d. CRT should be <3 sec and is inversely proportional to tissue perfusion; hypovolemia, shock, and hypothermia can prolong CRT.
    e. Weak central pulses and decreased perfusion should prompt rapid management.
8. Hemorrhage or bleeding may be visible or covert.
    a. Sources/sites of blood loss include, but are not limited to: subgaleal bleeding, lacerations, gastrointestinal tract, intracranial, intradermal (purpura, petechiae), and coagulopathy.
    b. Emergent management may be needed to prevent the development of hypotension and shock.
9. Neonates should be evaluated for signs and symptoms of congenital heart disease/heart failure, as well as heart murmurs or other adventitious cardiac sounds (rubs, gallops, clicks). It may be necessary to differentiate between innocent murmurs and pathologic murmurs.

D. Other considerations
1. Skin color
    a. Acrocyanosis is common in the first 24 hours; beyond this time period, cyanosis of extremities may be due to shock, sepsis, or congestive heart failure.
    b. Vasomotor instability after birth may cause mottling (cutis marmorata), which can be benign; if accompanied by other signs of cardiovascular compromise (bradycardia, decreased perfusion), it can signify a more serious condition.
    c. Pallor suggests blood loss or poor perfusion.
    d. Cyanosis is never normal and may indicate pulmonary disease, shock, or cardiac defect.

e. True mottling, pallor, and cyanosis suggest life-threatening problems and should prompt rapid intervention before further evaluation proceeds.
2. Hypothermia
   a. Hypothermia is life threatening in VLBW infants.
   b. If low temperature is detected, interrupt the evaluation and perform interventions to prevent heat loss.
   c. Place the neonate in a neutral thermal environment.
3. Glucose levels
   a. Hypoglycemia can lead to hypothermia and hypoxia.
   b. Serum glucose measurement is essential within 30–60 min of birth to detect the need for supplemental glucose.
4. Birth defects
   a. Birth defects may be minor or life threatening.
   b. Conditions that require immediate attention to prevent further injury or harm include: cyanotic heart disease, choanal atresia, meningomyelocele, encephalocele, omphalocele, gastroschisis, exstrophy of the bladder, diaphragmatic hernia, epidermolysis bullosa, ichthyosis, and seizures.
5. Jaundice appearing directly at birth is not normal and warrants management, evaluation, and possible treatment.

V. Secondary evaluation: When the neonate is stable and/or all appropriate interventions have been instituted

A. History
1. Frequently, the neonatal team obtains a comprehensive history prior to delivery.
2. In an emergency or unexpected delivery, it may be necessary to proceed with care without a complete history.
3. Regardless of when or where the history is obtained, the following elements should be included:
   a. Maternal history
      (1) Age
      (2) Obstetric and medical histories
      (3) History of present pregnancy: prenatal labs and testing, medications, antenatal management (cerclage, antibiotics, tocolysis, steroids, etc.)
      (4) Events surrounding labor and delivery: length of ruptured membranes, electronic fetal monitoring, analgesia/anesthesia, type of delivery, use of instrumentation (forceps, vacuum)

(5) Family history: chronic illnesses, hereditary diseases, genetic abnormalities
(6) Comprehensive physical examination

B. Neonatal examination
  1. Weight, measurements (head circumference, length)
  2. Gestational age (GA) evaluation
     a. GA evaluation is important to help determine particular neonatal risk factors and establish treatment plans.
     b. There are medical, ethical, and social issues that necessitate accurate GA assessment, especially for extremely low birth weight (ELBW) babies born at or near the threshold of viability.
     c. Data regarding mortality and morbidity are frequently used to advise parents in deciding on treatment options.
  3. Head-to-toe examination
     a. Extremely premature infants will have physical characteristics that are uniquely different from a term baby.
     b. Breast buds are often imperceptible or barely perceptible.
  4. Head, eyes, ears, nose, throat (HEENT)
     a. Petechiae of the face and facial bruising may be seen with trauma and venostasis, as in vertex deliveries or with tight nuchal cords.
     b. Fusion of eyelids may be noted in neonates <23 weeks gestation, precluding examination of the eyes.
     c. Ears are usually flat and, when you fold them, will stay folded.
  5. Cardiovascular system (CVS)/respiratory
     a. Soft murmurs may be audible prior to ductal closure and should be evaluated clinically and re-evaluated at 24 hours of age.
  6. Respiratory
     a. Coarse crackles, tachypnea, grunting and retracting may be present until lung fluid clears or with respiratory distress syndrome (with or without cyanosis) and must be monitored.
     b. Respiratory rates of 30–60/min are normal after transition and higher rates should be evaluated.

7. Gastrointestinal/abdomen
   a. Bowel sounds are absent at birth but begin to be audible at ~15 min–1 hour of age
8. Genitalia and anus
   a. Discoloration of the testes may be a hematoma or torsion and should be evaluated immediately. Keep in mind, however, that in VLBW neonates the testes may be completely undescended or in the inguinal canal.
   b. Attention should be paid to findings that are suggestive of ambiguous genitalia.
   c. Extremely premature males will have flat, smooth scrotum or only faint rugae with testes in the canals.
   d. Extremely premature female infants will have a prominent clitoris and flat labia; as they mature, the labia minora will be small and increase in size with age.
9. Musculoskeletal: extremities, back
10. Skin
    a. Jaundice at birth is always abnormal and requires immediate further investigation and follow-up.
    b. The dermis and epidermis in ELBW neonates are thin and fragile. Gentle handling is necessary to avoid denuding areas of skin by drying or rubbing.
       (1) The skin may be sticky, friable, and transparent or gelatinous, red, and translucent; based on gestational age.
11. Neurologic
    a. The neurologic examination (state, tone, posture, reflexes, etc.) differs according to gestational age. ELBW and VLBW neonates have different neurologic characteristics, which should be appreciated when performing assessment of this system. Refer to texts listed in the references for more details.
    b. The ELBW infant has poor tone with little to no posture.
       (1) There is no arm recoil in premature infants when the arm is extended.
       (2) The heel can easily be brought up to the ears and the knee has full flexion.
       (3) The elbow crosses easily over the chest with little resistance.

C. Physical findings of concern (also see Section IV.D.):
   1. Blue sclerae (osteogenesis imperfecta)

a. Sclerae may appear bluish in premature infants, but osteogenesis imperfecta should be ruled out if sclerae are deep blue.
2. Scaphoid abdomen (diaphragmatic hernia)
3. Dysmorphic features (trisomies, congenital anomalies, ambiguous/abnormal genitalia, syndromic features)
   a. Discovery should prompt a thorough assessment of other possible associated anomalies.
   b. Consider obtaining a genetics consult once the neonate is clinically stable. Speak to parents to inform them of the concerns.
4. Birth trauma (phrenic nerve injury, brachial plexus palsy, facial palsy, fractures)
5. Cleft lip and palate
6. Immobile cranial sutures (craniosynostosis)
7. Skeletal abnormalities: short limbs, syndactyly

VI. Diagnostic tests
A. Diagnostic tests assist in establishing a definitive diagnosis, identifying the presence and severity of cardiorespiratory problems and metabolic imbalances.
B. Some of these tests will have been done earlier in the neonate's life.
C. There is no ideal timing for performing these tests; the time will vary according to the individual situation and unit protocol.
D. Baseline testing should be based on the infant's condition and may include arterial blood gas (ABG), chest x-ray, complete blood count with differential, pulse oximetry, or invasive arterial monitoring.
E. Electrolytes are more helpful when obtained at 18–24 hours of age, although NICU policies may vary.

References

Annibale DJ, Bissinger RL. The golden hour. *Adv Neonatal Care.* 2010;10(5):221-223.

Askin D. Chest and lungs assessment. In: Tappero EP, ME Honeyfield ME, eds. *Physical Assessment of the Newborn: A Comprehensive Approach to the Art of Physical Examination.* 4th ed. Petaluma, CA: NICU Ink; 2009:75-86.

Bissinger RL. Golden hour of care for very low-birth-weight infants. *National Association of Neonatal Nurses E-news.* 2010;2(4):1-3. http://www.nann.org/pdf/enews/2010jul.pdf.

Bissinger RL, Annibale DJ. Thermoregulation in very low-birth-weight infants during the golden hour: results and implications. *Adv Neonatal Care.* 2010;10(5):230-238.

Cavaliere TA, Sansoucie DA. Assessment of the newborn and infant. In Kenner CA, Lott JW, eds. *Comprehensive Neonatal Nursing Care.* 5th ed. New York, NY: Springer; 2014:71-112.

Chameides L, Samson RA, Schexnayder SM, Hazinski MF, eds. *Pediatric Advanced Life Support: Provider Manual.* American Heart Association and American Academy of Pediatrics; 2012.

Conway-Orgel M. Management of hypotension in the very low-birth-weight infant during the golden hour. *Adv Neonatal Care.* 2010;10(5):241-245.

Fletcher MA. *Physical Diagnosis in Neonatology.* Philadelphia, PA: Lippincott Williams & Wilkins; 1997.

Schwengel, DA, Paidas, CN, Yaster M. Initial assessment. In: Nichols DG, Yaster M, Schleien CL, Paidas CN, eds. *Golden Hour: The Handbook of Advanced Pediatric Life Support.* 3rd ed. Philadelphia, PA: Mosby Elsevier; 2011:1-7.

Tappero, EP, Honeyfield, ME, eds. *Physical Assessment of the Newborn: A Comprehensive Approach to the Art of Physical Examination.* 4th ed. Petaluma, CA: NICU Ink; 2009.

Textbook of Neonatal Resuscitation. 6th ed. American Academy of Pediatrics and American Heart Association; 2011.

Vargo L. Cardiovascular assessment. In: Tappero EP, Honeyfield ME, eds. *Physical Assessment of the Newborn: A Comprehensive Approach to the Art of Physical Examination.* 4th ed. Petaluma, CA: NICU Ink; 2009:87-104.

Vargo L, Seri I. *The Management Of Hypotension in the Very-Low-Birth-Weight Infant: Guideline for Practice.* Glenview, IL: National Association of Neonatal Nurses; 2011:1-13.

4

Transition at Birth and Umbilical Cord Blood Gas Analysis

Gautham K. Suresh

I. Fetal circulation
A. The placenta is responsible for the respiratory, nutritional, and excretory functions during fetal life.
B. The umbilical vessels are part of the fetal circulation and are named as such.
   1. Veins carry blood back to the heart (umbilical vein).
   2. Arteries carry blood from the fetal heart (umbilical arteries).
C. The umbilical vein carries oxygenated blood from the placenta to the fetal inferior vena cava (bypassing much of the liver through the ductus venosus).
D. Blood in the umbilical vein has a partial pressure of oxygen (PO_2) of 30–35 torr.
E. A major portion of the oxygenated blood from the placenta is streamed through the foramen ovale into the left atrium and preferentially circulated to the head and upper extremities.
F. Highly oxygenated blood is therefore supplied to organs with the highest oxygen demand: the brain and myocardium.
G. Pulmonary blood flow is minimal, secondary to increased pulmonary artery pressure and reduced need for such flow.
H. 13%–25% of right-ventricular output flows to the lungs; the rest bypasses the lungs through the ductus arteriosus into the descending aorta (because the lungs are not active organs of respiration in the fetus).
I. *In utero*, the ductus remains open due to the hypoxic fetal environment, nitric oxide, and high circulating levels of prostaglandins.
J. The two umbilical arteries carry blood from the fetal aorta to the placenta; this blood has a PO_2 of ~20 torr.

II. Changes at birth
A. Overall, parallel (fetal) circulation (**Fig. 4-1**) transitions to a series (neonatal) circulation (**Fig. 4-2**).
B. The lungs take over as the organs of respiration during transition; they expand and fill with air as the newborn infant cries and breathes.

C. Pulmonary vascular resistance drops rapidly, pulmonary artery pressure decreases, and pulmonary blood flow increases.
D. Alveolar oxygen tension and arterial oxygen tension both increase.
E. Oxygen is a potent pulmonary vasodilator.
F. Umbilical arteries constrict soon after birth, primarily due to an increase in oxygen tension.
G. The constriction, combined with the clamping of the umbilical cord, which removes the low-resistance circulation of the placenta, causes an increase in systemic vascular resistance.
H. The systemic vascular resistance rises above the pulmonary vascular resistance, which reverses the direction of blood flow in the ductus arteriosus, changing the flow from left to right.
I. Three fetal shunts close after birth.

FIGURE 4-1
Fetal Circulation (Parallel)

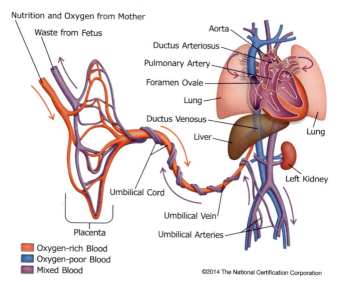

The umbilical vessels are part of the fetal circulation. The umbilical vein carries oxygenated blood from the placenta to the fetal inferior vena cava (bypassing much of the liver through the ductus venosus). A major portion of the oxygenated blood from the placenta is streamed through the foramen ovale into the left atrium and preferentially circulated through to the head and upper extremities. The two umbilical arteries carry blood from the fetal aorta to the placenta.

1. The ductus arteriosus usually closes functionally within 12–24 hours after birth, secondary to:
   a. The increase in oxygen related to the onset of spontaneous respirations
   b. The removal of the placenta, which is the site of prostaglandin E2 (PGE_2) production, and the increase in blood flow to the lungs where PGE_2 is metabolized, leading to a fall in PGE_2

FIGURE 4-2
Neonatal Circulation (Series)

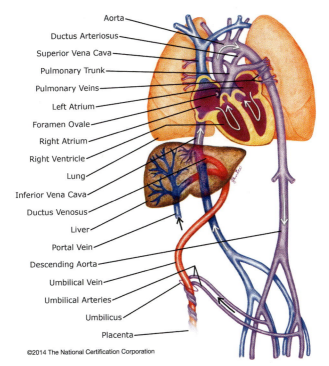

Overall, parallel (fetal) circulation transitions to a series (neonatal) circulation at birth. The lungs take over as the organs of respiration during transition. Umbilical arteries constrict soon after birth. The systemic vascular resistance rises above the pulmonary vascular resistance, which reverses the direction of the blood flow in the ductus arteriosus from left to right. Three fetal shunts — the ductus arteriosus, the ductus venosus, and the flap mechanism of the foramen ovale — close shortly after birth.

2. The ductus venosus closes functionally soon after birth, passively collapsing due to decreased blood flow following cord clamping and the removal of the placental bed.
3. Functional closure of the flap mechanism of the foramen ovale occurs, primarily due to the increased pressure in the left atrium (due to increased pulmonary venous return) and a decreased pressure in the right atrium (due to closure of the ductus venosus and the clamping of the umbilical cord).

III. Later changes

A. Between 6 and 8 weeks after birth, a slow fall in pulmonary vascular resistance and pulmonary artery pressure occur, due to the thinning of the medial layer of the pulmonary arterioles.

B. A further decrease occurs after the first two years, possibly related to the increase in number of alveolar units and their associated vessels.

C. Permanent closure of fetal shunts occurs.
1. Anatomic closure of the ductus venosus takes up to 3 weeks after birth and occurs by thrombosis, fibrosis, and muscle contraction.
2. The ductus is replaced by the ligamentum arteriosum.
3. Anatomic closure of the foramen ovale typically is complete by age 3; a small, hemodynamically insignificant shunt remains in many adults.

IV. Obtaining umbilical cord blood gas samples

A. At every delivery, immediately after the infant is born, a 10- to 20-cm segment of umbilical cord should be double-clamped, divided, and placed aside (**Fig. 4-3**).

B. This sample of cord ensures that cord blood is available for testing if necessary.

C. A clamped segment of cord is stable for pH and blood gas assessment for at least 60 min; a cord blood sample in a pre-heparinized syringe is stable for up to 60 min.

D. Delivery room personnel need to be skilled at obtaining adequate and accurate cord blood samples.

E. If the infant is vigorous and the Apgar scores at 1 and 5 min are ≥7, the cord sample can be discarded.

F. Cord blood samples should be drawn from the cord segment and sent for analysis if:

1. There are known risk conditions, such as suspected fetal compromise, abnormal fetal heart rate tracing, severe growth restriction, maternal thyroid disease, intrapartum fever, or multifetal gestations.
2. There is a problem during the delivery process.
3. The neonate's condition at 5 min after birth is not satisfactory (see Section IV.E).

G. Umbilical arterial values provide the most accurate information regarding fetal and newborn acid-base status.

H. If blood specimens are required, both umbilical venous and arterial specimens should be obtained to be sure that an umbilical artery specimen is sampled and to clarify the source of any pathophysiology.

I. The umbilical vein is larger and less muscular than umbilical arteries.

J. The samples should be unambiguously labeled and reported (e.g., "umbilical arterial" rather than "umbilical").

K. If there is difficulty obtaining an arterial blood specimen from the cord, the sample can be drawn from an artery on the chorionic surface of the placenta.

FIGURE 4-3
Umbilical Cord Arteries and Vein

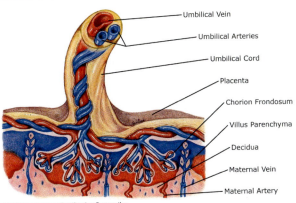

©2014 The National Certification Corporation

Immediately after the infant is born, a 10- to 20-cm segment of umbilical cord should be double-clamped, divided, and placed aside to ensure that a cord blood sample is available for testing if necessary. Delivery room personnel must be skilled in obtaining adequate and accurate cord blood samples. If the infant is vigorous and Apgar scores at 1 and 5 min are ≥7, the cord sample can be discarded.

1. These arteries are relatively easy to identify because they cross over the veins.
2. However, these samples are subject to rapid degradation and are far less reliable; they must be obtained as soon as possible after delivery.

V. Interpretation of umbilical cord blood gas values

A. Umbilical cord blood gas analysis can provide important information about the status of the infant during the intrapartum period and delivery; it can also contribute to predicting the infant's future health status.
B. Umbilical arterial cord blood acid-base and gas assessment remains the most objective determination of the fetal metabolic condition at the moment of birth.
C. All interpretations should be made in light of the fact that cord blood gas analysis is a static measure, indicating the acid-base status in the umbilical cord blood at a given point in time.
D. Umbilical cord blood gas values should always be interpreted in context with the obstetric history, prenatal course, events during delivery, and the neonate's condition at and after birth.
E. Normally, because fetal carbon dioxide is removed from the umbilical arterial blood in the placenta, umbilical venous blood has a slightly higher pH and lower partial pressure of carbon dioxide (PCO_2) than umbilical arterial blood.
F. When the sample is processed, pH, PCO_2, and PO_2 are directly measured.
   1. The bicarbonate, base deficit, and oxygen saturation are all calculated from the measured parameters.
   2. The base deficit reflects metabolic acidosis or alkalosis better than bicarbonate in the face of either high or low PCO_2 (**Table 4-1**).

VI. Identifying improperly collected and mislabeled specimens (quality-related issues)

A. Sample obtained from unclamped vs. clamped cord
   1. Immediately after delivery, placental metabolism and gas exchange continue.
   2. Any umbilical cord blood that stays in continuity with the placenta will have progressive changes in blood gas and pH values; for example, the cord arterial or venous pH can decrease by 0.2 units over the first hour after delivery.

a. Progressive changes do not occur if the sample is obtained from a cord segment isolated between two clamps.
b. If the analyzed specimen came from an unclamped cord, the timing in relation to delivery must be determined.

B. Umbilical arterial specimen labeled as venous or vice-versa
1. Mislabeling reportedly occurs ~10% of the time.
2. If the sample labeled as an arterial sample has a higher pH, lower PCO_2, and higher PO_2 than the sample labeled venous, then it is likely that the labels of the two samples were accidentally exchanged.
3. The bicarbonate and the base excess are approximately the same in umbilical venous and arterial blood, but if one has more severe metabolic acidosis, it is the arterial blood.

C. Both samples obtained from the same blood vessel
1. Duplicate sampling reportedly occurs ~10% of the time.
2. If the two samples have very similar values, they probably came from the same blood vessel.
3. Inadvertently obtaining two samples from the umbilical vein is quite common because the vein is easy to access.
4. If this occurs and the two samples show relatively normal values, it is still possible that the fetus had abnormal values in the umbilical arterial blood.

D. Air bubble in the specimen
1. An air bubble in the specimen can cause an erroneous reading.
2. Air bubbles can raise pH, lower PCO_2, and raise PO_2.
3. Modern blood gas analyzers usually identify air bubble contamination.

TABLE 4-1
Reference Values for Umbilical Cord Blood Gas Values

	pH	Base Excess	PCO_2	PO_2
Umbilical arterial blood (reflects fetal status)	7.26 [0.07]	-4.0 [3.0]	53 [10]	17 [6]
Umbilical venous blood (reflects maternal and placental status)	7.34 [0.06]	-3.0 [3.0]	41 [7]	29 [7]

Values are expressed as mean and standard deviation.

(Adapted from Helwig JT, Parer JT, Kilpatrick SJ, Laros RK Jr. Umbilical cord blood acid-base state: what is normal? *Am J Obstet Gynecol.* 1996;174(6):1807-1812.)

VII. Interpretation of true findings

A. Evidence of fetal compromise on cord blood gas analysis
1. If fetal umbilical arterial cord blood measures pH <7 and base deficit ≥12 nmol/L, there is evidence of metabolic acidosis.
2. In rare cases, both venous and arterial gases are normal, even in the face of fetal asphyxia and perinatal depression (see Section VII.C.4).
3. A low cord pH in infants who are vigorous at birth and free of cardiopulmonary compromise does not indicate an increased risk of adverse outcome.
4. Infants with pH <7 at birth who are not vigorous are at high risk of adverse outcome.

B. Uteroplacental insufficiency
1. The hallmarks of uteroplacental insufficiency are elevated PCO_2 and decreased venous PO_2, together with approximately equal derangements of both umbilical venous and arterial base deficits.
2. When there is impaired perfusion to the placenta, such as with placental abruption, differences between arterial and venous blood are small.

C. Cord compression
1. Intrinsic compression
   a. The umbilical cord vessels can become compressed if the cord becomes stretched.
   b. Intrinsic cord compression may occur with:
      (1) A short umbilical cord, particularly when the fetus descends during labor
      (2) A relatively short cord with fundal implantation
      (3) Wrapping of the cord around the fetal neck or other fetal part
      (4) Shoulder dystocia following delivery of the head
      (5) Breech delivery with a trapped head
      (6) True knot in the cord
2. External compression
   a. Cord compression can also occur from external factors.
   b. Factors can occur in the following conditions:
      (1) Cord prolapse (compression of the cord between the presenting part and the lower uterine segment); can be overt or occult
      (2) Breech presentation with entrapment of the aftercoming head

(3) Cord doubles back on itself (kinked)
(4) True knot in the cord (knot becomes tight due to fetal movement or fetal descent)
(5) Torsion of the cord
(6) Entwining of the cords with monoamniotic twins
3. Clinical impact of cord compression
   a. Observed effects depend on whether there is compression and occlusion of the thin-walled (and more easily compressed) umbilical vein alone, or of the umbilical vein and the umbilical arteries.
   b. If blood flow slows down but continues to flow through the umbilical vein with no alteration in umbilical arterial flow, the only effect on the cord blood gases might be an increase in the PO_2 of the umbilical venous blood.
      (1) Due to slower circulation through the placenta, more oxygen diffuses from the mother to the fetus.
      (2) This results in higher PO_2 in the blood flowing through the umbilical vein.
   c. Severe cord obstruction can lead to terminal fetal bradycardia, fetal acidosis, and neurological injury.
   d. The sequence of events with cord occlusion and terminal fetal bradycardia is described in **Table 4-2**.
   e. If only a venous blood sample is obtained from an obstructed cord, severe umbilical arterial acidosis may be missed.
4. Fetal compromise with normal cord blood gas values
   a. Even with acute intrapartum asphyxia, normal cord venous and arterial pH can occur in some situations.
   b. When fetal asphyxia occurs before delivery, the cord blood gas values may be normal because the fetus has had time to recover from the insult, although it may have neurologic injury.
   c. Sudden, complete cord occlusion may result in severe fetal compromise or death. In these cases, cord blood samples obtained at delivery merely provide a "snapshot" of the fetal acid-base status just prior to the obstruction, and not the true picture of the compromised fetus.
   d. Although extremely rare, fetal death with normal cord gases can also occur with fetal cardiac arrest.

D. Fetal circulatory failure
1. Typically, chronic fetal circulatory failure is not associated with a fetal metabolic acidosis.
2. Umbilical venous cord gases are usually normal or near normal.
3. Severe fetal circulatory failure with elevated right-heart pressures may result in interruption of umbilical venous flow while umbilical arterial flow continues.
4. Like cord occlusion (Section VII.C.), the result is a widened difference between the umbilical venous and arterial pH and PCO_2.
5. If fetal circulatory failure worsens and blood pressure falls below a critical level, blood no longer flows through the umbilical artery.
6. In this situation, umbilical arterial blood does not reflect the fetal status.

TABLE 4-2
Sequence of Events with Cord Occlusion

Anatomy	Changes in Blood Flow	Duration	Effect on Cord Gases
Narrowing of UV	UV: slowed UAs: no change	0 to a few sec	UV: increased PO_2 UAs: no change
Complete occlusion of UV and UAs	UV: no flow UAs: no flow (reflex decrease in fetal heart rate → reflex increase in fetal arterial BP)	1 to a few min	UV: no change UAs: no change
UV: completely occluded UAs: regain partial patency (secondary to increased BP)	UV: no flow UAs: partial restoration of flow (secondary to increased BP) → increasing fetal hypovolemia → increasing tissue ischemia	A few sec (rare) to <15 min	UV: no change UAs: increasing respiratory and metabolic acidosis
Resumption of complete occlusion of UV and UAs	UV: no flow UAs: no flow (secondary to increasing occluding forces, increasing hypovolemia, and/or decreasing BP)	0 to many min (depending on timing of delivery)	UV: no change UAs: no further change (continued increasing respiratory and metabolic acidoses at fetal tissue level)

BP = blood pressure; UAs = umbilical arteries; UV = umbilical vein
(Adapted from Pomerance JJ. *Interpreting Umbilical Cord Blood Gases for Clinicians Caring for the Fetus or Newborn*. 2nd ed. Glendora, CA: BNMG; 2012.)

References

ACOG Committee on Obstetric Practice. ACOG committee opinion no 348: umbilical cord blood gas and acid-base analysis. *Obstet Gynecol.* 2006;108(5):1319-1322.

Armstrong L, Stenson BJ. Effect of delayed sampling on umbilical cord arterial and venous lactate and blood gases in clamped and unclamped vessels. *Arch Dis Child Fetal Neonatal Ed.* 2006;91(5):F342-345.

Armstrong L, Stenson BJ. Use of umbilical cord blood gas analysis in the assessment of the newborn. *Arch Dis Child Fetal Neonatal Ed.* 2007;92(6):F430–F434.

Duerbeck NB, Chaffin DG, Seeds JW. A practical approach to umbilical artery pH and blood gas determinations. *Obstet Gynecol.* 1992;79(6):959-962.

Dyer A, Ikemba C. Core concepts: fetal cardiac physiology. *NeoReviews.* 2012;13(10):e583-e589.

Helwig JT, Parer JT, Kilpatrick SJ, Laros RK Jr. Umbilical cord blood acid-base state: what is normal? *Am J Obstet Gynecol.* 1996;174(6):1807-1812.

Johnson JW, Richards DS. The etiology of fetal acidosis as determined by umbilical cord acid-base studies. *Am J Obstet Gynecol.* 1997;177(2):274-280.

Nakamura KT, Smith BA, Erenberg A, Robillard JE. Changes in arterial blood gases following cardiac asystole during fetal life. *Obstet Gynecol.* 1987;70(1):16-17.

Pomerance JJ. *Interpreting Umbilical Cord Blood Gases for Clinicians Caring for the Fetus or Newborn.* 2nd ed. Glendora, CA: BNMG; 2012.

Pomerance JJ. Umbilical cord blood gases casebook: interpreting umbilical cord blood gases, VII. *J Perinatol.* 2000;20(5):338–339.

Riley RJ, Johnson JW. Collecting and analyzing cord blood gases. *Clin Obstet Gynecol.* 1993;36(1):13–23.

Strickland DM, Gilstrap LC 3rd, Hauth JC, Widmer K. Umbilical cord pH and PaCO2: effect of interval from delivery to determination. *Am J Obstet Gynecol.* 1984;148(2):191–194.

Westgate J, Garibaldi JM, Greene KR. Umbilical cord blood gas analysis at delivery: a time for quality data. *Br J Obstet Gynaecol.* 1994;101(12):1054-1063.

Basic Management of the Airway

Catherine Theorell

I. Overview
A. Process of resuscitation and stabilization after delivery involves:
1. Rapid, systematic evaluation of infant's condition
2. Management decisions based on evaluation
3. Performance of intervention or action
4. Re-evaluation after infant's response

B. All infants, whether they require only initial stabilization or complete resuscitation, deserve skilled, timely, and appropriate responses by resuscitators.

C. Parents may be present and should be thoroughly informed of the need for intervention and involved in the care of their infant.

II. Preparation
A. Assemble appropriate equipment in delivery room.
B. Make sure staff is trained and skilled. Review infant's anticipated needs with all team members.
1. Mock codes and simulation scenarios are useful training tools to improve individual skills as well as teamwork required for effective resuscitation.
2. Good communication between obstetrics and neonatal team is essential in anticipating need for resuscitation.

C. Review antepartum and intrapartum history to identify at-risk infants.
D. Identify high-risk situations before delivery to allow time to prepare and assemble appropriate equipment and personnel.

III. Equipment
A. Every delivery room should have a designated newborn resuscitation area that contains:
1. Adequate space
2. Radiant warmer
3. Pulse oximeter
4. Source of blended oxygen
5. Adequate suction
6. Drugs and supplies as specified in the resuscitation guidelines outlined by the American Academy of Pediatrics (AAP)

7. Neonatal Resuscitation Program (NRP) guidelines placed in code cart or resuscitation bag for easy accessibility
- B. Supplies and equipment should be routinely checked to ensure everything is complete and in working order.
- C. For every delivery, there should be at least one person present who has skills and knowledge to perform complete resuscitation.
- D. There should be two or three people available to assist if the infant is compromised.

IV. Management
- A. Full-term infant
  1. Resuscitation of full-term infants is not a focus of this book; readers are referred to NRP guidelines.
- B. Preterm infant
  1. While the provider attending any delivery should be prepared for resuscitation, the delivery of preterm infants presents increased risk of requiring such intervention.
  2. In triage, infants should be rapidly evaluated for:
     - a. Passage of meconium *in utero*
     - b. Difficulty breathing
     - c. Decreased tone
     - d. Vigorous activity and normal behavior
  3. Place infant on radiant warmer and conduct thorough and systematic assessment.
  4. Skin color at birth is not usually helpful in determining status of a newborn; it may take several minutes for even healthy term infants to reach oxygen-saturation levels >90%.
  5. Tactile stimulation
     - a. Drying and suctioning infant usually initiates respiration.
     - b. If infant does not begin regular respiration after drying and suctioning, flick the soles of infant's feet or rub infant's back.
     - c. If these actions fail to initiate sustained or sufficient respirations, or if respirations are gasping or insufficient to sustain a heart rate of >100 beats/min (bpm), quickly initiate positive-pressure ventilation (PPV).
     - d. In this situation, continued tactile stimulation is not useful, and may be harmful, as it allows infant's depressed respiratory state to persist longer.

V. Oxygen needs during resuscitation
A. Oxygen therapy
  1. Use of oxygen in neonatal resuscitation has generated significant discussion over the last several years.
  2. Recent research has advised against routine use of oxygen for transient cyanosis and to avoid high concentrations of oxygen whenever possible. The application of a pulse oximeter is recommended for all infants who are not vigorous at birth.
  3. Resuscitation of term newborns may begin with 21% oxygen.
  4. Resuscitation of preterm newborns may begin with somewhat higher concentrations of oxygen.
  5. If infant is breathing spontaneously and heart rate is >100 bpm, but infant remains cyanotic at 2–3 min of life, oxygen may be administered through a free-flow system.
  6. Management with oxygen therapy
     a. Delivery of high amounts of oxygen is not associated with increased neonatal saturation during transition to extrauterine life.
     b. Physiology is similar to cardiac anomalies with right-to-left shunt.
     c. As transition progresses, targeted saturations increase during early adaptation, impacting oxygen delivery.
  7. Targeted saturations should take into account disease process and changing saturation goals (see Section IV.B.4). Recent studies of normal-term newborns demonstrate that it takes almost 10 min or longer for healthy infants to reach an oxygen saturation of >90%.
  8. If saturations remain below targeted goal:
     a. Progressively higher concentrations of oxygen can be delivered by adjusting oxygen concentration on blender and holding oxygen mask firmly over infant's face to create a seal.
     b. Alternatively, an oxygen tube cupped in the hand may be used.
     c. Attention to the infant's underlying pathophysiological condition might dictate more aggressive management.
  9. A flow-inflating bag can deliver high concentrations of blow-by oxygen.

10. Caution: Self-inflating bags only deliver oxygen when the bag is compressed; they cannot be used for blow-by oxygen delivery or continuous positive airway pressure (CPAP).
11. High concentrations of oxygen are generally not necessary.
    a. Room-air resuscitation can be effective in the absence of available oxygen.
    b. Hyperoxia should be avoided, particularly in preterm infants.
    c. Oxygen should be considered and managed as a drug with beneficial and adverse effects.
12. Except in emergencies, oxygen should be delivered heated and humidified.
13. It is reasonable to provide heated, humidified oxygen as soon as the need for continuous oxygen is identified.

B. Pulse oximetry
   1. Determines the amount of oxygen the infant requires.
   2. Is essential to understanding adequate oxygenation.
      a. Reliance on color is inaccurate.
      b. Pulse oximetry should be available in all high-risk deliveries and rapidly available for unanticipated resuscitations.
      c. Availability of pulse oximetry should not delay resuscitation.
   3. Resuscitation priorities are to stabilize ventilation, heart rate, and oxygenation.
   4. Pre-ductal saturation should be measured by placing probe on newborn's right hand or wrist.
      a. The right hand reflects the saturation of the blood perfusing the heart, brain, and muscle.
      b. The NRP recommends placing the probe prior to turning on the pulse oximeter to obtain the most rapid signal.
   5. Using pulse oximetry, supplemental oxygen concentration should be adjusted to achieve target values for pre-ductal saturation.
   6. Oxygen concentration should be adjusted up or down to achieve a saturation that gradually increases toward targeted saturation goals.
   7. Oxygen saturations in the low 90s are not, on average, expected until 10 min of age.

C. Persistent cyanosis
  1. Confirm persistent cyanosis with pulse oximetry.
  2. Adjust supplemental oxygen concentration on the blender to achieve target values for pre-ductal saturations (**Table 5-1**).
  3. If the concentration of oxygen does not affect the infant's level of oxygen saturation, consider presence of cyanotic heart disease.

VI. Asphyxia: physiological considerations

A. Resuscitation goals: Reverse the pathologic process of asphyxia as soon as possible and avoid death or permanent injury.
B. Hypoxia and acidosis, regardless of duration, increase vasoconstriction of pulmonary vascular bed, resulting in increased risk of persistent pulmonary hypertension.
C. Intrapartum asphyxia can be divided into two categories:
  1. Acute, near-total asphyxia
     a. Abrupt onset, lasting from 5 to 30 min
     b. Results in complete or near complete cessation of blood flow to the fetus
     c. Caused by uterine rupture, complete abruption, or severe cord compression
  2. Partial, prolonged asphyxia
     a. Slower onset, over many hours
     b. Usually caused by a variety of factors, resulting in uteroplacental insufficiency

TABLE 5-1
Targeted Saturation Goal in the First 10 Min of Life

Time	Saturations	Provide or Increase Oxygen
1 min	60%–65%	If <60% at 1 min
2 min	65%–70%	If <65% at 2 min
3 min	70%–75%	If <70% at 3 min
4 min	75%–80%	If <75% at 4 min
5 min	80%–85%	If <80% at 5 min
10 min	85%–95%	If <85% at 10 min

Note: Once a decision is made to provide oxygen, wean or discontinue it as tolerated to keep saturations in acceptable ranges after they reach 85%.

(Adapted from MacDonald MG, Mullett MD, Seshia MMK, eds. *Avery's Neonatology: Pathophysiology and Management of the Newborn*. 6th ed. Philadelphia, PA: Lippincott Williams & Wilkins; 2005.)

      c. Fetus undergoes classic diving reflex in attempt to preserve circulation
      d. Diving reflex involves increased non-cerebral peripheral vascular resistance, increasing blood flow to head, heart, and adrenal glands and decreasing flow to non-vital organs
- D. During early stages of asphyxia, oxygen content of blood is low, yet amount of oxygen delivered to heart and head is maximized by greater cardiac output (resulting from increased heart rate) and increased flow.
- E. Increased peripheral vascular resistance and greater cardiac output cause blood pressure (BP) to rise in early asphyxia.
- F. BP remains stable as long as myocardium can sustain output.
- G. If hypoxia and acidosis get worse, myocardium fails and cardiac output and BP decrease.
- H. Decreased cardiac output results in significant damage to brain and other organs.
- I. In most cases, infants are born with a heart rate, although it may be <100 bpm.
- J. Unlike resuscitation of adults or older children, adequate ventilation is a mainstay of neonatal resuscitation.
- K. Throughout this time, characteristic changes in infant's respiratory pattern start with gasping respirations; each of these changes may or may not have occurred *in utero*.

VII. Apnea
- A. Primary apnea
  1. Asphyxia continues.
  2. Respirations cease.
  3. Tactile stimulation may stimulate respirations.
- B. Secondary apnea
  1. Asphyxia is not corrected.
  2. Infant begins to gasp irregularly again.
  3. Respirations cease entirely.
  4. Tactile stimulation does not restore respirations.
  5. PPV and successful resuscitation are required immediately.
- C. Differentiation may not be possible during resuscitation
- D. General approach is to treat all apnea as secondary, providing PPV

VIII. CPAP and assisted ventilation
- A. CPAP

1. Controversy persists regarding most comparative effectiveness between CPAP and PPV in the initial stabilization of preterm infants.
2. CPAP may be effective in the stabilization of lung expansion and functional residual capacity (FRC).
   a. Diminished FRC is characteristic of respiratory distress syndrome and other pathological conditions encountered in the delivery room.
   b. Supporting FRC might reduce the need for mechanical ventilation.
      (1) Stabilization of alveolar expansion
      (2) Preservation of surfactant function that is lost in atelectasis
      (3) Hence, the terminology "minimally invasive respiratory support" has been used to describe this philosophical approach to care
3. CPAP may be indicated if the infant displays any of these symptoms:
   a. Spontaneous breathing but insufficient respirations
   b. Heart rate >100 bpm
   c. Labored respirations
   d. Evidence of inadequate oxygenation (**Table 5-1**)
4. CPAP training is necessary for resuscitators.
5. Required equipment:
   a. Either a flow-inflating bag and mask or a T-piece resuscitator and mask
   b. Cannot be given with a self-inflating bag or nasal cannula

B. PPV
1. Indicated if infant displays any of these symptoms:
   a. Apneic: gasping or inadequate respiratory effort
   b. Heart rate <100 bpm, even if breathing
   c. Low oxygen saturation despite free-flow oxygen at 100%
2. Required equipment:
   a. Self-inflating bag with oxygen reservoir, flow-inflating bag, or T-piece resuscitator with mask that is attached to source of oxygen
   b. Bag size should be between 200 mL and 750 mL for all newborns
   c. Appropriately sized face mask able to create tight seal to infant's face

d. Source of blended oxygen or available compressed oxygen tank
   e. All equipment, including self-inflating and flow-inflating bags, as well as T-piece resuscitators, should have integral pressure gauge or pressure manometer and a pressure release or "pop-off" valve attached
3. Rising heart rate and audible breath sounds indicate effective ventilation.
4. Heart rate may increase without visible chest movement, particularly in preterm infants. For term infants, once the heart rate has improved, ventilation may need to be continued based on the respiratory rate and the quality of the infant's spontaneous ventilation.
5. Start with inspiratory pressures of ~12–20 cm of H_2O and at 40–60 bpm.
6. Bag at a rate of 40–60 breaths/min.
7. Avoid excessive chest inflation; use lowest inflation pressure necessary to maintain the heart rate >100 bpm while gradually improving oxygen saturation.
8. Assess infant for rising heart rate and improving oxygen saturation.
9. If heart rate is not increasing or saturation is not improving after 5–10 breaths of PPV, assistant should assess if bilateral breath sounds and chest movement are present.
10. If bilateral breath sounds are not present and chest does not rise, perform ventilation-corrective steps as outlined by the NRP:
    a. For infants undergoing PPV, reassess respiratory effort, heart rate, and oxygen saturation as outlined by the NRP.
    b. If ventilation is still not effective, consider alternative airway access (intubation or laryngeal mask if infant's weight allows).
    c. If the infant requires bag mask ventilation for longer than several minutes, place an 8-Fr orogastric tube or larger, based on the size of the infant, to decompress the stomach and avoid lung compression and gastric content aspiration.
C. Alternative airway access
   1. Intubation is recommended when tracheal suctioning is required in the non-vigorous, meconium-stained newborn.

2. Intubation indicated if the following measures fail:
   a. PPV does not result in adequate clinical improvement.
   b. Ventilation with a mask is ineffective despite corrective steps.
   c. Need for PPV lasts beyond a few minutes or is necessary to improve the efficacy of assisted ventilation.
   d. Chest compressions are necessary to facilitate coordination of ventilation and maximize the efficiency of each positive-pressure breath.
   e. Special indications exist, such as extreme immaturity, drug administration, or suspected diaphragmatic hernia.
3. Intubation procedure should ideally take no longer than 30 sec.
4. Use number-1 blade of laryngoscope for term infants, number-0 for preterm newborns, number-00 for extremely preterm newborns.
5. Laryngeal mask is indicated:
   a. If facial or upper airway malformations make ventilation by face mask ineffective
   b. If PPV with face mask fails to achieve effective ventilation
   c. If intubation not possible
6. Alternative airway considerations
   a. Available sizes of laryngeal mask airways are too large for very small preterm babies or those less than ~32 weeks of gestation.
   b. Device cannot be used to suction meconium from the airway, limiting its usefulness in certain circumstances.
   c. Air leak at the mask-larynx interface may result in insufficient inflation pressure in the lungs.
   d. Insufficient evidence exists to recommend the laryngeal mask airway for medication administration or for prolonged assisted ventilation in newborns.

D. If infant **fails to respond** to any of the above measures:
   1. Additional expertise might be needed for chest compressions, insertion of umbilical catheters, or pleural drainage of air or fluid.
   2. Consider other complications, like hypovolemia and pneumothorax.
   3. If heart rate is <60 bpm despite 30 sec of effective PPV, begin chest compressions.

IX. Suction

A. Setup
 1. Bulb syringe and suction should be available.
 2. Always suction the mouth first, then the nose, to avoid aspiration if the infant gasps.
 3. Although 12- to 14-Fr suction catheters are recommended for term babies, it is more appropriate to use a 10 Fr in very low birth weight (VLBW) infants.
 4. Suction should be set at 80–100 mmHg.

B. If infant is vigorous and responsive, suctioning is not indicated. However, if secretions are interfering with ventilation:
 1. Gently clear airway with bulb syringe.
 2. Suction mouth first in case the infant gasps when nose is suctioned.
 3. Vigorous suctioning and stimulation of the posterior pharynx may induce bradycardia.
 4. If using suction catheter, insert no more than 5 cm from the lips; limit suctioning to no more than 5 sec.

C. If meconium is found in amniotic fluid, management is parallel to that for term infants:
 1. All non-vigorous infants with thick or thin meconium should undergo direct laryngoscopy and tracheal suctioning.
 2. It is possible that meconium entered the mouth of the fetus and was aspirated into the lungs prior to delivery.
 3. Aspiration of meconium in the lungs may result in ball-valve obstruction of airways, causing gas trapping and air leaks.
 4. Suction trachea only if infant is not vigorous or requires PPV or intubation.
 5. If intubation is anticipated and required for a non-vigorous infant:
    a. Attach meconium aspirator adapter to endotracheal tube.
    b. Apply regulated wall suction at ~80–100 mmHg as endotracheal tube is withdrawn.
    c. Trachea can be re-intubated and suctioned again if necessary.
    d. Guidelines for intubation can be found in the NRP toolbox.

6. Some infants with thick meconium are severely asphyxiated; it may be impossible to clear the trachea completely of meconium before beginning PPV.
7. Clinical judgment must be used to determine the number of re-intubations necessary, based on the condition of the infant.

X. Special considerations for VLBW infants during the Golden Hours

A. If breathing is spontaneous and the heart rate is >100 bpm, allow the infant time to transition.
B. For low birth weight infants with labored respirations, use either early application of CPAP or intratracheal surfactant to improve lung volume.
C. It is normal for saturations to fluctuate from the high 80s to the 90s in the first few days of life.
D. Consider CPAP of 4–6 cm H_2O in these infants.
E. If the infant does not respond to 6 cm H_2O of CPAP, then PPV should be considered.
F. If PPV is required, initial peak pressures should result in adequate, but not excessive, lung expansion.
   1. Pressures depend on lung disease and compliance.
   2. Peak pressures may vary from peak pressures of 12–20 cm, or perhaps as high as 25 cm, H_2O and positive end-expiratory pressure (PEEP) pressures of 2–6 or higher.
      a. Infants with surfactant deficiency require high levels of peak pressure and CPAP/PEEP.
      b. Infants with more mature lungs require lower pressures.
   3. Excessive peak pressures and PEEP may result in pneumothoraces or air leaks.

XI. Ventilators

A. Decision to initiate mechanical ventilation is complex; take into account:
   1. Severity of respiratory depression and pulmonary pathology
   2. Severity of blood gas abnormalities
   3. Natural history of perinatal asphyxia
   4. Degree of cardiovascular and other physiologic instabilities
B. Pressure-controlled ventilators
   1. Commonly used in neonatal care
   2. Time cycled and pressure limited
   3. Control flow, pressure, and rate of each delivered breath

4. Ventilator rate and peak airway pressure delivered per ventilator settings
5. Air-oxygen mixtures heated and humidified for delivery through continuous-flow circuit attached to airway
6. Ventilatory rates adjusted with tidal volume to ensure adequate ventilation
7. Inspiratory times vary from 0.2 to 1 sec; commonly 0.25–0.5 sec
8. Inspiratory times must allow adequate expiration to avoid over-inflation of lungs
9. Delivered tidal volume depends on peak-inspired pressure and airway leaks
10. Peak-inspired pressure adjusted to achieve optimal tidal volume (5–7 mL/kg), minute ventilation, and effective gas exchange based on blood gas analysis
11. PEEP stabilizes airway, preventing alveolar collapse
12. PEEP settings range from 2 to 6 cm of H_2O pressure, depending upon disease process
13. Peak airway pressure of 4–20 cm of H_2O used as pressure-control ventilator

C. Volume-control ventilators
1. Deliver set tidal volume.
2. Rates for volume ventilation and pressure-control ventilation vary.
3. Monitoring mechanical and spontaneous tidal volume allows for distinction between machine and infant minute ventilation.
4. Make sure inspiratory time allows for adequate volume delivery.
5. Short inspiratory time (<0.32 sec) reduces volume delivery.
6. Peak inspiratory pressure varies automatically with changing lung compliance and minimizes risk of lung over-distention after surfactant therapy.
7. PEEP is the same for volume and pressure-control ventilation.

D. Synchronized intermittent mechanical ventilation
1. Useful if infant is breathing spontaneously but irregularly
2. Available for pressure-control, volume-control, and assisted-control ventilators
3. Requires lower peak inspiratory pressure settings, yet achieves optimal tidal volume and maintains adequate minute ventilation

4. Provides greater comfort
5. Requires less sedation of infants
E. High-frequency ventilation
 1. A variety of strategies and devices that provide ventilation at rapid rates and very low tidal volumes, reducing the risk of barotrauma.
 2. Indicated if:
    a. Conventional mechanical ventilation does not result in adequate oxygenation or ventilation.
    b. Infant requires very high airway pressures.
 3. Oxygenation and ventilation change rapidly after initiating high-frequency ventilation; repeat chest radiographs and frequent blood gases are required (**Fig. 5-1**).
 4. There are three types of high-frequency ventilators:
    a. High-frequency jet ventilator injects high-velocity stream of gas into endotracheal tube.

FIGURE 5-1
Radiograph of Newborn with Diffuse Surfactant Deficiency on High-Frequency Ventilation

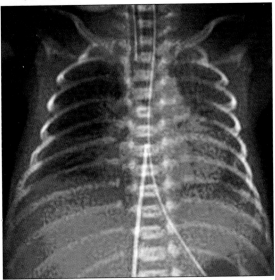

High-frequency ventilation includes a variety of strategies and devices that provide ventilation at rapid rates and very low tidal volumes, reducing the risk of barotrauma. It is indicated if conventional mechanical ventilation does not result in adequate oxygenation or ventilation, or if the infant requires very high airway pressures. Oxygenation and ventilation change rapidly after initiating; repeat chest radiographs and frequent blood gases are required.

b. High-frequency flow interrupter operates at high frequencies but has passive exhalation.
c. High-frequency oscillatory ventilator:
(1) Generates tidal volume less than or equal to dead space by means of an oscillating piston or diaphragm.
(2) Mechanism creates active exhalation and inspiration.

XII. Arterial blood gas assessment
A. Initial management of ventilation, oxygenation, and changes in acid-base balance is most accurately determined by arterial blood gas studies.
B. Assessing blood gas immediately after birth must take into account the time required for the effect of cardiopulmonary interventions to be translated into improved gases in the low birth weight infant.
C. Arterial blood gas
1. Standardized index accepted as a measure of respiratory status, especially for the oxygenation of low birth weight infants.
2. Invasive monitoring procedure requires arterial puncture or placement of indwelling arterial catheter.
3. Results may vary according to gestational age of infant, age at time of sampling, and ongoing ventilatory care.
4. Arterial oxygen values range from 80–95 mmHg for a term infant to 45–60 mmHg for a preterm infant (<30 weeks gestation).
5. Arterial carbon dioxide values range from 35–45 mmHg for a term infant to 38–50 mmHg for a preterm infant (<30 weeks gestation).
6. Arterial blood gas values are also used to calculate indexes for determining progression of respiratory disease in infants.
D. Venous blood gases
1. Cannot be interpreted in the same way as arterial blood gases.
2. pH values are slightly lower in the venous blood from higher carbon dioxide levels.
3. Venus oxygen values are of little value in the NICU.
E. Capillary blood gases

1. "Arterialize" capillary blood by simply warming the infant's heel just before sampling.
2. pH is usually slightly lower and partial pressure of carbon dioxide ($PaCO_2$) values are slightly greater than arterial values and vary considerably depending on sampling technique.
3. Capillary partial pressure of oxygen (PaO_2) levels are not useful measures.

References

Berghella V, ed. *Maternal-Fetal Evidence Based Guidelines*. 2nd ed. New York, NY: Informa Healthcare; 2011.

Cloherty JP, Eichenwald EC, Hansen AR, Stark AR. *Manual of Neonatal Care*. 7th ed. Philadelphia, PA: Wolters Kluwer Health/Lippincott Williams & Wilkins; 2012.

Gardner SL, Carter BS, Enzman-Hines MI, Hernandez JA. *Merenstein and Gardner's Handbook of Neonatal Intensive Care*. 7th ed. St. Louis, MO: Mosby Elsevier; 2011.

Gomella TL, Cunningham MD, Eyal FG, eds. *Neonatology: Management, Procedures, On-Call Problems, Diseases, and Drugs*. 7th ed. New York, NY: McGraw Hill/Lange; 2013.

Instructor Manual for Neonatal Resuscitation. 6th ed. American Academy of Pediatrics and American Heart Association; 2011.

MacDonald MG, Mullett MD, Seshia MMK, eds. *Avery's Neonatology: Pathophysiology and Management of the Newborn*. 6th ed. Philadelphia, PA: Lippincott Williams & Wilkins; 2005.

Martin RJ, Fanaroff AA, Walsh MC. *Fanaroff and Martin's Neonatal-Perinatal Medicine: Diseases of the Fetus and Infant*. 9th ed. St. Louis, MO: Mosby Elsevier; 2011.

6

Cardiac Support

Catherine Theorell

I. Overview
A. According the American Heart Association, ~10% of newborns require some assistance to begin breathing.
B. About 1% require cardiac resuscitation.
C. If the infant does not respond to initial stabilization (warming, clearing the airway, stimulation) or to effective ventilation, it may be necessary to begin cardiac resuscitation.
D. Providers should provide 30 sec of positive-pressure ventilation (PPV) before beginning chest compressions for infants with heart rates <60 beats/min (bpm), moving to medication if chest compressions are not sufficient.
E. Throughout the process, monitor respiration, heart rate, and oxygenation saturation.

II. Chest compressions
A. Effective ventilation must be ensured for 30 sec prior to commencing chest compressions.
   1. If ventilation is not effective, ensure corrective actions are taken.
      a. Adjust the mask.
      b. Reposition the head to assure midline and sniffing position.
      c. Suction the mouth, then the nose.
      d. Open the mouth during ventilation.
      e. Increase the pressure provided.
   2. If ventilation is still not effective, consider an alternate airway such as intubation.
B. Initiate chest compressions to help maintain cardiac output.
C. Compressions are indicated whenever the heart rate is <60 bpm despite at least 30 sec of effective PPV.

III. Heart rate assessment
A. Assess heart rate by palpating pulsations at the base of the umbilical cord or by auscultating the heart while palpating peripheral pulses.
B. An assistant should use finger gestures or finger tapping to represent the heart rate; the representation should be visible to members of the resuscitation team.

1. Count the number of beats for 6 sec and multiply by 10 to get the rate.
2. Verbal communication using closed-loop communication methods described in such sources as TeamSTEPPS® is probably more effective than visual cues such as tapping a finger to demonstrate a heart rate.

C. As an adjunct to counting, a pulse oximeter may be used to detect pulse wave.
1. In low perfusion states, the oximeter may not detect a consistent pulse.
2. If the oximeter is functioning or if the pulse is easily palpated at the base of the cord, ventilation can continue while heart rate is determined.
3. If unable to palpate pulsations at the base of the umbilical cord or if the pulse oximeter is not functioning, both compressions and ventilation may need to be stopped for a few seconds to auscultate the heart rate.
4. Interruption of chest compressions to check the heart rate may result in decreased perfusion pressure in the coronary arteries.

D. Chest compressions with coordinated ventilation should be continued for at least 60 sec (one cycle) before stopping briefly to assess heart rate.
E. Discontinue chest compressions when the heart rate is >60 bpm.
F. During chest compression, PPV is provided after every three compressions at a rate of 30 bpm; after compressions are stopped, PPV should be continued at a rate of 40–60 bpm.
G. Heart rate, respiratory status, and oxygen saturation should be assessed continuously, or at least every 30 sec.
H. If the heart rate rises >100 bpm and the newborn begins to breathe spontaneously, PPV rate should be gradually decreased and post-resuscitation care should be provided.

IV. Chest compression technique

A. Apply compression over the lower third of the sternum, just below an imaginary line drawn across the nipples.
B. Avoid compressing the xiphoid process.
C. The two techniques — thumb and two-finger — are shown in **Fig. 6-1**.
1. The thumb technique is preferred.
   a. Results in greater mean arterial pressure
   b. Can be used in most situations

c. The thumb technique: Press sternum with thumbs while encircling chest with fingers
    2. The two-finger technique is less effective.
        a. Useful during umbilical line placement
        b. Only if space does not allow for thumb technique to be performed
D. Compress the sternum to a depth of approximately one-third of the anterior-posterior diameter of the chest.
E. Make the compression phase shorter than the relaxation phase of each stroke to allow for greater cardiac filling and improved blood flow.
F. There should be three compressions plus one ventilation in each 2-sec cycle; ~120 events for every minute of life.
G. One breath should be interposed every three compressions.
H. Assess effectiveness.
    1. Palpate peripheral pulses or umbilical cord pulse; this method may provide erroneous findings.
    2. A transducer connected to an umbilical or peripheral arterial catheter is the most accurate evaluation method; however, this equipment is not usually available in delivery rooms and there may not be time to obtain.

FIGURE 6-1
Chest Compression Techniques — Thumb and Two-Finger

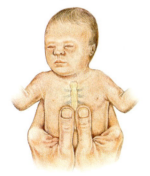
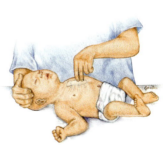

©2014 The National Certification Corporation

Of the two techniques, the thumb technique is preferred because it results in greater mean arterial pressure and can be used in most situations. To perform the thumb technique: Press the sternum with the thumbs while encircling the chest with the fingers. The two-finger is less effective, but it can be useful during umbilical line placement or if space does not allow for thumb technique. Compress the sternum to a depth of approximately one-third of the anterior-posterior diameter of the chest. Make the compression phase shorter than the relaxation phase of each stroke. Interpose one breath for every three compressions.

I. Pulse oximeter
   1. Infants may have pulse oximeter probes already in place.
   2. If the heart rate is <60 bpm, the oximeter may have a low signal strength and not work well when the infant has poor perfusion.
   3. Increase the oxygen concentration to 100% until the oximeter gives a reliable signal.
   4. Use the data to adjust supplemental oxygen.
J. Intubation
   1. Strongly recommended when chest compressions commence; helps ensure effective ventilation.
   2. Correct placement of the endotracheal tube should be confirmed with a CO_2 detector.
   3. CO_2 detectors will only "read" the presence of CO_2 if the infant has adequate perfusion and blood flow to the lungs; poorly perfused infants may have no change in the CO_2 detector despite a properly placed endotracheal tube (false negative).
   4. Provides stable airway and prevents gas from entering the stomach.
   5. Gas in the stomach can raise the diaphragm, making ventilation difficult.
   6. Place an oral gastric tube to ensure stomach decompression.

V. Medications

A. The most common cause of neonatal cardiac depression is from respiratory etiologies; thus, the adequacy of respiratory resuscitation is essential in the sequence of resuscitation for most neonates with bradycardia or cardiac arrest.
B. If the infant is born with no detectable heartbeat or if chest compressions and ventilation do not increase the heart rate to >60 bpm within 30 sec, the infant may require medications to support cardiovascular function.
C. Preferably, administer medication through an umbilical venous catheter.
   1. When using an umbilical venous catheter, insert the catheter ~2–4 cm into the umbilical vein just beneath the skin for a term infant (less for a preterm infant) until blood flow is established.
   2. If the catheter is inserted too deeply, the tip may lodge in the liver and may result in necrosis from medication administration directly into the liver.

3. If an umbilical catheter is not available, epinephrine may be administered through the endotracheal tube, though this route is less preferred.
4. Intratracheal administration of epinephrine is not as reliable or as effective as intravascular administration.

D. Epinephrine is indicated if the heart rate remains <60 bpm after 30 sec of effective assisted ventilation and at least another 45–60 sec of coordinated chest compressions and effective ventilation.
1. The recommended concentration of epinephrine is 1:10,000 (0.1 mg/mL).
2. Administer the dose rapidly.
3. The recommended IV dose of epinephrine is 0.1–0.3 mL/kg of 1:10,000-solution in a 1-mL syringe.
4. The recommended intratracheal dose of epinephrine is 0.5–1.0 mL/kg of 1:10,000-solution in a 3-mL to 6-mL syringe; follow dosing with PPV.
5. Assess the newborn's heart rate ~1 min after administering IV epinephrine (intratracheal-administrated doses may take longer).
6. Additional epinephrine can be administered every 3–5 min.

E. Respiratory depression
1. Respiratory depression may be seen in infants with brain injuries or other abnormalities, or because the mother received narcotic analgesia or other sedative drugs prior to delivery that crossed the placenta prior to birth.
2. If respiratory depression is only related to the anesthesia and there is no asphyxia, the infant usually has a good heart rate and simply needs ventilatory assistance.
3. If respiratory depression is due to inhaled anesthetic, ventilation of the infant usually removes the anesthetic from the infant's circulation.
4. If the baby can be adequately ventilated, naloxone hydrochloride (Narcan) administration should not be used.
5. If respiratory depression continues and there is a history of maternal narcotic administration within 4 hours of the delivery, naloxone may be considered.
6. Limitations related to half-life and potential adverse effects limit the utility of this drug.

a. Naloxone does not reverse the effects of inhaled anesthetics, magnesium sulfate, or nonnarcotic analgesics.
b. Naloxone is not the first choice of drug given in a resuscitation and is rarely used in the delivery room.
c. The dose of naloxone is 0.1 mg/kg, preferably given intravenously.
d. If the effects of the narcotic last longer than the naloxone, the infant may slip back into respiratory depression; close observation is mandated and repeated doses of naloxone may be necessary.
e. Naloxone should never be given to an infant of a narcotic-addicted mother; it causes acute withdrawal symptoms, including seizures, in the neonate.

References

Berghella V, ed. *Maternal-Fetal Evidence Based Guidelines*. 2nd ed. New York, NY: Informa Healthcare; 2011.

Cloherty JP, Eichenwald EC, Hansen AR, Stark AR. *Manual of Neonatal Care*. 7th ed. Philadelphia, PA: Wolters Kluwer Health/Lippincott Williams & Wilkins; 2012.

Gardner SL, Carter BS, Enzman-Hines M, Hernandez JA. *Merenstein and Gardner's Handbook of Neonatal Intensive Care*. 7th ed. St. Louis, MO: Mosby Elsevier; 2011.

Gomella TL, Cunningham MD, Eyal FG, eds. *Neonatology: Management, Procedures, On-Call Problems, Diseases, and Drugs*. 7th ed. New York, NY: McGraw Hill/Lange; 2013.

Instructor Manual for Neonatal Resuscitation. 6th ed. American Academy of Pediatrics and American Heart Association; 2011.

Martin RJ, Fanaroff AA, Walsh MC. *Fanaroff and Martin's Neonatal-Perinatal Medicine: Diseases of the Fetus and Infant.* 9th ed. St. Louis, MO: Mosby Elsevier; 2011.

Thermoregulation

Robin L. Bissinger

I. Temperature regulation
  A. Balance between heat loss and heat production
  B. Care requires multiple initiatives to improve outcomes
  C. Expands on and supports the Neonatal Resuscitation Program (NRP) guidelines to maintain warmth in delivery room and during the first hours to days of the infant's life, ensuring the unique needs of the very low birth weight (VLBW) infant are met

II. Pathophysiology
  A. The fetus produces heat as a product of metabolism, not for thermogenesis, and cannot regulate temperature *in utero*.
  B. Heat from the fetus moves by both conduction and convection (**Fig. 7-1**).
    1. The majority of heat moves by conduction from the fetal skin surface into the amniotic fluid and uterus and then to the mother.

FIGURE 7-1
Thermoregulation *In Utero*

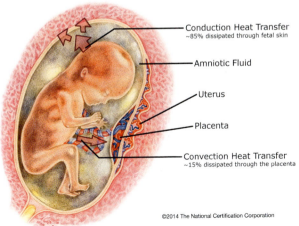

A fetus cannot regulate temperature *in utero*. The majority of heat from the fetus moves by conduction from the fetal skin surface into the amniotic fluid and uterus and then to the mother. To a lesser extent, heat moves by convection from the fetal blood into the placenta and then to the maternal blood.

2. To a lesser extent, heat transfers by convection from the fetal blood to the placenta and then to the maternal blood.
C. Fetal temperature is ~0.5°C–1.0°C (0.9°F–1.8°F) higher than the maternal temperature, due to this endogenous heat production by the fetus and the surrounding core temperature of the mother.
D. This temperature gradient between the mother and the fetus remains despite changes in maternal temperature.
   1. For example, if the mother becomes hyperthermic, the fetal temperature will become elevated secondary to a decreased ability to dissipate heat across a temperature gradient.
   2. The fetal temperature must remain higher than the maternal temperature to maintain the thermal gradient to offload fetal heat.
E. Heat flows down a gradient; if the fetus generates a significant amount of heat, it must be dissipated via the mother.
   1. Fetal temperature is directly related to maternal temperature and may be hypo- or hyperthermic at birth, based on the temperature of the mother.
   2. Fetal thermogenesis is suppressed *in utero*.
   3. Fetal hyperthermia can occur with maternal fever because heat dissipation becomes limited in this situation.
   4. Following birth, in the immediate transitional period, rapid changes in neonatal temperature occur (see Section III).
F. At birth, the neonate transfers from an aqueous intrauterine environment to a gaseous postnatal environment with considerable differences in temperatures.
G. Without intervention at birth the infant will cool, using 150 kcal of energy/min to keep warm.
H. The infant's body temperature can drop 0.2°C –1.0°C (0.36°F–1.8°F)/min.
I. The goal is to achieve a neutral thermal state.
   1. Neither gain nor lose heat
   2. Oxygen consumption and energy utilization minimal
   3. Core-to-skin gradient small
   4. Normothermia: Axillary temperature of 36.5°C–37.5°C (98°F–100°F)
   5. Temperatures outside this range require clinical response (**Table 7-1**)
J. Mechanisms of heat production after birth:
   1. Non-shivering thermogenesis

a. Primary mode of heat production in neonates and infants up to one year of age
b. Produces heat through oxidation of free fatty acids from brown adipose tissue (BAT) cells.
   (1) BAT cells are activated at birth with the clamping of the umbilical cord.
   (2) At birth the temperature falls, initiating heat production.
c. Requires an increase in norepinephrine and thyroid-stimulating hormone; norepinephrine is stimulated by the separation of the placenta and as a response to cooling.
d. Sympathetic nervous system mediates the reaction to cold.
   (1) An immature system in VLBW infants, the sympathetic nervous system mediates vasomotor control and matures with gestation and postnatal age.
   (2) It stimulates the peripheral vascular, leading to vasoconstriction that reduces blood flow and heat loss through conduction.
      (a) VLBW infants have immature vasomotor control during the first 12 hours to few days of life, even when faced with extreme cold stress.
      (b) They may not be able to conserve heat.
   (3) It stimulates the release of norepinephrine from nerve endings on the surface of brown fat.

TABLE 7-1
Recommended Axillary Temperatures in Infants ≤1,500 Grams

Ranges	Temperature	Action Needed
Normal	36.5°C–37.5°C (98°F–100°F)	Continue
Potential cold stress	36°C–36.5°C (97°F–98°F)	Cause for concern
Moderate hypothermia	32°C–36°C (90°F–97°F)	Danger; immediate warming of baby needed
Severe hypothermia	<32°C (90°F)	Outlook grave; skilled care urgently needed

Note: The American Heart Association and the American Academy of Pediatrics in 2006 stated that the goal (of the first temperature) should be an axillary temperature of 36.5°C (98°F). Goal is to achieve normothermia and avoid hyperthermia, which is associated with progressive cerebral injury.

(Adapted from Bhatt DR, White R, Martin G, et al. Transitional hypothermia in preterm newborns. *J Perinatol.* 2007;27(suppl 2):S45-S47.)

                (a) Brown adipose tissue breaks down to glycerol and non-esterified fatty acids, releasing heat.
                (b) This processes is dependent on oxygen.
            (4) It increases thyroid-stimulating hormone.
        e. Thyroid surge occurs at birth and augments the sympathetic response.
            (1) This surge is stimulated by:
                (a) Cooler extrauterine environment that stimulates thermal skin receptors
                (b) Clamping of the umbilical cord
                (c) Catecholamine surge at birth
            (2) Thyroid-stimulating hormone increases thyroxine (T4) and conversion to iodothyronine, which increases fat oxidation and heat production.
            (3) This results in a breakdown of BAT, producing heat.
        f. VLBW infants have limited ability to generate heat with non-shivering thermogenesis due to immaturity and inefficient brown fat metabolism.
    2. Shivering
        a. Shivering thermogenesis can occur as a response to extreme thermal stress, but this capacity is diminished in neonates.
        b. Due to immature skeletal muscles, infants are unable to shiver, resulting in decreased heat production.
  K. Thermogenic process requires oxygen and glucose; there is an increased need for thermogenesis at birth.
  L. Premature infants with an immature thermogenic response and decreased brown fat will have increased respiratory distress, poor tissue perfusion, and metabolic acidosis from cold stress.

III. Mechanisms of heat loss
  A. At birth, heat is lost rapidly.
  B. Core body temperatures drop 2°C–3°C (3.6°F–5.4°F) in first 30 min of life.
  C. Heat transfer must be continuously modified to maintain core temperature in very narrow range.
  D. In neonates, heat losses are larger and must be reduced.
  E. Controlling thermal environment maintains normal body temperature and can eliminate thermal stress in infants.

F. VLBW infants are often exposed to multiple procedures, cold rooms, cold infusions, and cold equipment, which may lead to hypothermia in the first minutes to hours of life.
G. Heat loss exceeds heat production at birth and occurs between the infant and environment through convection, radiation, conduction, and evaporation.
    1. Convection
        a. Amount of heat transferred from the infant's skin to the environment.
            (1) Moving air or water currents carry heat away from the body.
            (2) Heat is conducted from the body surface to the surrounding air.
        b. Infants lose heat to the air very rapidly in cooler rooms. Ambient air temperature is often documented as 27°C (81°F).
        c. Warm air rises from the newborn's body and is replaced with cooler air.
            (1) Natural convection is related to the difference between the infant's skin temperature and the air temperature.
                (a) Warm air rises from the skin's surface and carries heat and body moisture with it.
                (b) This air then cools and falls back on the baby.
            (2) Forced convection is based on air movement, with an increased heat loss when more air movement is at the level of the baby.
        d. Minimizing risk
            (1) Select one person in the delivery room to be responsible for thermal management.
            (2) Control airflow and air temperature in the delivery room.
                (a) Use air diverters from vents
                (b) Use wraps
                (c) Use hats
                (d) Strategic design of delivery and resuscitation areas
            (3) Decrease movement of personnel and opening/closing of doors until the infant is in a secure environment.
            (4) Cover with warm towels and blankets when moving the infant.

(5) Swaddle the infant.
(6) Provide warmed, humidified air.
(7) Warm all hoods, shields, and walls that are near the infant.
(8) Use double-walled incubators and transporters.
(9) Keep porthole doors closed.

2. Radiation
    a. Cooler nearby objects, like doors and windows, may absorb heat even though they are not in direct contact with the infant.
    b. Radiant energy transfers from surfaces.
    c. Infant will radiate heat to the nearest solid object.
    d. Rate of heat loss is based on the temperature differences of the nearby surfaces and the infant's skin.
    e. Minimizing risk
        (1) Use radiant warmers since they radiate heat to the infant.
        (2) Use double-walled incubators that warm the air between the walls to reduce temperature gradient and supply heat to the outside environment.
        (3) Warm environmental surfaces (plastic surfaces such as hoods, walls, windows, etc.) to prevent transfer of body heat to walls and windows in the unit.
    f. Research demonstrates that the use of radiant warmers leads to a significant increase in insensible water loss, which can lead to increased oxygen consumption and gradients in body temperature, dependent on location relative to the radiant heat source.

3. Conduction
    a. Objects of different temperatures that come into contact with each other exchange heat; hotter objects give heat to cooler objects.
    b. Infants lose body warmth to anything they come into contact with that is colder.
    c. Surfaces and equipment usually have a temperature equal to that of ambient air at 27°C (81°F); infants lose heat upon contact, even at 36°C (97°F).
    d. Minimizing risk
        (1) Pre-warm all equipment, towels, blankets, scales, and sterile fields.
        (2) Pre-warm fluids if possible.

4. Evaporation
   a. Water loss from the skin or respiratory tract, in which water is converted from a liquid to a gas
   b. Skin is covered with amniotic fluid; as liquid evaporates from skin, the infant loses heat
   c. Major source of heat loss in premature infants
   d. Minimizing risk
      (1) Dry the infant and/or place in plastic wrap to decrease heat loss.
      (2) Keep wet linens away from the infant; remove them as quickly as possible.
      (3) Use double-walled incubators.
      (4) Initially provide at least 60% humidity.

IV. Neonatal considerations: Innate protective mechanisms for prevention of heat loss in VLBW infants are limited and, in many cases, ineffective.

A. Disproportionate body-mass-to-surface ratio; contributes to excess amounts of water and heat loss
B. Exposed body posture with decreased ability to alter positions; contributes to rapid heat loss through radiation
C. Decreased subcutaneous fat
D. Lack of adequate brown fat stores to fully initiate non-shivering thermogenesis
E. Decreased ability to convert thyroxine for heat production
F. Poor vasomotor control
G. Structurally and functionally immature skin
   1. Poorly developed epidermis (**Fig. 7-2**)
      a. Only 2–3 cell layers thick
      b. Thin epidermis lies on the dermis, which lies directly on muscle due to lack of subcutaneous fat
      c. In VLBW infants, skin redness due to blood-rich dermis, easily visible through poorly developed epidermis
      d. Cells brushed off by contact with bedding, clothing, or washing
      e. Vapor barrier at birth further diminished with loss of cells, leading to increased water loss through skin
      f. Extremely low birth weight infants (ELBW, those <1,000 g) can look like severe burn victims; total skin disruption

2. Diminished barrier function
   a. One clinically significant difference between VLBW and term infants is development of stratum corneum.
   b. Poorly developed stratum corneum is a portal for infection and risk for toxicity from environmental toxins.
   c. There is high risk for fluid and electrolyte imbalances.
3. Barrier dysfunction with large trans-epidermal water loss (TEWL)
   a. Diminished heat regulation due to high TEWL leads to poor thermoregulation.
   b. Glistening skin of the VLBW infant is caused by high TEWL, which results in moist skin surface during the first hours of life.
   c. TEWL is the single most important channel of heat loss from the skin during the first days of life.
      (1) Water loss may be as great as 200 mL/kg/day.
      (2) For every 1 mL of water lost by evaporation, a premature baby can lose ~560 calories of heat (0.56 kcal of heat evaporation).
      (3) Maximum environmental temperature may not maintain the infant's temperature.
      (4) With loss of water goes loss of heat.

FIGURE 7-2
Epidermis and Dermis in Premature Infants

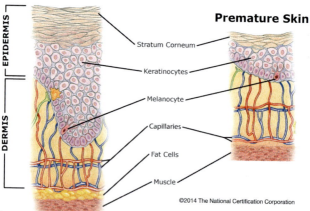

The premature infant's thin, poorly developed epidermis lies on the dermis, which lies directly on muscle due to lack of subcutaneous fat. The blood-rich dermis causes skin redness, which is easily visible through the epidermis.

     d. Massive water loss can lead to dehydration, electrolyte imbalances, and thermal instability.
     e. Hypernatremic dehydration may be seen in the first week of life.
     f. Stratum corneum matures rapidly during the first two weeks of life.
  4. Environment
     a. To decrease TEWL, provide humidity.
     b. TEWL is low when relative humidity is ~90%.
     c. Warmers may be able to overcome heat loss, but not fluid loss.
     d. Studies have **not** demonstrated increased infection with humidity.

V. Hypothermia
  A. Definition
     1. Heat losses exceed heat production.
     2. Hypothermia in infants is an independent risk factor for morbidity and mortality.
     3. Infant's temperature can drop 0.2°C–1.0°C (0.36°F–1.8°F)/min if there is no intervention in the delivery room.
  B. Causes
     1. Heat loss
     2. Infection
     3. Maternal hypothermia at birth
  C. Signs and symptoms
     1. Hypoxia (tachypnea, grunting, flaring, retracting, central cyanosis)
        a. Increased demand for oxygen for thermogenesis may decrease oxygen delivery to tissues and other vital organs, worsening respiratory distress and desaturation.
        b. Hypoxia can lead to anaerobic metabolism and pulmonary vasoconstriction.
        c. May lead to respiratory failure, pulmonary hemorrhage, and surfactant inactivation.
        d. Twice as much oxygen is needed if infant's temperature is 35°C (95°F), rather than 37°C (99°F).
     2. Hypoglycemia (lethargy, bradycardia, irritability, apnea, seizures)
        a. Increased metabolic rate to produce heat
        b. Increased glucose needs at a time when stores are diminished and glucose delivery is delayed

3. Respiratory and metabolic acidosis (apnea, seizures, pulmonary hemorrhage)
    a. Anaerobic metabolism with ongoing hypoxia leads to decreased cardiac output and acid-base abnormalities.
    b. Brown fat is converted to produce heat.
    c. Fatty acids and lactic acid from incomplete glucose breakdown result in a lower pH.
4. Cardiovascular compromise (tachycardia followed by bradycardia, hypotension)
    a. Decreased baseline heart rate, blood pressure, and perfusion
    b. Impaired contractility and function
5. Neurologic compromise (irritability, lethargy, unresponsiveness)
    a. Decreased circulation and increased permeability of the blood-brain barrier
    b. May increase the risk of intraventricular hemorrhage (IVH) in the first three days of life, with alterations in superior vena cava flow and hypoperfusion-reperfusion injury directly related to cost stress and inadequate vasomotor tone

D. Prevention and management
    1. Radiant warmers
        a. Radiant warmers alone cannot deliver enough heat to maintain normothermia in ELBW infants.
        b. Inadequate as a sole source of thermal care in the delivery room.
        c. Pre-warm radiant warmers to 37°C (99°F).
        d. Ensure the infant is warm prior to transporting to the NICU.
    2. Environmental temperatures in delivery room and stabilization areas (**Table 7-2**)
        a. Maintenance of normothermia in mother prior to delivery is essential, especially during cesarean deliveries.
        b. Cold operating rooms have been linked to increased incidences of serious infections such as tachycardia, increased blood loss, and in some cases, death.
        c. Warm the delivery room to at least 27°C (80°F) for ELBW infants.
        d. Warm the delivery room to 24°C–26°C (75°F –79°F) for all other infants.
        e. Eliminate drafts.

3. Occlusive wrap
   a. Prevents hypothermia — <36.5°C (98°F) — in premature infants <29 weeks gestation in the delivery room.
   b. Significantly improves admission temperatures (see **Fig. 7-3**).
   c. Reduces both convective and evaporative heat loss by 30%.
      (1) Permits heat to be gained by infant from radiant heat source and reduces amount of evaporative heat loss.
      (2) Blocks air currents and keeps preterm infants warmer.
   d. Decreases oxygen consumption.
   e. Choice of wrap should be based on thermal qualities, allowing net heat gain from heat source such as polyethylene plastic.
   f. Wrap should not be removed during resuscitation and care until the VLBW infant is in a pre-warmed, humidified environment set at a temperature that will control for wrap removal.
   g. Considerations
      (1) In ELBW infants, there is concern that skin may stick to the wrap and macerate on removal.

TABLE 7-2

Recommended Stabilization Room Temperatures Based on Post-Menstrual Age and Birth Weight

Estimated Post-Menstrual Age (weeks)	Estimated Birth Weight (g)	Delivery Room/Stabilization Area Temperature
≤26	≤750	27°C (80°F)
27–28	751–1,000	27°C (80°F)
29–32	1,001–1,500	≥22°C (72°F); goal 24°C (75°F)
33–36	1,501–2,500	≥22°C (72°F); goal 24°C (75°F)
37–42	≥2,501	≥21°C (70°F); goal 24°C (75°F)

Based on the American Society of Heating, Refrigerating and Air-Conditioning Engineers (ASHRAE) and World Health Organization recommendations for delivery room temperatures.

(Adapted from Bhatt DR, White R, Martin G, et al. Transitional hypothermia in preterm newborns. *J Perinatol*. 2007;27(suppl 2):S45-S47.)

(2) Hyperthermia has been reported when multiple means of maintaining temperature have been used.
(3) Wrap should be removed once the infant is stabilized in an incubator.
(4) Do not leave wrap on for long periods while infant is under radiant heat source.
4. Hats
   a. Woolen hats reduce heat loss.
   b. Tube-gauze or stockinet caps have been shown to be ineffective.
   c. Hats lined in plastic wrap may be most effective in reducing heat loss.
5. Transwarmer mattresses
   a. Reduce hypothermia
   b. May cause overheating, especially when used in combination with other products to prevent heat loss
E. Transport and admission to NICU
   1. Transport in closed radiant warmer or transport incubator to prevent drafts.
   2. Admit to pre-warmed, humidified incubator.
      a. At least 60% humidity or greater is required to decrease TEWL.

FIGURE 7-3
Occlusive Wrap and Hat Used to Prevent Hypothermia

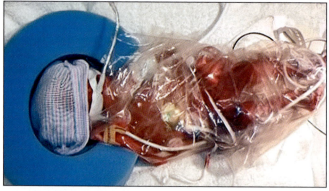

Occlusive wrap and hat helps prevent hypothermia — <36.5°C (98°F) — in premature infants <29 weeks gestation in the delivery room and significantly improves admission temperatures in the NICU. Wrap should be removed when infant is stabilized in incubator and during resuscitation and care.

b. Utilize sleeves on incubators; humidity is lost when portal doors are open.
   c. If 80% humidity is used, humidity will drop to ~60% with open portals.
3. If lines are not placed until NICU admission, make sure wrap is intact for line placement and radiant heat is utilized during the procedure.
4. Use clear drapes for the procedure to disperse the maximum amount of heat to the infant.
5. Monitor temperature throughout procedures.
6. Do not place anything into the infant's environment that has not been pre-warmed.
7. If possible, pre-warm IV fluid.
8. Ensure ventilator heaters are set at warm, 35°C–38°C (95°F–100°F); there are no randomized controlled studies that evaluate the exact temperature.

F. Management of hypothermia
   1. Rewarm at a rate of 0.5°C–1.0°C (0.9°F–1.8°F)/hour above the infant's current temperature until normal temperature is reached.
      a. Control the environment and eliminate potential heat loss.
      b. Maintain ambient temperature 1.0°C –1.5°C (1.8°F–2.7°F) higher than the infant's temperature.
      c. Increase the air temperature by 1°C (1.8°F) each hour until the infant is normothermic.
      d. Monitor the temperature of the infant every 15–30 min.
      e. Warm IV fluids.
   2. Increase humidity to reduce evaporative losses.
   3. Monitor the infant for apnea and hypotension; risk is greater with rapid rewarming.

G. Severe hypothermia
   1. Use humidified, warmed oxygen.
   2. Slow rewarming increases the exposure to hypothermia, but rapid rewarming will increase oxygen requirements and may lead to apnea and hypotension.

VI. Hyperthermia
A. Fever in a neonate defined as core body temperature >37.5°C (100°F)

B. Causes
 1. Iatrogenic due to overheating is the most likely cause of hyperthermia.
    a. Excessive heat from incubators, radiant warmers, or excessive swaddling
    b. Poor heat dissipation in newborns, with inability to effectively sweat
    c. Sweat glands develop ~30–32 weeks gestation
 2. Fever is uncommon in neonates.
    a. When present, it is often due to bacterial sepsis or viral toxins.
    b. Infants cared for with servocontrol need to have both their skin temperature and air temperature trends followed.
       (1) Since the environmental air will increase or decrease to maintain the infant's core temperature, the infant may appear stable.
       (2) Decreasing or increasing air temperature trends may indicate a developing infection.
    c. When assessing infants with fever, only 10% will have sepsis.
    d. The majority of septic infants present with hypothermia.
    e. The immunologic cascade is stimulated by exogenous pyrogens, which also stimulate prostaglandin E2 (PGE_2), leading to an increase in hypothalamic set point and resulting in fever.
 3. Evaluate for dehydration; infants exclusively breast-fed may develop a fever due to dehydration.
C. Signs and symptoms
 1. Respiratory distress (tachypnea, grunting, flaring, retracting, apnea); use of oxygen and calories because of increased metabolism.
 2. Cardiovascular compromise (tachycardia); increased metabolic rate with added stress.
 3. Some infants become hyperactive and irritable; others become lethargic.
 4. Active sweating may be noted in term infants.
D. Consequences: Increased metabolic and O_2 demand
E. Prevention
 1. Be sure any measures to prevent heat loss do not cause hyperthermia.

2. Use caution when combining wrap and transwarmer mattresses.
F. Management
1. Remove source of overheating.
2. Decrease air temperature by 1°C (1.8°F), allowing infant to cool off.

VII. Conclusion
A. Health care providers must provide meticulous thermal care immediately after birth, during resuscitation, and in the first hours to days of life.
B. A team member in the delivery room should have a lead role in thermal care as part of the resuscitation process.

References

Bhatt DR, White R, Martin G, et al. Transitional hypothermia in preterm newborns. *J Perinatol.* 2007;27(suppl 2):S45-S47.

Horn EP, Schroeder F, Gottschalk A, et al. Active warming during cesarean delivery. *Anesth Analg.* 2002;94(2):409-414.

Knobel R, Holditch-Davis D. Thermoregulation and heat loss prevention after birth and during neonatal intensive-care unit stabilization of ELBW infants. *J Obstet Gynecol Neonatal Nurs.* 2007;36(3):280-287.

Knobel RB, Holditch-Davis D, Schwartz TA, Wimmer JE Jr. Extremely low birth weight preterm infants lack vasomotor response in relationship to cold body temperatures at birth. *J Perinatol.* 2009;29(12):814-821.

MacDonald MG, Mullett MD, Seshia MMK, eds. *Avery's Neonatology: Pathophysiology and Management of the Newborn.* 6th ed. Philadelphia, PA: Lippincott Williams & Wilkins; 2005.

McCall EM, Alderdice F, Halliday HL, Jenkins JG, Vohra S. Interventions to prevent hypothermia at birth in preterm and/or low birthweight infants. *Cochrane Database of Systematic Reviews* 2010, Issue 3. Art. No.: CD004210. DOI: 10.1002/14651858.CD004210.pub4.

Power GG, Blood AB. Perinatal thermal physiology. In: Polin RA, Fox WW, Abman SH, eds. *Fetal and Neonatal Physiology.* 4th ed. Philadelphia, PA: Saunders Elsevier; 2011.

Rutter N. Clinical consequences of an immature barrier. *Semin Neonatol.* 2000;5(4):281-287.

Watkinson M. Temperature control of premature infants in the delivery room. *Clin Perinatol.* 2006;33(1):43-53.

World Health Organization, Maternal and Newborn Health/Safe Motherhood. *Thermal Protection of the Newborn: A Practical Guide.* Geneva: WHO/RHT/MSM/97.2:1997. WHO Web site. http://whqlibdoc.who.int/hq/1997/WHO_RHT_MSM_97.2.pdf. Accessed December 17, 2013.

8

Respiratory Diseases

Frances R. Koch

I. Overview

A. Most neonates admitted to the NICU present with respiratory symptoms. Clinical observations of the infant can play a significant role in providing important information about pulmonary function.

B. Respiratory rate: The respiratory rate is often elevated in neonatal respiratory diseases.

C. Retractions: Because the neonatal chest wall is very compliant relative to pulmonary compliance, retractions are easily visible. Retractions become more apparent as the lungs become stiffer; severe retractions are signs of complications from respiratory disease, obstruction, air leaks, or atelectasis.

D. Nasal flaring: An effort to decrease nasal airway resistance.

E. Grunting: The audible sound a neonate generates during expiration. The grunt occurs when the glottis is partially closed in order to hold gas in the lungs, which helps to generate increased airway pressure or maintain functional residual capacity and lung volume.

F. Cyanosis:
   1. An indicator of poor gas exchange, best observed by examining the oral mucosa
   2. Difficult to assess visually
   3. Dependent on the temperature spectrum of ambient light
   4. Should not be used, as pulse oximetry provides more objective, accurate data

II. Respiratory distress syndrome (RDS): An acute lung disease present at birth, associated with insufficient surfactant production. It almost exclusively affects infants born at <37 weeks of gestation.

A. Risk factors
   1. Decreasing gestational age
   2. Cesarean section without labor
   3. Male sex
   4. Caucasian
   5. Second-born twin
   6. Gestational diabetes and insulin-dependent mother

B. Pathophysiology
  1. Previously referred to as hyaline membrane disease based on pathological appearance
     a. Gross autopsy: diffuse lung atelectasis, congestion, edema
     b. Histologic examination: diffusely collapsed peripheral air spaces (atelectasis), over-distended proximal respiratory bronchioles lined with necrotic epithelium, hyaline membranes (fibrinous matrix of materials from the blood and injured epithelial cells); edema probably represents an acute inflammatory process
  2. Insufficient or delayed surfactant production resulting in decreased pulmonary function
     a. Reduced lung compliance and therefore increased work of breathing
     b. Reduced functional residual capacity
        (1) Law of Laplace and role of surfactant
        $$P = 2T/r$$
        Where
        P = Distending pressure or pressure needed for inflation or to avoid alveolar collapse
        T = Surface tension
        r = Radius of the alveoli
            (a) The pressure required to keep the alveoli distended is directly proportional to the surface tension and indirectly to the radii of the alveoli.
            (b) In surfactant deficiency, air tends to leave smaller alveoli (higher pressure) and go to larger alveoli where there is less pressure, thus causing collapse of smaller alveoli (atelectasis) and over-distension of the larger ones.
        (2) Role of surfactant as variable surface active agent
            (a) Surfactant decreases the surface tension and therefore decreases the amount of pressure needed for inflation or distension.
            (b) In the less distended alveoli (smaller radius), the surfactant becomes more concentrated on the surface. Lowering the surface tension diminishes the required pressure needed for inflation.

(c) In larger alveoli, the surfactant is spread more thinly, increasing the surface tension and therefore increasing recoil pressure.
- c. Reduced gas exchange
  - (1) Alveolar hypoventilation: Inability of lungs to eliminate carbon dioxide as a result of atelectatic lung or poorly ventilated areas
  - (2) Ventilation-perfusion (V/Q) ratio imbalance: Describes areas of lung depending on amount of ventilation and perfusion to each compartment (e.g., a V/Q of <1 indicates a poorly ventilated area with perfusion common in RDS)
    - (a) The V/Q ratio can refer to a single alveolus, a group of alveoli, or the entire lung; a V/Q ratio of 1 is for optimal lung exchange.
  - (3) Right-to-left shunts increased
- d. Reduced effective pulmonary blood flow

C. Diagnosis
  1. Clinical presentation
     a. Immediately after birth or within several hours
     b. Frequently worsens in severity as atelectasis progresses
     c. Almost always premature infants (with few exceptions)
     d. Often cyanotic with respiratory distress requiring supplemental O_2
     e. Pallor from anemia or peripheral vasoconstriction
     f. Expiratory grunting, nasal flaring, subcostal and intercostal retractions
     g. If uncomplicated course, recovery starts ~48 hours
        (1) Heralded by diuresis
        (2) Oxygen requirements usually decline rapidly after 72 hours
  2. Radiological
     a. Diffuse reticulogranular pattern giving a classic ground-glass appearance bilaterally with superimposed air bronchograms; appearance is result of alveolar atelectasis and aerated bronchioles on superimposed background of non-aerated alveoli (**Fig. 8-1**)
     b. Symmetric and homogenous unless there is unequal distribution of exogenously administered surfactant
     c. Complete "white out" of lungs in the most severe cases (**Fig. 8-2**)
     d. Lung volumes typically decreased, however, positive airway pressure can eliminate this finding

FIGURE 8-1
X-Ray of Respiratory Distress Syndrome (RDS)

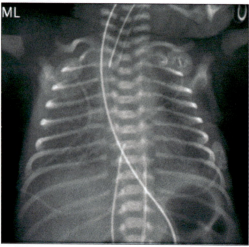

Diffuse reticulogranular pattern gives a ground-glass appearance bilaterally with superimposed air bronchograms. Appearance is result of alveolar atelectasis and aerated bronchioles on superimposed non-aerated alveoli.

FIGURE 8-2
X-Ray of Severe Respiratory Distress Syndrome (RDS)

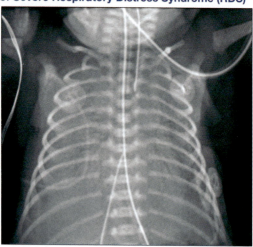

Severe RDS appears as a complete "white out" of lungs.

- e. Cardiac silhouette normal to slightly increased
- f. RDS cannot be reliably differentiated from neonatal pneumonia with chest x-ray
3. Laboratory – untreated
    a. Moderate to severe hypoxemia
    b. Hypercarbia (respiratory acidosis)
    c. Mild to severe metabolic acidosis
    d. Secondary effects of hypoxemia can complicate the picture in severe disease
D. Management
    1. Prevention
        a. Prevent premature birth — remains a challenge
            (1) Appropriate and early maternal-fetal medicine referral
            (2) Treatment of bacterial infections
            (3) Cerclage
            (4) Appropriate use of tocolytic therapy
            (5) Avoidance of "elective" early term delivery (<39 weeks)
        b. Prediction of RDS risk by antenatal testing of amniotic fluid
            (1) Testing to confirm fetal lung maturity (FLM) to electively deliver <39 weeks should be avoided. It is sometimes evaluated if the findings impact the balance between maternal-fetal risks of continuing the pregnancy vs. a preterm birth.
            (2) In a 2011 study, Kamath reported that infants <39 weeks gestation with documented FLM had significantly higher rates of neonatal morbidities compared to those infants born ≥39 weeks gestation.
            (3) FLM testing continues to decrease, probably because of stricter adherence to avoiding early elective deliveries as well as the unavailability of many of the FLM tests at many laboratories.
        c. Antenatal steroids to accelerate lung maturation
            (1) NIH recommendation for fetuses 24–34 weeks gestational age
            (2) Decreased risk or severity of RDS, death, and intraventricular hemorrhage
        d. Establish and preserve functional residual capacity (FRC) — delivery room interventions

(1) Prophylactic exogenous surfactant, given usually immediately after delivery in a selected group of premature infants to try and prevent the onset of RDS
(2) Early intervention with continuous positive airway pressure (CPAP) rapidly after delivery or immediately following delivery of exogenous surfactant

2. Management and diagnostic tools
   a. Appropriate resuscitative measures
   b. Alveolar recruitment
      (1) Secretion of surfactant is impaired by inadequate expansion.
      (2) Goal is to provide positive end-expiratory pressure (PEEP); centers vary on initial methods to provide pressure for recruitment.
         (a) Early intubation and surfactant in weight- or gestational age-targeted groups vs. early nasal CPAP with rescue intubation
         (b) If early intubation, prompt delivery of exogenous surfactant (within 15 min of birth) is associated with lower mortality and bronchopulmonary dysplasia
         (c) CPAP has been associated with increased risk of pneumothorax; providers need to be skilled in utilizing this lung-recruitment strategy
   c. Surfactant replacement therapy (see Section II.E)
   d. Blood gas monitoring
      (1) Frequency depends on severity of disease, including O_2 requirement.
      (2) Can expedite the weaning process.
      (3) Some centers have incorporated ventilation-weaning protocols relying on minute ventilation and desired tidal volume, which lessen the need for blood gas sampling, particularly in preterm infants without indwelling arterial access (**Table 8-1**).
   e. Continuous pulse oximetry
      (1) Noninvasive measure for indirectly determining oxygen saturation that could alleviate the need for arterial catheterization in infants with mild RDS.
   f. Thermal neutrality
      (1) Goal is to decrease overall caloric expenditure (55 calories/kg/day in first four days).

TABLE 8-1
Ventilation-Weaning Protocols

	Clinical Parameter	Wean	Tolerate	Evaluate	Weaning
From Ventilator	V_te (mL/kg)	5–6	3–4	<3 or >6	Decrease ΔP (usually by decreasing PIP).
	MV (mL/kg/min)	240–400	160–240	<160 or >400	Decrease ΔP or RR, with goal of reducing V_te first.
From Blood Gas	pH	7.28–7.35	7.28–7.27	<7.25 or >7.35	Based on expectation for arterial sample. May need to make adjustments if capillary or venous. If out-of-range pH is respiratory in origin (vs. metabolic) adjust MV as above. If PaO_2 or SpO_2 is less than desired, wean rate rather than PIP.
	$PaCO_2$ (mmHg)	41–56	56–60	<41 or >60	Wean MV as above. If PaO_2 or SpO_2 is less than desired, wean rate rather than PIP.
	PaO_2 (mmHg) (EGA 23–31 weeks)	51–65	41–50	<41 or >65	Adjust by manipulating MAP (primarily by adjusting PEEP, but also with PIP or inspiratory time) or FiO_2. Avoid PEEP <4 to avoid atelectrauma.
	PaO_2 (mmHg) (EGA 32–36 weeks)	56–70	51–55	<50 or >70	In general, do not wean PEEP until $FiO_2 < 0.40$.

ΔP = delta P (PIP-PEEP); EGA = estimated gestational age; FiO_2 = fraction of inspired oxygen; MAP = mean airway pressure; MV = minute ventilation; $PaCO_2$ = partial pressure of carbon dioxide; PaO_2 = partial pressure of oxygen; PEEP = positive end-expiratory pressure; PIP = peak inspiratory pressure; RR = respiratory rate; SpO_2 = pulse oximetry oxygen saturation; V_te = expired tidal volume

- (2) Minimize oxygen consumption and requirements.
- (3) In RDS patients, hypoxia may impact the infants' ability to increase their metabolic rates if they are cold.
- (4) Cold stress can inactivate surfactant.
g. Fluids, electrolytes, and nutrition
   - (1) RDS characterized by:
     - (a) High surface tension and high-permeability pulmonary edema and fluid retention
     - (b) High levels of arginine vasopressin with low levels of atrial natriuretic peptide (ANP), resulting in low urine output and fluid retention until increase in ANP at onset of diuretic phase
   - (2) Premature infants have an excess of extracellular fluid at birth and an expected 10% weight loss within the first week.
   - (3) It is not necessary to administer sodium in the first 1–5 days of life, as sodium will be a reflection of fluid status at this time and fluid intake should be adjusted accordingly.
     - (a) In the extreme premature infant, sodium levels may rise >150 mEq/L as a result of increased insensible losses.
     - (b) In this situation, liberal use of fluids and humidification is essential.
     - (c) Monitor for hyperglycemia as the fluid rate is increased.
   - (4) Potassium should also be restricted secondary to hyperkalemia from decreased urinary output in the first few days of life.
   - (5) Close attention to nutritional support is paramount.
     - (a) Total parenteral nutrition is supplied on the first day of life to include amino acids, glucose, and in many cases, lipids. It is important to establish a positive nitrogen balance from the beginning.
     - (b) Minimal enteral nutrition via gavage feeds is often initiated within the first 24 hours of life, but may vary by institution.

E. Surfactant replacement: Several natural formulations of surfactant from bovine or porcine lungs are available for prevention and rescue therapy for RDS.
   1. Timing
      a. Institution sets guidelines for prophylactic surfactant therapy.
         (1) Example: At <1,000 g or <28 weeks gestational age, delivery of exogenous surfactant should be given within 15–30 min of birth.
         (2) A study by Dunn suggested delivering exogenous surfactant within 15–30 min of birth if infant is <26 weeks.
      b. For larger infants not within prophylactic guidelines, it is preferable to give surfactant within 2 hours of life.
      c. Infants may be able to rapidly extubate to CPAP after exogenous surfactant, therefore decreasing the need for mechanical ventilation.
   2. Dosing and administration
      a. Dosing interval depends on the brand that is used at your institution.
      b. The drug is given quickly in 2–4 aliquots through a catheter passed into the end of the endotracheal tube.
      c. Each aliquot is followed by providing mechanical breaths with ambu bag, T-piece apparatus, or ventilator to ensure even distribution.
      d. Peak inspiratory (PIP) pressure and oxygen may have to be increased during administration.
      e. Slow administration results in poor distribution because of the effects of gravity.
   3. Response
      a. Improved oxygenation as a result of V/Q matching
      b. Increased lung volume and stabilization of functional residual capacity
      c. Increased lung compliance; rapidity might depend on surfactant used
      d. Decreased incidence in air leaks
      e. Improved mortality from RDS
   4. Complications
      a. Bradycardia and desaturations
      b. Endotracheal tube obstruction

c. Possible mildly increased risk of pulmonary hemorrhage, usually in first 72 hours of life (controversial; literature not consistent)
d. Air leaks could result if accompanied by rapid change in lung compliance without change in pressure setting

F. Mechanical ventilation
1. See Chapter 5.
2. Current conceptual approaches aim to preserve lung expansion (open lung) and FRC.
3. Major sources of pulmonary parenchymal damage:
   a. Volutrauma (excessive tidal volumes resulting in excessive expansion)
   b. Atelectasis resulting from inadequate distending pressure and cyclical recruitment or loss of recruitment
   c. Rapid inspiratory rise

III. Transient tachypnea of the newborn

A. Pathophysiology
1. At birth, for effective gas exchange to take place, there must be 1) clearance of excess of fetal lung fluid, and 2) increased pulmonary blood flow for V/Q matching.
   a. Failure can result in retained fetal lung fluid with transient pulmonary edema causing transient tachypnea.
   b. Process of clearing fluid begins 2–3 days prior to birth with a decrease in lung fluid production, from 25 to 18 mL/kg.
   c. The onset of labor accentuates the clearing of fluid from the lungs.
   d. Experiments on fetal lambs show two-thirds of total clearance during this time period.
2. The key process in movement of fluid from the fetal lung is transport of sodium across the pulmonary epithelium.
3. After birth, lung epithelium switches from a membrane that predominantly secretes chloride to one that absorbs sodium. The developmental changes in ion and fluid movement across the lung membranes (**Fig. 8-3**) can be described as follows:
   a. In the fetal stage, chloride is actively secreted via Cl- channels in the lung epithelium; sodium reabsorption is low.

b. Near the time of labor, there is reversal of the chloride and sodium ions and water movement. There is a predominance of positive sodium reabsorption across epithelial Na+ channels (ENaC), followed by water. ENaC are developmentally regulated and reach peak expression at term gestation. Therefore, preterm infants are born with decreased expression of these channels.
   (1) First, there is passive movement of sodium from the lumen across the apical membrane into the cell via sodium channels.
   (2) Second, sodium is actively transported from the cell across the basolateral membrane into the serosal space.
c. Factors influencing ENaC
   (1) Exogenous glucocorticoids
      (a) Stimulate the transcription of ENaC in the lung
      (b) Increase the number of available channels
      (c) Enhance the responsiveness of lungs to β-adrenergic agents and thyroid hormones

FIGURE 8-3
Ion Transport Across Alveolar Epithelial Cells

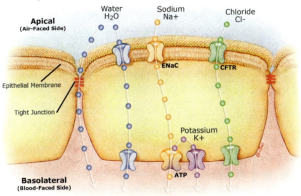

©2014 The National Certification Corporation

Na+ ions enter the apical membranes of alveolar epithelial (both type II or type I cells) via a variety of ENaC and non-ENaC channels. K+ ions, brought into the cells by the pump in exchange of Na+ ions, leave the cells passively through basolaterally located K+ channels. To maintain neutrality, Cl- ions enter cells through CFTR-type channels and exit basolaterally via a Na, K, or Cl cotransporter. The combined movement of Na+ and Cl- ions creates an oncotic gradient leading to the reabsorption of alveolar fluid.

- (2) Endogenous catecholamines
  - (a) Increased levels at birth are important for alveolar fluid clearance by increasing the activity of sodium channels.
  - (b) However, recent studies of exogenous catecholamines did not show similar findings. The result is increased activity of the channels and not an increase in the number of ENaC available.
- (3) Air interface environment; increase in oxygen tension influences assembly of ENaC

B. Diagnosis and clinical presentation
  1. Initially, many thought transient tachypnea was limited to term or late preterm infants. However, smaller preterm infants are also at risk of retained fetal lung fluid. Retained lung fluid may complicate their respiratory course, which may already include RDS, thus increasing need for supplemental oxygen and ventilation.
  2. Often history of:
     a. Maternal diabetes
     b. Heavy maternal sedation
     c. Delivery by elective cesarean section without labor
        (1) Vaginal-birth-after-cesarean rates have fallen secondary to fear of trial of labor associated with more perinatal morbidity and mortality.
        (2) More recently, efforts have been made to deliver via elective cesarean at ≥ 39 weeks or waiting for the onset of labor to avoid the higher risk of transient tachypnea, RDS, and persistent pulmonary hypertension unrelated to gestational age.
  3. Clinical presentation
     a. May be mildly depressed at birth
     b. Tachypnea with respiratory rates from 60 to 120 breaths/min; may have grunting, nasal flaring, and retractions
     c. May have little or no requirement for supplemental oxygen
     d. Excessive oxygen requirement (>0.40) should suggest possibility of alternate diagnosis
  4. Radiologic
     a. Chest x-ray may show hyperinflation/hyperaeration (often with mild cardiomegaly)

b. "Sunburst pattern" of prominent vascular markings stemming from the hilum secondary to retained fluid in the perivascular cuffs (**Fig. 8-4**)
c. Fluid within the widened interlobar fissures
d. Seldom appearance of coarse fluffy densities indicating alveolar edema
e. Resolution of radiographic abnormalities over 2–3 days

5. Laboratory
   a. Blood gas often reveals respiratory acidosis that normalizes within 24 hours
   b. Mild to moderate hypoxemia by blood gases or oximetry

C. Management
   1. Often benign, self-limiting disease
   2. Seldom requires >40% supplemental oxygen
      a. Highest O_2 requirement is at the onset of disease.
      b. O_2 requirement progressively decreases.
      c. Most infants need only room air within 24 hours.
   3. Infants respond rapidly to nasal CPAP if needed
   4. If uncomplicated course, infants recover quickly with no residual pulmonary disabilities

FIGURE 8-4
X-Ray of Retained Fetal Lung Fluid

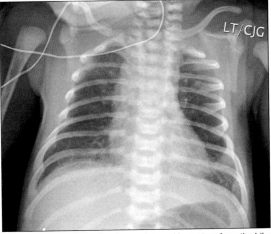

The "sunburst pattern" of prominent vascular markings stem from the hilum secondary to retained fluid in the perivascular cuffs.

5. Studies have shown that although this disease is a result of retained lung fluid, diuretics were not effective
6. From preterm animal and human data, exogenous glucocorticoids

D. Differential diagnoses
1. RDS
2. Pneumonia
3. Sepsis
4. Polycythemia
5. Amniotic fluid aspiration
6. Congenital malformations
7. Congenital heart disease

IV. Apnea of prematurity

A. Diagnosis
1. A diagnosis of apnea of prematurity can only be made after the elimination of other causes for apnea.
2. Incidence is inversely related to gestational age.
3. It is usually stated that apnea of prematurity begins subsequently to the first day of life; however, in reviewing polygraphic recordings of bradycardia or desaturations reported by staff in that initial day, apnea usually precedes those events.
4. Most apneas occur during active sleep in which there is decreased arousal, muscle tone, absence of respiratory drive and upper airway adductor activity, irregular breathing, and chest wall distortion during inspiration.

B. Definition
1. Varies widely among different studies, but most accepted is cessation of breathing for >15–20 sec, usually accompanied by desaturations and bradycardia.
   a. 15- to 20-sec cessations in respiratory activity result in decreased exchange of oxygen and carbon dioxide.
   b. Shorter episodes of periodic breathing may also be associated with bradycardia or desaturations.
2. Three categories based on presence of upper airway obstruction:
   a. Central: Total cessation of respiratory effort with no evidence of obstruction
   b. Obstructive: Upper airway obstruction (usually in the pharynx) presents, resulting in chest wall movement or respiratory effort, but no airflow

c. Mixed: Obstructed respiratory efforts usually following central pauses in breathing; accounts for 50% of long apneic spells
C. Periodic breathing vs. apnea
  1. Periodic breathing: Cycles of regular respiratory effort of 10–15 sec that are interrupted by pauses of ≥ 3 sec
     a. Considered benign and no treatment needed.
     b. Respiratory pauses are usually self-limited and respiration continues, whereas infants with true apnea may fail to reinitiate respiratory efforts fully or do so suboptimally.
D. Pathophysiology
  1. Proposed mechanisms by which apnea of prematurity manifests: decreased response to hypercarbia, hypoxic depression, and enhancement of inhibitory reflexes
  2. Ventilation response to CO_2
     a. The chemosensitive region of the ventrolateral surface of the medulla is a key area in regulating respiratory and ventilation activity in response to CO_2 levels.
     b. After birth it is presumed that infants depend on an adequate ventilation response to abnormally high CO_2 levels.
     c. This is directly related to advancing gestational age.
        (1) Term neonates are able to increase their tidal volume and frequency of respirations in response to increased CO_2.
        (2) Preterm infants, however, do not increase their frequency of respirations and are also associated with a prolonged expiratory phase that is mediated at the brainstem level.
        (3) At a similar CO_2 level, a preterm infant with apnea vs. a control with no apnea will have decreased minute ventilation. With all pulmonary parameters the same, this evidence points to central immaturity for respiratory neural output, but the cause and effect have yet to be identified.
     d. There appears to be a decrease in diaphragm activity with central and mixed apnea in preterm infants. Diaphragmatic failure can also occur from the increased work needed to generate adequate tidal volume secondary to a very compliant chest wall.

3. Response to hypoxia
   a. Typical finding after an apneic event is a decrease in arterial partial pressure of oxygen (PaO_2) and oxygen saturation in preterm infants.
      (1) Decreases in saturation may be greater in obstructive apnea vs. central apnea.
      (2) Bradycardia that follows has been related to stimulation of the carotid body chemoreceptors in response to the hypoxia.
   b. After birth, PaO_2 rises and peripheral chemoreceptors, which respond to hypoxia to stimulate breathing, are quiet.
      (1) In preterm infants exposed to hypoxia, there exists a biphasic response:
         (a) Phase 1: Initial increase in ventilation for 1–2 min likely secondary to stimulation of peripheral chemoreceptors
         (b) Phase 2: Then a decline in ventilation below baseline due to decreased respiratory frequency
      (2) Not well understood; may last for weeks.
   c. Though hypoxic ventilator depression has been thought to be an underlying cause for apnea of prematurity, hypoxia usually does not precede the apneic event.
      (1) PaO_2 is usually normal at baseline.
      (2) Hypoxia can worsen apnea.
      (3) The role of hypoxia and its role in the underlying cause of ventilation depression are unknown.
   d. Increased inhibitory reflexes
      (1) Laryngeal stimulation can cause apnea in the preterm infant secondary to this exaggerated reflex.
      (2) Mediated through the superior laryngeal nerve.
      (3) Precise mechanism for the exaggerated reflex is not known, but may be related to decreased central neural output.

E. Evaluation
   1. All infants at risk should have continuous cardiopulmonary monitoring; pulse oximetry monitoring is common.
   2. Consideration for other causes of apnea is warranted.

- a. Infections
- b. Intracranial hemorrhage
- c. Asphyxia
- d. Anemia
- e. Metabolic disorders (e.g., hypoglycemia)
- f. Thermoregulation instability
- g. Medications (e.g., prostaglandins to maintain a patent ductus arteriosus, opiates)
- h. Brain malformations and spinal cord injury
3. Gastroesophageal reflux
   - a. Though it is often discussed as a culprit in causing apnea, evidence shows that apnea precedes reflux, rather than the reverse.
   - b. This suggests that the loss of neural respiratory output is accompanied by a decrease of lower esophageal tone, and then the infant refluxes.
   - c. Therefore, treatment of reflux with antacids will not resolve apnea.

F. Management
1. Other causes of apnea should be eliminated as clinically indicated and treated accordingly.
2. Methylxanthines
   - a. Action
     - (1) Mainstay pharmacologic therapy (theophylline and caffeine)
     - (2) Increases respiratory neural output
     - (3) Blocks adenosine receptors; adenosine, an inhibitory neuroregulator in the central nervous system, released during hypoxia
   - b. Effects
     - (1) Increased minute ventilation
     - (2) Improved CO_2 sensitivity
     - (3) Enhanced diaphragmatic activity
     - (4) Decreased second phase of hypoxia-induced ventilation depression
     - (5) Decreased periodic breathing
     - (6) Decreased apnea and mechanical ventilation
   - c. Dosing
     - (1) Loading dose followed by maintenance
     - (2) Caffeine: Oral and IV; load with 20 mg/kg followed in 24 hours with 5–8 mg/kg once every 24 hours

(a) Caffeine has higher therapeutic index, so lower toxicity compared to theophylline, therefore levels less critical
    (3) Theophylline: Oral; load with 5–6 mg/kg followed by 1–2 mg/kg every 8–12 hours; serum levels monitored
  d. Adverse effects (usually with toxic levels, less likely with caffeine)
    (1) Tachycardia
    (2) Cardiac dysrhythmias
    (3) Feeding intolerance
    (4) Seizures (infrequent)
  e. Potential neuroprotective effects
    (1) Though an inhibitory neuroregulator, adenosine has been shown to protect the brain from cell death during periods of hypoxia and ischemia in animal modes.
    (2) A multicenter study published in 2007 looked at long-term neurodevelopmental outcomes at 18–21 months.
      (a) Infants were 500–1,250 g and assigned to either receive caffeine or placebo for apnea of prematurity until caffeine was no longer needed (median postmenstrual age of 35 weeks).
      (b) Results indicated an improved rate of survival without neurodevelopmental disability.
        i. An important intermediate variable was the discontinuation of positive airway pressure one week earlier in infants on caffeine. Ventilator injury can lead to bronchopulmonary dysplasia, which is an independent risk factor for neurodevelopmental delay.
3. CPAP
  a. Is safe and effective, especially in longer events of apnea that also have an obstructive component
  b. Stents open the upper airway
  c. Increases functional residual capacity, therefore improving oxygenation
  d. High-flow nasal cannula
  e. Nasal intermittent positive-pressure ventilation (NIPPV) can be considered prior to intubation and ventilation for refractory events

(1) Currently not able to deliver synchronized in the United States, but may change in the future; rates up to 20 beats/min (or higher at some institutions) may be used
(2) Inconsistent conclusions regarding whether NIPPV reduces the risk of BPD
(3) Commonly used in several countries in extremely low birth weight (ELBW) infants

G. Discharge management
1. Most apnea of prematurity resolves ~36–40 weeks postconceptual age, but the course might be more prolonged in ELBW infants.
2. The most extreme premature infants may have events extending past 40 weeks, but will usually resolve ~43–44 weeks.
3. An apnea-free period is usually required prior to discharge and may range from 3 to 10 days.
4. Some infants who are ready for discharge may continue to have events of periodic breathing with desaturations and bradycardias, with apnea of >20 sec the rarity.
   a. Institutions may vary as to method of discharge preparedness:
      (1) Discontinue methylxanthine but observe for cessation of events prior to discharge.
      (2) Continue caffeine and set up patient for home cardiopulmonary monitoring; continue to monitor until cessation of events (e.g., for 48–72 hours).
         (a) Usually in infants that are still premature or were of extreme prematurity
         (b) Offers alternative to a prolonged hospital stay
         (c) American Academy of Pediatrics (AAP) recommends home monitoring not be used as a crutch in order to discharge patient early; patient must demonstrate an event-free period

References

Baird TM, Martin RJ, Abu-Shaweesh JM. Clinical associations, treatment, and outcomes of apnea of prematurity. *NeoReviews*. 2002;3:e66-e69.

Bancalari E, ed. *The Newborn Lung: Neonatology Questions and Controversies*. 2nd ed. Philadelphia, PA: Saunders Elsevier; 2012.

Bland R. Lung fluid balance during development. *NeoReviews*. 2005;6(6):e255-e267.

Dunn MS, Shennan AT, Zyack D, Possmayer F. Bovine surfactant replacement therapy in neonates of less than 30 weeks' gestation: a randomized controlled trial of prophylaxis versus treatment. *Pediatrics*. 1991;87(3):377-386.

Gleason CA, Devaskar S, eds. *Avery's Diseases of the Newborn*. 9th ed. Philadelphia, PA: Saunders Elsevier; 2012.

Goldsmith JP, Karotkin EH, eds. *Assisted Ventilation of the Neonate*. 5th ed. St. Louis, MO: Saunders Elsevier; 2011.

Jain L, Eaton DC. Physiology of fetal lung fluid clearance and the effect of labor. *Semin Perinatol*. 2006;30(1):34-43.

Kamath BD, Marcotte MP, DeFranco EA. Neonatal morbidity after documented fetal lung maturity in late preterm and early term infants. *Am J Obstet Gynecol*. 2011;204(6):518.e1-e8. doi: 10.1016/j.ajog.2011.03.038.

MacDonald MG, Mullett MD, Seshia MMK, eds. *Avery's Neonatology: Pathophysiology and Management of the Newborn*. 6th ed. Philadelphia, PA: Lippincott Williams & Wilkins; 2005.

Martin RJ, Abu-Shaweesh JM, Baird TM. Pathophysiological mechanisms underlying apnea of prematurity. *NeoReviews*. 2002;3:e59-e64.

Martin RJ, Fanaroff AA, Walsh MC. *Fanaroff and Martin's Neonatal-Perinatal Medicine: Diseases of the Fetus and Infant*. 9th ed. St. Louis, MO: Mosby Elsevier; 2011.

Schmidt B, Roberts RS, Davis P, et al. Long-term effects of caffeine therapy for apnea of prematurity. *N Engl J Med*. 2007;357(19):1893-1902.

Vermont-Oxford Network DRM Study Group. Randomized trial comparing 3 approaches to the initial respiratory management of preterm neonates. *Pediatrics*. 2011;128(5):e1069-e1076.

Pulmonary Emergencies

Cheryl A. Carlson

I. Aspiration syndromes

A. Overview
   1. Meconium is the most commonly aspirated material, but it is not generally seen in very low birth weight (VLBW) infants.
   2. VLBW infants may aspirate blood; it is important to differentiate aspiration from pulmonary hemorrhage.
   3. Amniotic fluid may be aspirated. This is complicated by the presence of vernix caseosa, dead cells, or infectious agents.

B. Etiology may occur:
   1. *In utero* secondary to hypoxic event, as a result of hypoxia-induced respiration
   2. In the immediate perinatal period
   3. Postnatally

C. Pathophysiology
   1. Presence of foreign substance in lungs can lead to:
      a. Obstruction and atelectasis
      b. Obstruction with distal overexpansion
      c. Lung inflammation
      d. Surfactant inactivation
   2. Infants with pulmonary hemorrhage vs. maternal blood aspiration often have severe cardiopulmonary compromise.

D. Clinical presentation
   1. Includes grunting, subcostal and intercostal retractions, cyanosis, poor respiratory effort, or severe respiratory failure.
   2. Suctioning of blood from stomach may indicate maternal blood aspiration as the etiology of blood in the lungs.

E. Management
   1. For VLBW infants ≥28–29 weeks gestation, continuous positive airway pressure (CPAP) may be effective.
   2. Infants with severe respiratory distress and increased oxygen requirements require intubation, surfactant administration, and ventilator support.

3. Surfactant-associated proteins may be important in moderating the inflammatory response in the premature lung due to aspiration.

II. Infections
A. Congenital pneumonia
   1. Incidence: Between 5% and 20%
   2. Increased susceptibility due to immaturity of respiratory and immune systems
   3. Increased risk of neonatal infection with decreasing gestational age
B. Etiology
   1. Congenital pneumonia
      a. Acquired transplacentally via intrauterine infection
   2. Perinatal pneumonia
      a. Occurs during birth process from organisms in birth canal
      b. May follow premature rupture of membranes
C. Pathophysiology
   1. Invasion of neonatal lung with organisms present in amniotic fluid
   2. Congenital or transplacental infection
      a. Related to maternal systemic illness
      b. Rubella: Results from primary maternal infection
      c. Varicella, herpes simplex virus (HSV), and cytomegalovirus (CMV): May be primary or recurrent maternal illness
   3. Perinatal infection
      a. Occurs during process of labor and delivery
      b. Organism present in genital tract after rupture of membranes or during passage through the birth canal
         (1) Group B *streptococcus* (GBS)
         (2) *Escherichia coli (E. coli)*
         (3) *Listeria monocytogenes*
         (4) *Klebsiella*
         (5) *Enterobacter*
         (6) *Proteus mirabilis*
   4. Clinical presentation
      a. Respiratory distress, including grunting, subcostal and intercostal retractions
      b. Cyanosis
      c. Poor or ineffective respiratory effort
      d. Severe respiratory failure

5. Management
    a. For VLBW infants ≥28–29 weeks gestation, initial management with CPAP may be effective.
    b. Infants with severe respiratory distress and increased oxygen requirements require intubation, surfactant administration, and ventilator support.

III. Air leak syndromes
A. Overview
1. Alveoli rupture with presence of air in non-pulmonary airspace (**Fig. 9-1**).
    a. Pulmonary interstitial emphysema (PIE)
    b. Pneumomediastinum
    c. Pneumothorax
    d. Pneumopericardium
    e. Pneumoperitoneum
    f. Subcutaneous emphysema
    g. Air embolism

FIGURE 9-1
Air Leak Syndromes

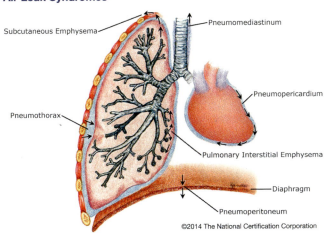

©2014 The National Certification Corporation

Pneumothorax is the most commonly seen air leak syndrome immediately after birth. Others are often seen with continued ventilator support. Air leak syndromes occur when alveoli rupture and air enters the perivascular and peribronchial spaces. Air can be trapped, leading to pulmonary interstitial emphysema (PIE). A pneumomediastinum occurs when air dissects the mediastinum. Air that ruptures into the pleural space causes a pneumothorax. Air that travels along the great vessels and ruptures into the pericardial space causes a pneumopericardium. Air that ruptures into the posterior peritoneum and peritoneal cavity causes a pneumoperitoneum. If air ruptures under very high pressure and enters the pulmonary capillaries, an air embolism occurs.

2. Pneumothorax is the most commonly seen air leak syndrome immediately after birth.
3. Other air leak syndromes are often seen with continued ventilator support.

B. Etiology
 1. Rupture of alveoli due to high ventilator pressures and structural immaturity of alveolar cells, leading to accumulation of air in non-ventilated spaces
 2. Excessive tidal volumes and overexpansion that may result from high peak inspiratory pressures (PIP) and high mean airway pressure, and/or prolonged inspiratory time used with manual or mechanical ventilation
 3. Aspiration syndromes and pulmonary hypoplasia increase incidence of pneumothorax
 4. Increased incidence with respiratory distress syndrome (RDS)
    a. Surfactant deficiency leads to high surface tension, unequal aeration, and collapse of alveoli
    b. High pressures used with manual or mechanical ventilation
 5. Increased incidence with inexperienced personnel
 6. Pneumothorax may occur spontaneously

C. Pathophysiology
 1. Alveoli rupture and air enters the perivascular and peribronchial spaces.
    a. Air can be trapped, leading to PIE.
       (1) Air moves into loose connective tissue and travels along the sheaths or the arterioles, moving into the hilum of the lungs.
       (2) Interstitial air can dissect around blood vessels or along lymphatics.
       (3) Air collects as small distinct bubbles of extra-alveolar air and acts as a pulmonary splint, stiffening the lungs and compromising ventilation.
    b. Air can also dissect the mediastinum, leading to a pneumomediastinum.
       (1) Isolated disorder that often occurs spontaneously
       (2) Air can rupture up into the neck, leading to subcutaneous emphysema
 2. Air that ruptures into the pleural space causes a pneumothorax.
    a. Collapse of lung by air accumulation in pleural space
    b. Shift of mediastinum to opposite side of air leak

c. Shift of trachea and point of maximal impulse (PMI) to opposite side of air leak
3. Air that travels along the great vessels and ruptures into the pericardial space causes a pneumopericardium.
   a. Pathophysiology is often unknown.
4. Air can also rupture through the sheaths of the aorta and vena cava into the posterior peritoneum and then into the peritoneal cavity, causing a pneumoperitoneum.
5. If air ruptures under very high pressure it can enter the pulmonary capillaries, causing an air embolism.

D. Clinical presentation
   1. PIE
      a. Usually gradual onset
      b. Increased oxygen requirement due to decreasing lung compliance
      c. Increased carbon dioxide retention
      d. Decreasing ability to ventilate
   2. Pneumomedisatinum
      a. Usually asymptomatic
      b. May cause minimal respiratory distress
   3. Pneumothorax
      a. Acute decompensation after use of CPAP or positive-pressure ventilation
      b. Decrease or absence of breath sounds on affected side
      c. Decreased pulse pressure
      d. Respiratory distress: grunting, intercostal/subcostal retractions, cyanosis
      e. In VLBW infants, acute presentation may include bradycardia, hypotension, increased oxygen requirement, persistent cyanosis
   4. Pneumopericardium
      a. Sudden cyanosis
      b. Sudden, profound hypotension
      c. Distant heart sounds
      d. Metabolic acidosis
      e. Rapid death
      f. Can also be asymptomatic
   5. Pneumoperitoneum
      a. Delayed gastric emptying and emesis
      b. Bloody stools
      c. May compress inferior vena cava, decreasing blood return to heart and causing severe acidosis

6. Subcutaneous emphysema
   a. Air present in subcutaneous layer of skin
   b. Crackle feeling upon palpitation
   c. Usually a symptom of a more severe diagnosis
7. Air embolism
   a. Sudden cyanosis and circulatory collapse
   b. Bradycardia
   c. Air seen mixed with blood from umbilical arterial catheter

E. Diagnosis and management
   1. Preliminary diagnosis by transillumination using fiber optic light source for a pneumothorax
   2. Definitive diagnosis by chest x-ray
      a. PIE demonstrates unilateral or bilateral hyperinflation; small, cyst-like lucencies that may be round, linear, or oval; and a uniform distribution in the affected area (**Fig. 9-2**).
      b. Pneumomediastinum may demonstrate a well-outlined thymus or a halo around the heart (**Fig. 9-3**).

FIGURE 9-2
Pulmonary Interstitial Emphysema (PIE)

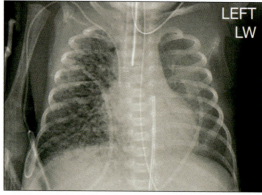

PIE on x-ray demonstrates unilateral or bilateral hyperinflation; small, cyst-like lucencies that may be round, linear, or oval; and a uniform distribution in the affected area. Onset is usually gradual. Presentation includes increased oxygen requirement and carbon dioxide retention and decreasing ability to ventilate. Selective intubation of the unaffected side may assist with reabsorption of interstitial air and effective ventilation of the unaffected lung. Gentle ventilation should be used before considering high frequency ventilation.

FIGURE 9-3
Pneumomediastinum

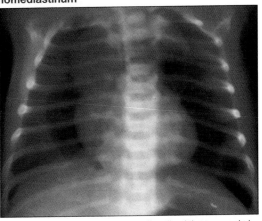

Pneumomediastinum may demonstrate a well-outlined thymus or a halo around the heart. The infant is often asymptomatic and pathophysiology is often unknown. Pneumomediastinum may cause minimal respiratory distress and usually resolves spontaneously.

FIGURE 9-4
Pneumothorax

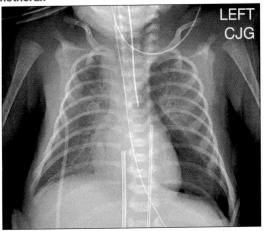

Pneumothorax demonstrates air in the pleural space along the apical or lateral margins of the hemithorax. The line shows the interface between the air in the pleural space and the collapsed lung. Pneumothorax presents with acute decompensation after CPAP or positive-pressure ventilation, a decrease or absence of breath sounds on the affected side, decreased pulse pressure, and respiratory distress. In VLBW infants, acute presentation may include bradycardia, hypotension, increased oxygen requirement, and persistent cyanosis.

c. Pneumothorax demonstrates air in the pleural space along the apical or lateral margins of the hemithorax. A line will show an interface between the air in the pleural space and the collapsed lung (**Fig. 9-4**).

d. Pneumopericardium shows air around the heart; sometimes a broad radiolucent halo completely surrounds the heart (**Fig. 9-5**).

e. Discuss x-ray of pneumoperitoneum (**Figs. 9-6A and 9-6B**).

f. Air embolism demonstrates intracardiac and intravascular air and air in the portal veins.

3. Management
   a. PIE
      (1) Consider placing affected side down for 24–48 hours.

FIGURE 9-5
Pneumopericardium

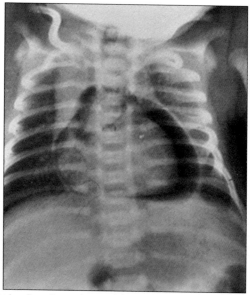

Pneumopericardium shows air around the heart. In some cases, a broad radiolucent halo completely surrounds the heart. Pneumopericardium may be asymptomatic or present with sudden cyanosis, sudden and profound hypotension, distant heart sounds, and metabolic acidosis. Treat with pericardiocentesis to prevent rapid death.

FIGURE 9-6A
Pneumoperitoneum (Anterior-Posterior View)

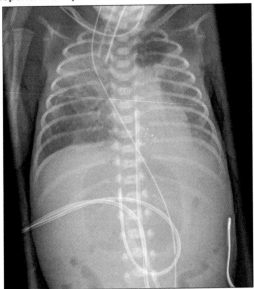

FIGURE 9-6B
Pneumoperitoneum (Left Lateral Decubitus)

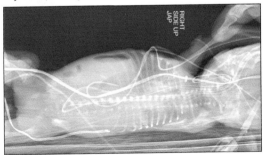

X-rays showing pneumoperitoneum require discussion. Pneumoperitoneum presents with delayed gastric emptying and emesis and with bloody stools. It may compress the inferior vena cava, decreasing blood return to the heart and causing severe acidosis. In Fig. 9-6A, air is centralized mid-abdomen. In Fig. 9-6B, air is layered above the liver. Treat with paracentesis.

    (2) Selective intubation of the unaffected side may assist with reabsorption of interstitial air and effective ventilation of the unaffected lung.
    (3) Use gentle ventilation.
    (4) Consider changing to high frequency ventilation.
  b. Pneumomediastinum
    (1) Conservative
    (2) Usually resolves spontaneously
  c. Pneumothorax
    (1) In acute presentation, after preliminary diagnosis with transillumination
    (2) Needle aspiration
    (3) Placement of chest tube with negative-pressure drainage system
    (4) Often requires intubation and ventilator support
  d. Pneumopericardium: pericardiocentesis (see Chapter 23)
  e. Pneumoperitoneum: paracentesis (see Chapter 23)
  f. Air embolism: no beneficial treatment known

IV. Pulmonary hypoplasia/agenesis

A. Overview
  1. Abnormal development of the lung
  2. May be complete agenesis of one or more lobes of one lung or abnormal development leading to pulmonary hypoplasia of one or both lungs
  3. Arrest or delay of lung development reduces branching of airways and vessels, which reduces air exchange units
  4. Failure of branching of the respiratory tree is not reversible
  5. May be associated with other congenital anomalies
B. Etiology
  1. Pulmonary hypoplasia due to primary failure of lung development or to secondary factors affecting the fetus *in utero*
  2. Affects development of both the pulmonary vasculature and alveoli
  3. May be associated with oligohydramnios from early rupture of fetal membranes, abnormal renal development, placental abnormalities, or intrauterine growth restriction
  4. Space-occupying lesions in the chest, such as diaphragmatic hernia, congenital cystic adenomatoid malformation (CCAM), or pulmonary sequestration

C. Pathophysiology
   1. Decreased amount of lung mass, abnormal pulmonary vasculature and alveoli
   2. Primary factors
      a. Intrinsic failure of the lungs to develop
      b. May be due to deficiencies in transcription factors, growth factors, or lack of receptors
   3. Secondary factors
      a. Decreased thoracic volume from space-occupying lesions in chest
         (1) Congenital diaphragmatic hernia (CDH)
         (2) Pulmonary sequestration
         (3) CCAM
         (4) Pleural effusions and fetal hydrops
      b. Decreased amniotic fluid volume
         (1) Renal dysgenesis or agenesis, other renal abnormalities
         (2) Early rupture of membranes
      c. Congenital heart disease
         (1) Associated with poor pulmonary blood flow
D. Clinical presentation
   1. Acute decomposition at birth if bilateral hypoplasia/agenesis
   2. Inadequate ventilation and oxygenation
   3. Chest radiograph may be helpful in determining degree of pulmonary expansion
E. Management
   1. Intubation and use of minimal ventilator settings to oxygenate and ventilate
   2. Gentle ventilation strategies to prevent air leak syndromes
   3. Note that with hypoplasia, minute ventilation must be maintained for adequate gas exchange, resulting in lower total tidal volumes and higher rates
   4. Use of high frequency ventilation

V. CDH
A. Etiology
   1. Failure of the diaphragm to close during embryonic development, allowing for displacement of abdominal contents such as small intestines, liver, and stomach into the chest cavity
      a. More commonly seen on left (85%) but may occur on right (13%), or, rarely, bilateral (2%)

b. Defect varies in size
2. Degree of pulmonary hypoplasia dependent on fetal age when defect occurs and size of defect on affected side
3. About 40% associated with other congenital anomalies
4. Pulmonary hypoplasia is associated with this entity but the exact etiology is not completely delineated; it is thought that abdominal organs in the chest prevent lungs from developing
5. 50%–60% diagnosed prior to birth using fetal ultrasound

B. Incidence
   1. 1:5,000 live births
   2. Termination rates ~60%–70%
   3. Fetal surgery
      a. Repositioning of the liver led to increasing fetal deaths.
      b. New surgery using endotracheal occlusion appears to prevent the loss of lung fluid and allows lung stretching and growth.
         (1) Studies report increased survival in these infants.
         (2) Complications include premature rupture of membranes in almost 50% of these pregnancies.

C. Pathophysiology
   1. Pulmonary compression by the herniated organs leads to:
      a. Pulmonary hypoplasia
      b. Abnormalities in alveoli number
      c. Abnormal and pulmonary vasculature
         (1) Thickened alveolar septum
         (2) Increased arterial wall thickness
      d. Airway muscular hyperplasia
         (1) Extension of the muscle layer in the preacinar arteries
   2. Another hypothesis is an insult in the lungs not related to the diaphragm.

D. Clinical presentation
   1. Clinical signs of respiratory distress, but small or late defects might be relatively asymptomatic
   2. Most infants have severe pulmonary hypoplasia and hypertension leading to respiratory failure with the inability to oxygenate or ventilate
   3. Scaphoid abdomen
   4. Displacement of heart sounds

E. Management
   1. For known CDH, intubate immediately, provide gentle ventilator management, and consider use of high frequency ventilator with persistent hypercapnia.
   2. With the use of gentle ventilation, surgical repair should be delayed.
   3. Severe pulmonary hypertension may require the use of inhaled nitric oxide (iNO) to regulate vascular tone.
      a. Some providers will add sildenafil for improved therapy with iNO.
   4. Placement of vented oral/nasogastric tube with low, continuous suction allows for decompression of intestinal contents in chest cavity.
   5. If conventional therapy fails, extracorporeal membrane oxygenation (ECMO) should be considered based on criteria.
F. Outcomes
   1. Survival is reported to be 60%–90% in term infants, with variability noted between institutions.
   2. Poorest outcomes are noted in premature infants, with the lowest survival for infants <29 weeks (31%), followed by those 29–32 weeks (~35%). Survival for infants >32 weeks only increases to 40%.
   3. These lower survival rates are probably related to prematurity as well as the CDH, in addition to the inability to use ECMO in these patients.
   4. Overall survival for all infants is based on the severity of pulmonary hypoplasia and hypertension, and is often center-specific due to differences in management styles.
   5. Infants with additional abnormalities have the lowest survival rates.

VI. Choanal atresia
A. Overview
   1. Etiology unknown
   2. Abnormal soft tissue, membrane, or bony tissue blocks the back of the nasal passage, known as the choana
   3. Occurs during fetal development, when membrane that separates nose and mouth fails to rupture
   4. May be unilateral or bilateral
B. Pathophysiology
   1. Infants are obligate nose breathers for the first 4–6 weeks of life.

2. Blockage of the airway prevents infants from breathing through the nose.
C. Clinical presentation
   1. Acute presentation of respiratory distress with bilateral atresia, relieved by infant crying
   2. Unilateral atresia generally not diagnosed by respiratory distress
   3. Inability to pass nasogastric tube down the nares
D. Management
   1. If bilateral, intubation and ventilator support required prior to surgical intervention
   2. Surgical intervention also for unilateral obstruction
   3. May not be evident until infant is extubated or there is failure to pass an oral gastric tube through one of the nares
   4. Oral airway

VII. Pierre Robin syndrome
A. Overview
   1. Congenital disorder (facial abnormality)
   2. Associated with other anomalies
      a. Mandibular deficiency (micronathia or small jaw)
      b. Presence of U-shaped or V-shaped cleft palate
      c. Airway obstruction due to backwards displacement of the tongue
   3. Severity of symptoms may vary
   4. May occur as isolated defect, part of a recognized syndrome, or part of a complex of multiple congenital anomalies
   5. Diagnosis of possible syndrome often critically important for correct management of newborn with Robin sequence
B. Etiology
   1. Blockage of nasal passages as seen with choanal atresia, may be unilateral or bilateral
   2. Three essential components:
      a. Micrognathia/retrognathia
      b. Cleft palate
      c. Relative glossoptosis
   3. Airway distress common immediately after delivery, due to micrognathia and relative glossoptosis
C. Pathophysiology
   1. May be associated with other congenital anomalies, including CHARGE syndrome

2. Cleft palate (usually U-shaped, but V-shape also possible)
3. Glossoptosis, often accompanied by airway obstruction
   a. Tongue not actually larger than normal, but because of small mandible, is large for airway and causes obstruction
   b. Rarely, tongue is smaller than normal
D. Clinical presentation
   1. Generally appears after extubation, ranging from cyanosis to severe asphyxia with bottle- or breast-feeding
   2. Should be suspected with micrognathia
E. Management
   1. In VLBW infants, intubation and surfactant administration due to concurrent RDS
   2. Infant should not be positioned on back to prevent airway obstruction from the tongue falling back
   3. Placement of nasopharyngeal airway or tube to maintain patency of airway
   4. Mandibular distraction surgery done at later date

VIII. Abdominal distension: Elevation of diaphragm due to increased intra-abdominal pressure

A. Etiology may be due to:
   1. Abdominal mass, including renal tumors
   2. Ascites due to hydrops or other etiologies
   3. Liver or intestinal mass
   4. Massive intestinal dilation due to obstruction or severe ileus
B. Pathophysiology
   1. Difficulty in providing adequate lung expansion due to abdominal distension
   2. Persistent hypoventilation and hypoxia in spite of adequate positive-pressure ventilation
C. Clinical presentation
   1. Severe abdominal distension
   2. Inability to ventilate and oxygenate infant
D. Management
   1. Intubation with positive-pressure ventilation (might require high airway pressures)
   2. Paracentesis with suspected abdominal ascites
   3. Follow-up abdominal ultrasound to determine defect

References

Bancalari E, *The Newborn Lung: Neonatology Questions and Controversies*. 2nd ed. Philadelphia, PA: Elsevier Saunders; 2012.

Cloherty JP, Eichenwald EC, Hansen AR, Stark AR. *Manual of Neonatal Care*. 7th ed. Philadelphia, PA: Wolters Kluwer Health/Lippincott Williams & Wilkins; 2012.

Cole A, Lynch P, Slator R. A new grading of Pierre Robin sequence. *Cleft Palate Craniofac J*. 2008;45(6):603-606.

MacDonald MG, Mullett MD, Seshia MMK, eds. *Avery's Neonatology: Pathophysiology and Management of the Newborn*. 6th ed. Philadelphia, PA: Lippincott Williams & Wilkins; 2005.

Martin RJ, Fanaroff AA, Walsh MC. *Fanaroff and Martin's Neonatal-Perinatal Medicine: Diseases of the Fetus and Infant*. 9th ed. St. Louis, MO: Mosby Elsevier; 2011.

Olasoji HO, Ambe PJ, Adesina OA. Pierre Robin syndrome: an update. *Niger Postgrad Med J*. 2007;14(2):140-145.

Polin RA, Fox WW, Abman SH, eds. *Fetal and Neonatal Physiology*. 4th ed. Philadelpia, PA: Saunders Elsevier; 2011.

Pruzansky S. Not all dwarfed mandibles are alike. *Birth Defects*. 1969;5(2):120-129.

Tsao KJ, Allison ND, Harting MT, Lally PA, Lally KP. Congenital diaphragmatic hernia in the preterm infant. *Surgery*. 2010;148(2):404-410.

Van Mieghem T, DeKoninck P, Sandaite I, et al. Congenital diaphragmatic hernia. In: Copel JA, ed. *Obstetric Imaging*. Philadelphia, PA: Saunders Elsevier; 2012:137-142.

Cardiovascular Stability and Shock

Lyn Vargo

I. **Assessment in the delivery room**
   A. Review of maternal history and specific delivery information are imperative to initial assessment of possible shock.
   B. Possible etiologies of shock in delivery room:
      1. Hypovolemic shock (acute blood loss)
         a. Fetal-maternal transfusion (acute)
         b. Abnormal umbilical cord insertion
         c. Placental abruption (primarily caused by maternal trauma)
      2. Distributive shock (vasodilation)
         a. Placental abruption
         b. Placenta previa
         c. Umbilical cord prolapse or accident
         d. Tight nuchal cord
         e. Fetal infection
      3. Cardiogenic shock
         a. Asphyxia (may also be a common pathway for several kinds of shock)
         b. Chronic fetal-maternal transfusion
         c. Twin-to-twin transfusion
         d. Arrhythmias
         e. Cardiomyopathy
         f. Congenital heart defects
   C. A clinical assessment of the infant may indicate hypovolemia and possible shock demonstrated as:
      1. Continued bradycardia without improvement in circulatory status despite adequate ventilatory management, chest compressions, and epinephrine
      2. Extreme pallor
      3. Delayed capillary refill
      4. Weak pulses
   D. Direct or indirect blood pressure (BP) measurement is generally not done in the delivery room.
      1. There is little evidence on how to determine specific BP parameters that affect long-term outcomes, morbidity, and mortality in very low birth weight (VLBW) infants.

2. Due to the unique physiology of the VLBW infant in the period immediately following delivery, management of hypotension during the first three postnatal days of life should be approached differently.
3. If possible, the etiology of the hypotension should be determined and used to guide treatment of hypotension and shock.

II. Management of hypovolemia in the delivery room

A. Volume expansion is indicated during resuscitation only when blood loss is demonstrated and the infant is not responding to resuscitation.
B. Volume must be given intravascularly, emergently via umbilical venous catheter (**Table 10-1**).
C. Isotonic crystalloid solution is recommended using either 0.9% NaCl (normal saline) or Ringer's lactate.
    1. Recommended dose at 10 mL/kg
    2. Type O, Rh-negative paced red blood cells (RBCs) should be considered with severe fetal anemia
D. Rate of volume expander administration is very important; rapid administration may increase the risk of intraventricular hemorrhage in premature infants.
E. Administer volume expander over at least 5–10 min (in code situation).
    1. If possible, administration should be over 20–30 min, especially in VLBW infants.

TABLE 10-1
Recommended Volume Expanders in the Delivery Room

Volume Expander	Dosage	Repeat	Notes
0.9% NaCl	10 mL/kg	Once	Give over at least 5–10 min or slower if possible
Ringers lactate	10 mL/kg	Once	Give over at least 5–10 min or slower if possible
Blood – maternal crossmatch	10 mL/kg	Once	Use judiciously in infants with *in utero* anemia; rapid administration may cause heart failure
Blood – type O, Rh-negative	10 mL/kg	Once	Use judiciously in infants with *in utero* anemia; rapid administration may cause heart failure

Note: In critically unstable infants with evidence of large blood loss, additional volume may be considered.

2. Rapid administration rates might increase the risk of complications such as altered cerebral blood flow and central nervous system injury.
F. Rate may need to be accelerated in urgent, unstable situations where volume loss is preventing effective resuscitation.

III. Assessment in the NICU
A. BP should be evaluated immediately upon admission to the NICU and thereafter as determined by status of infant and unit protocol.
B. Many VLBW infants require continuous BP monitoring.
 1. Oscillometer measurement
   a. If the infant is stable, BP may be monitored noninvasively via an oscillometer placed on an extremity.
   b. Accurate measurement with an oscillometer requires an appropriately sized cuff.
   c. The cuff should be 25%–55% wider than the diameter of the limb being measured.
   d. The inflatable bladder should encircle the extremity being measured without overlapping.
 2. Umbilical artery catheter measurement
   a. If the infant is not stable, an umbilical artery catheter provides more accurate readings.
   b. The catheter tip must be placed in the thoracic aorta (T6–T9) or the distal aorta (L3–L4), or a peripheral artery catheter should be placed.
   c. The transducer must be positioned at the level opening of the catheter and zeroed correctly.
   d. If the catheter is too small, systolic readings may be low; this measurement error is an important consideration in VLBW infants.
   e. Damping caused by air bubbles and clots in the system may decrease systolic readings and increase diastolic readings.
C. Hypotension
 1. Hypotension indicates that auto-regulation of blood flow to vital organs may be compromised — there is lack of agreement on a numerical value or definition in the VLBW infant.
   a. The most common definition for hypotension in the early postnatal days is mean BP ≤ the infant's gestational age in weeks.

b. Others define hypotension as a mean arterial pressure of <30 mmHg in postnatal days 1–2.
c. Clinicians should be aware that these are at least somewhat arbitrary conventions on the first day of life and the condition of the infant should be included in any evaluation of hypotension.
d. It is important to note that most VLBW infants >23–26 weeks gestation have a mean arterial pressure of >30 mmHg by postnatal day three.

2. To understand hypotension, one must look beyond BP value.
   a. End-organ perfusion, systemic blood flow, and tissue oxygenation in individual patients are among the many other variables that need to be considered, though are difficult to assess (see Section III.C.1).
   b. Additional studies are needed to elucidate appropriate postnatal hemodynamic assessment and management in VLBW infants.

3. Parameters that may provide nonspecific guidelines include:
   a. Decreased urine output may indicate circulatory compromise, but this may not be reflected in the first 24 hours of life. Low urine output generally occurs in VLBW infants in postnatal day one.
   b. Presence of metabolic acidosis (assessed by measurements of bicarbonate, lactate, and anion gap) may indicate circulatory compromise, but lactic acidosis must be differentiated from bicarbonate wasting in the VLBW infant.
   c. Capillary refill time (measured by blanching one area of the skin and measuring the time required for baseline color to return to that area) may be helpful if BP is <30 mmHg and capillary refill time is ≥3 sec in VLBW infants; may be altered in presence of pressors.
   d. A definitive increase in heart rate (from a clearly established baseline) may be useful in an infant with marginal BP values. However, be aware that many factors may affect heart rate beside circulatory compromise.

4. Although not widely practical or available at this time, functional echocardiography, near infrared spectroscopy (NIRS), and cerebral-function monitoring with amplitude-integrated EEG are all being investigated as tools to better understand acceptable cardiac parameters in VLBW infants.

IV. Assessment of shock

A. Definition: A state in which oxygen supply to the tissues does not meet the oxygen demand of the tissues
B. Three phases of shock
 1. Compensated phase: Blood flow and oxygen delivery to vital organs, such as the heart, brain, and adrenal glands, are maintained at the expense of blood flow and oxygen delivery to non-vital organs.
    a. BP is maintained.
    b. Heart rate increases.
    c. Myocardial contractility increases.
    d. Stroke volume decreases.
    e. Central venous pressure decreases.
    f. Urine output decreases.
    g. Extremities feel cool.
    h. Capillary refill is delayed.
 2. Uncompensated phase: Compensatory mechanisms begin to fail.
    a. BP decreases.
    b. Stroke volume decreases.
    c. Myocardial contractility decreases.
    d. Organ (vital and non-vital) perfusion decreases.
    e. Lactic acidosis develops.
 3. Ischemic or irreversible phase: Tissue damage and death occur.
C. Assessing phases of shock in the VLBW infant
 1. It is not possible to determine the phases of shock by BP alone; as discussed in Section IV.B, a host of factors need to be considered, including urine output, metabolic acidosis, capillary refill time, and heart rate.
 2. Shock is not generally recognized in the compensatory phase because BP and other measures appear normal.
 3. Shock is usually identified in the uncompensated phase.
 4. Failure to recognize and intervene during uncompensated shock can result in progression to irreversible shock, organ damage, and death.

5. If effective treatment in the uncompensated phase is not initiated, cellular function and integrity are compromised and shock may progress to the irreversible phase.
6. The BP parameters that define hypotension during each of the phases of shock are not known.

V. Agents to treat hypotension and shock: The known or suspected cause of hypotension should assist in making a decision for treatment (Table 10-2)

A. Volume
1. Volume — normal saline, lactated ringers, or blood products — may be used to treat hypotension caused by hypovolemia; note that significant anemia might require emergent transfusion of packed RBCs.
2. See **Table 10-1** for information on volume administration in the delivery room.
3. Assuming euvolemia, volume is less effective than inotropes in increasing BP.

TABLE 10-2
Treatment of Hypotension

Cause of Hypotension	Volume	Dopamine	Dobutamine	Epinephrine	Hydrocortisone
Acute blood loss or hypovolemia	1st choice (blood may be preferred)	Consider if volume correction doesn't work			
Myocardial dysfunction		Add if dobutamine is not effective alone	1st choice	If both dobutamine and dopamine do not work in combination, discontinue dopamine and add epinephrine	
Chorioamnionitis or sepsis/sudden inflammatory response syndrome (SIRS)		1st choice		Consider 2nd if dopamine doesn't work	If refractory hypotension, consider low dose (obtain baseline serum cortisol)
Unknown		1st choice	Add as 2nd choice	If adding dobutamine is ineffective, consider switching to epinephrine	If refractory hypotension, consider low dose (obtain baseline serum cortisol)

4. Albumin is not generally recommended if volume is needed for the initial treatment of hypotension — it is less readily available (resulting in delays in treatment), may increase risk of infection, and costs more than normal saline.
5. If volume is used for the initial treatment of hypotension post delivery room, begin with one dose of 10–20 mL/kg of normal saline over 30–60 min.
6. Excessive use of volume beyond the above amount should be avoided.

B. Dopamine
1. An endogenous catecholamine, dopamine is the most common sympathomimetic amine use to treat hypotension.
2. It is a precursor to epinephrine and norepinephrine.
3. It stimulates the alpha- and beta-adrenergic and dopaminergic receptors.
4. At low doses, it increases myocardial contractility, but at high doses (>10 mcg/kg/min), peripheral vasoconstriction and increased afterload play a primary role in increasing BP.
5. When the cause of hypotension is not known, dopamine is an effective method to increase systolic and mean BP and does not appear to be associated with adverse effects.
6. Dopamine is more effective than dobutamine, hydrocortisone, or colloid in increasing BP.
7. Most infants respond to dopamine at a dose of ≤20 mcg/kg/min, the majority responding to ≤10 mcg/kg/min.
8. Dopamine should be increased in cautious stepwise increases. It is not necessary to wait more than 3–5 min when titrating the drug, as long as the pump has been set up correctly and appropriate line priming has occurred.

C. Dobutamine
1. Dobutamine is a synthetic inotropic sympathomimetic amine.
2. Dobutamine increases myocardial contractility by stimulating myocardial adrenergic receptors. It also has a variable degree of peripheral vasodilatory effect via stimulation of cardiac beta-adrenergic receptors.
3. The vasodilatory and peripheral effect of dobutamine make it a good drug for treating hypotension related to low cardiac output and myocardial insufficiency in the VLBW infant during the first postnatal day of life.

4. During the first postnatal day of life, when there is a sudden increase in peripheral vascular resistance at birth caused by removal of the low-resistance placenta, dobutamine may increase cardiac output by creating systemic vasodilation and improving low systemic blood flow.
5. Low-dose dopamine can be added to dobutamine if BP decreases with the use of dobutamine.
6. Response to dobutamine has been demonstrated with doses as low as 5 mcg/kg/min. Dobutamine will also increase systemic blood flow and cardiac output at doses of 10–20 mcg/kg/min.
7. Dobutamine should be increased in cautious stepwise increases. It is not necessary to wait more than 3–5 min when titrating the drug, as long as the pump has been set up correctly and appropriate line priming has occurred.

D. Epinephrine
1. Epinephrine is an endogenous catecholamine, which is secreted by the adrenal gland in response to stress.
2. Epinephrine has strong beta-adrenergic effects and slightly weaker alpha-adrenergic effects.
3. Epinephrine increases BP and tissue perfusion by increasing systemic vascular resistance and increasing cardiac output.
4. There is little evidence present for any known association between the use of epinephrine in VLBW infants and adverse outcomes.
5. Epinephrine is a more potent vasoconstrictor than dopamine; therefore, it should be increased with cautious stepwise increases only.
6. At higher doses, epinephrine's vasoconstrictive effects may be especially helpful when treating hypotension and shock related to sepsis, characterized by a state of vasodilation.
7. The dose range for epinephrine in newborns is generally between 0.05 and 2.6 mcg/kg/min.

E. Corticosteroids
1. Hypotension with vasopressor resistance and dependence is often associated with relative adrenal insufficiency in the VLBW infant.
2. Some hypotension in VLBW infants may be related to down-regulation of cardiovascular adrenergic receptors. Corticosteroids may also increase BP in some infants by up-regulation of these receptors.

3. Hydrocortisone may be as effective as dopamine in increasing BP related to relative adrenal insufficiency and down-regulation of cardiovascular receptors. However, long-term safety data is not known.
4. Short-term use of hydrocortisone for refractory or vasopressor-resistant hypotension is not associated with adverse consequences; long-term safety data is not known.
5. Hydrocortisone should not be used with indomethacin. There is an increase in spontaneous ileal perforations with the use of these drugs concurrently.
6. Doses of hydrocortisone as low as 1 mg/kg/day have been demonstrated to increase BP; some studies have used doses as high as 2–3 mg/kg/day.
7. Dexamethasone is not recommended for treatment of hypotension due to adverse neurodevelopmental outcomes.

F. Milrinone
1. Milrinone inhibits phosphodiesterase-III. Its use increases cyclic adenosine monophosphate concentration, which potentiates the access of calcium to myocardial contractile tissue.
2. Milrinone is a positive inotrope and has a vasodilatory effect through the inhibition of phosphodiesterase-III.
3. It is unknown at this time whether milrinone has this effect in VLBW infants during the first 24 hours of life, when it is useful for the myocardial insufficiency seen in these infants.
4. At present, there is little evidence to support the use of milrinone in this population.

VI. Other considerations for treatment

A. Infants with patent ductus arteriosus (PDA) often have hypotension due to low diastolic BP.
B. Use volume expansion with caution in these infants; it may increase symptoms associated with a significant PDA.
C. Rather than volume or vasopressors, treatment of the PDA itself is recommended to manage hypotension.

References

Cayabyab R, McLean CW, Seri I. Definition of hypotension and assessment of hemodynamics in the preterm neonate. *J Perinatol.* 2009;29(suppl 2):S58-S62.

Engle WD. Definition of normal blood pressure range: the elusive target. In: Kleinman CS, Seri I, eds. *Hemodynamics and Cardiology: Neonatology Questions and Controversies.* 2nd ed. Philadelphia, PA: Saunders Elsevier; 2012:49-77.

Fernandez EF, Cole CH. The preterm neonate with cardiovascular and adrenal insufficiency. In: Kleinman CS, Seri I, eds. *Hemodynamics and Cardiology: Neonatology Questions and Controversies.* 2nd ed. Philadelphia, PA: Saunders Elsevier; 2012:293-309.

Heckmann M, Trotter A, Pohlandt F, Lindner W. Epinephrine treatment of hypotension in very low birth weight infants. *Acta Paediatr.* 2002;91(5):566-570.

Higgins S, Friedlich P, Seri I. Hydrocortisone for hypotension and vasopressor dependence in preterm infants: a meta-analysis. *J Perinatol.* 2010;30(6):373-378.

Ibrahim H, Sinha IP, Subhedar NV. Corticosteroids for treating hypotension in preterm infants. *Cochrane Database of Systematic Reviews* 2011, Issue 12. Art. No. CD003662. DOI: 10.1002/14651858.CD003662.pub4.

Kluckow M, Seri I. Clinical presentation of neonatal shock: the very low birth weight neonate during the first postnatal day. In: Kleinman CS, Seri I, eds. *Hemodynamics and Cardiology: Neonatology Questions and Controversies.* 2nd ed. Philadelphia, PA: Saunders Elsevier; 2012:237-267.

McLean CW, Cayabyab RG, Noori S, Seri I. Cerebral circulation and hypotension in the premature infant: diagnosis and treatment. In: Perlman JM, Polin RA, eds. *Neurology: Neonatology Questions and Controversies.* Philadelphia, PA: Saunders Elsevier; 2008:3-26.

Osborn DA, Evans N, Kluckow M. Clinical detection of upper body flow in very premature infants using blood pressure, capillary refill time, and central-peripheral temperature difference. *Arch Dis Child Fetal Neonatal Ed.* 2004;89(2):F168-F173.

Park MK. *Pediatric Cardiology for Practitioners.* 5th ed. Philadelphia, PA: Mosby Elsevier; 2008:9-39.

Sassino-Higgins S, Friedlich P, Seri I. A meta-analysis of dopamine use in hypotensive preterm infants: blood pressure and cerebral hemodynamics. *J Perinatol.* 2011;31(10):647-655.

Soleymani S, Borzage M, Seri I. Hemodynamic monitoring in neonates: advances and challenges. *J Perinatol.* 2010;30(suppl):S38-S45.

Subhedar NV, Shaw NJ. Dopamine versus dobutamine for hypotensive preterm infants. *Cochrane Database of Systematic Reviews* 2003, Issue 3. Art. No. CD001242. DOI: 10.1002/14651858.CD001242.

Textbook of Neonatal Resuscitation. 6th ed. American Academy of Pediatrics and American Heart Association; 2011.

Vargo L, Seri I. *The Management of Hypotension in the Very-Low-Birth-Weight Infant: Guideline for Practice.* Glenview, IL: National Association of Neonatal Nurses; 2011:1-13.

11

Cardiac Emergencies
Julie R. Ross

I. Adaptation to extrauterine environment

A. Fetal circulation is characterized by low systemic vascular resistance (SVR) and high pulmonary vascular resistance (PVR) (**Fig. 11-1**).

B. *In utero* environment offers stability and protects cardiac output from alteration by external factors.

C. Transition from fetal circulation to neonatal circulation following the birth of a very low birth weight (VLBW) infant results in potential for cardiac instability; cardiac output can be negatively affected by multiple factors.
   1. Increased SVR
   2. Presence of systemic→pulmonary shunts — ductal- and atrial-level left-to-right shunting can result in up to 50% of recirculation of normal cardiac output

FIGURE 11-1
Fetal Circulation

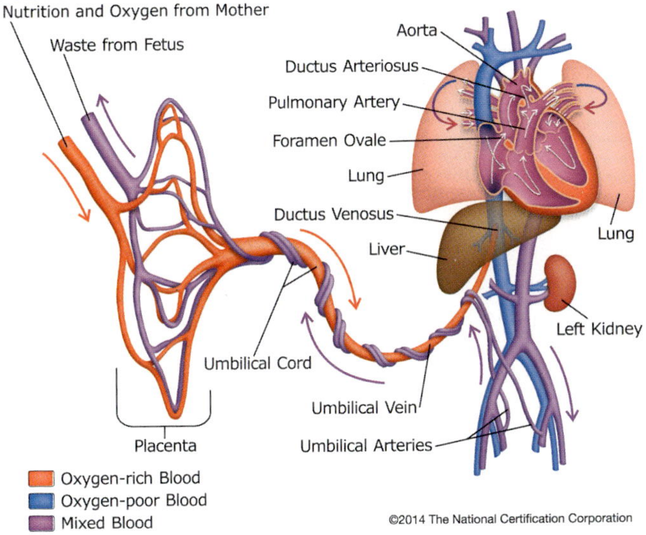

Before birth, oxygen-poor blood is carried from the fetus to the placenta via the umbilical arteries. Oxygen-rich blood returns to the fetus via the umbilical vein. Fetal circulation is characterized by low SVR and high PVR. Transition from fetal to neonatal circulation following the birth of a VLBW infant results in potential for cardiac instability.

3. Positive-pressure ventilation decreasing preload
4. Immature myocardium — fewer mitochondria and less energy stores

II. Neonatal shock
A. Pathophysiology
 1. Shock occurs when delivery of oxygen does not meet the tissue demands, resulting in energy failure.
 2. Oxygen delivery (Do_2)
    Do_2 = Cardiac output x Arterial oxygen content (CaO_2)
    Where:
    Cardiac output = Stroke volume x Heart rate (HR)
    Stroke volume determined by afterload, preload, and contractility
    CaO_2 = [1.34 x Hemoglobin (Hb) x O_2 saturations (SaO_2)] + [0.003 x Arterial partial pressure of oxygen (PaO_2)]
B. Phases of shock
 1. Compensated
    a. Vital organ function is maintained.
    b. Blood flow is redistributed to heart, brain, and adrenal glands.
    c. Key clinical signs
       (1) Blood pressure is preserved.
       (2) HR and contractility increase to maintain cardiac output.
       (3) Urine output may be decreased.
 2. Uncompensated
    a. Follows unrecognized and untreated compensated shock.
    b. Decreased blood flow to vital organs results in hypoperfusion and lactic acidosis.
 3. Irreversible
    a. Multisystem organ failure as result of cellular damage, resulting in death
C. Etiologies of shock
 1. Hypovolemia
    a. Decreased preload leads to reduction in cardiac output, resulting in hypotension and decreased tissue perfusion.
    b. Causes
       (1) Absolute hypovolemia (uncommon cause of neonatal shock)
          (a) Intrapartum fetal blood loss

        i. Placental abruption on fetal side of placenta
        ii. Acute fetomaternal hemorrhage
        iii. Tight nuchal cord
    (b) Postnatal hemorrhage
        i. Variety of causes, including birth trauma (cord avulsion, subgaleal hemorrhage) and disseminated intravascular coagulation
  (2) Relative hypovolemia
    (a) Vasodilation
    (b) Systemic inflammatory response syndrome with capillary leak; abdominal surgical conditions, sepsis
    (c) Reduced venous return secondary to mechanical ventilation and increased intrathoracic pressure

2. Myocardial dysfunction
   a. Immature myocardium in preterm neonates increases risk of dysfunction in immediate transitional period.
      (1) Limited ability to increase contractility
         (a) SVR increases following delivery, which results in increased afterload, placing strain on immature myocardium.
         (b) Leads to decreased cardiac output and hypotension.
      (2) Adaptation to postnatal hemodynamic changes occurs quickly over first 12–24 hours of life.
   b. Causes
      (1) Perinatal asphyxia
         (a) Decreased oxygen delivery to myocardium associated with perinatal depression can lead to significant myocardial dysfunction.
            i. Worsened by associated metabolic acidosis.
            ii. Cardiac enzymes can be marker of severity of insult.
      (2) Septic shock
      (3) Acquired and congenital heart disease (CHD)
         (a) Ductal-dependent structural heart defects, cardiomyopathies, and tachyarrhythmias may result in myocardial dysfunction and shock (see Section III).

3. Peripheral vasodilation
   a. Relaxation of peripheral vasculature resulting in decreased blood pressure, low cardiac output, and decreased venous return, resulting in shock
   b. Causes
      (1) Sepsis
         (a) Inflammatory cytokines are stimulated, which results in vasodilation and resulting hypotension.
      (2) Other causes of increased systemic inflammatory response syndrome
         (a) Maternal chorioamnionitis
         (b) Respiratory distress syndrome (RDS)
         (c) Asphyxia
         (d) Major surgery

D. Treatment
   1. Volume expanders (only if known blood loss)
      a. Blood transfusion preferable, although isotonic solutions may be used if blood is unavailable.
      b. Limit fluid resuscitation in shock secondary to myocardial dysfunction and peripheral vasodilation.
   2. Inotrope therapy
      a. Dopamine
         (1) Endogenous catecholamine that stimulates dopaminergic and α- and β-adrenergic receptors
            (a) Increased heart rate and contractility via β-adrenergic and dopaminergic receptors
            (b) Peripheral vasoconstriction via α-adrenergic receptors at higher doses
            (c) Increased renal blood flow at low doses secondary to renal dopaminergic receptors
         (2) Indications
            (a) Shock related to peripheral vasodilation (e.g., sepsis)
            (b) Myocardial dysfunction and cardiogenic shock
         (3) Dose
            (a) Typical starting dose for blood pressure response is 5 mcg/kg/min.
            (b) May be increased up to 20 mcg/kg/min.
         (4) Side effects
            (a) Tachycardia
            (b) May become less effective with prolonged use

b. Dobutamine
    (1) Synthetic catecholamine that exerts its effects with mainly β-adrenergic stimulation
      (a) Increased contractility and HR
      (b) No vasoconstriction/increase SVR
    (2) Indications
      (a) Ideal for myocardial dysfunction/cardiogenic shock
      (b) Less effective for shock secondary to vasodilation due to no vasoconstrictive properties
    (3) Dose: 2–20 mcg/kg/min
    (4) Side effects
      (a) Tachycardia (less than with dopamine)
      (b) Decrease in SVR; may result in decreased coronary perfusion
3. Systemic steroid therapy
  a. Hydrocortisone therapy has been shown to be effective in vasopressor-resistant hypotension.
    (1) Relative adrenal insufficiency may occur in critically ill VLBW neonates.
    (2) Glucocorticoids aid in reducing desensitization to catecholamines.
    (3) Increase in blood pressure may occur as soon as 2 hours after first dose with decreasing pressor requirement by 8–12 hours after first dose.
  b. Dose: 1mg/kg/dose three times a day has been shown to increase blood pressure and decrease vasopressor requirement.
  c. Side effects:
    (1) Spontaneous gastrointestinal perforation if given in conjunction with indomethacin
    (2) Transient hyperglycemia

III. CHD
A. Incidence
  1. Overall incidence is ~8 in 1,000 live births.
  2. Serious CHD (requiring surgery or catheterization in first year of life) is 2.4 in 1,000 live births.
  3. Increased incidence in VLBW infants, at 8.9 in 1000 live births; mortality rate is increased in preterm population.
  4. Increased incidence may be related to increased risk of preterm birth, intrauterine growth restriction, and associated extracardiac malformations.

B. Evaluation
   1. History
      a. If not diagnosed prenatally, birth history is typically unremarkable.
      b. Family history of CHD in siblings or parents increases the risk to the fetus.
   2. Physical examination
      a. Vital signs
         (1) Four extremity blood pressures; lower extremity less than upper extremity increases suspicion for coarctation of aorta
         (2) Pre-ductal and post-ductal oxygen saturations
            (a) Differential cyanosis
               i. Post-ductal saturations lower than pre-ductal saturations indicate R→L shunting at patent ductus arteriosus (PDA) with increased PVR
               ii. Critical coarctation with increased PVR
               iii. Etiology may also be non-cardiac (e.g., pulmonary hypertension, severe lung disease, pneumothorax)
            (b) Reverse differential cyanosis
               i. Pre-ductal saturations lower than post-ductal saturations
               ii. Transposition of great arteries (TGA) with intact ventricular septum, PDA, and either pulmonary hypertension, interrupted aortic arch, or coarctation of aorta
      b. Inspection
         (1) Level of distress
         (2) Presence/absence of cyanosis
         (3) Dysmorphic features present
         (4) Respiratory pattern often a comfortable tachypnea; however, in preterm infants, may be complicated by presence of RDS
      c. Palpation
         (1) Femoral and brachial pulses
         (2) Capillary refill/perfusion assessment
         (3) Presence of hyperdynamic precordium
         (4) Palpation for hepatomegaly (right-sided failure), location of liver
      d. Auscultation

(1) Evaluation of second heart sound (S2); single S2 suggestive of absence or malpositioning of aortic/pulmonary valves
(2) Location of heart sounds; displacement to right side of chest sign of CHD
(3) Murmurs
    (a) Location
    (b) Many serious defects may not present with a murmur
    (c) Harsh murmurs more indicative of pathologic process
   3. Diagnostic evaluation
      a. Oxygen challenge (hyperoxia) test
         (1) Measure PaO_2 levels before and after providing 100% oxygen for minimum of 5 min.
            (a) PaO_2 <100 mmHg in absence of severe lung disease increases likelihood of CHD.
            (b) PaO_2 of 100–200 mmHg may indicate complete mixing defect.
            (c) PaO_2 >250 mmHg indicates CHD unlikely.
      b. Chest x-ray: Evaluate heart size and shape, positioning, border contours, pulmonary vascular markings, presence of thymic shadow
      c. EKG
      d. Echocardiography/cardiology consultation
C. Categories of structural heart defects
   1. Cyanotic heart disease
      a. TGA
         (1) Pathophysiology: Aorta arises from right ventricle and pulmonary artery arises from left ventricle, resulting in parallel circulations.
         (2) Clinical presentation: Severe cyanosis, murmurs are rare, loud single S2.
         (3) Chest x-ray: Normal heart size, "egg-on-a-string" appearance.
         (4) Management: Prostaglandin infusion should be started immediately if suspected.
      b. Tetralogy of Fallot (**Fig. 11-2**)
         (1) Pathophysiology: ventricular septal defect (VSD), right ventricular outflow tract (RVOT) obstruction, overriding aorta, right ventricular hypertrophy
         (2) Clinical presentation

(a) Possible cyanosis
    i. Pink Tetralogy of Fallot: Mild RVOT obstruction results in normal saturations early in life.
    ii. Blue Tetralogy of Fallot: Severe RVOT obstruction results in early cyanosis.
(b) Systolic murmur
(c) Single, loud S2 (anterior aorta)
(d) TET spell
    i. Occurs at times of agitation, crying, stooling.
    ii. Increased PVR and decreased SVR leads to increased R→L shunt, decreased pulmonary blood flow, and resulting desaturations, cyanosis, acidosis.
(3) Chest x-ray
    (a) Pulmonary vascular markings decreased with worsening obstruction.
    (b) Later in life, may have "boot-shaped" heart.
(4) Management
    (a) TET spell
        i. Knee-chest position
        ii. Morphine
        iii. Isotonic fluid bolus
    (b) Prostaglandins may be required if severe outflow tract obstruction.

FIGURE 11-2
Tetralogy of Fallot

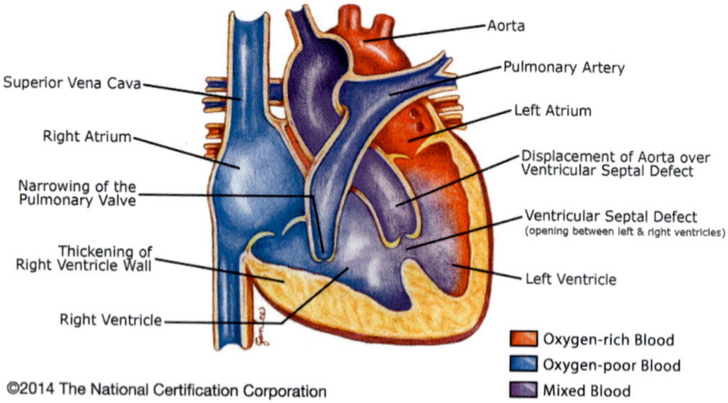

©2014 The National Certification Corporation

Combination of four abnormalities that results in oxygen-poor blood to flow out of the heart and into the body.

c. Pulmonary atresia with intact ventricular septum
   (1) Pathophysiology
      (a) Abnormal pulmonary valve when leaflets do not form or fuse.
      (b) Results in hypoplastic right ventricle with hypertrophied wall; pulmonary arteries are typically normally formed.
      (c) May have right ventricular-dependent coronary circulation due to high right ventricular pressures.
      (d) Requires the presence of R→L communication — atrial septal defect (ASD), patent foramen ovale (PFO), and PDA — to survive.
   (2) Clinical presentation
      (a) Severe cyanosis at birth
      (b) Single S2, murmur uncommon
   (3) Chest x-ray: Decreased pulmonary vascular markings
   (4) Management
      (a) Prostaglandins immediately to maintain ductal patency
      (b) Requires further evaluation of coronary anatomy prior to surgical repair
d. Truncus arteriosus (**Fig. 11-3**)
   (1) Pathophysiology
      (a) Single arterial vessel gives rise to systemic, pulmonary, and coronary circulation.

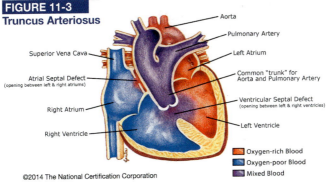

FIGURE 11-3
Truncus Arteriosus

©2014 The National Certification Corporation

A single arterial vessel gives rise to systemic, pulmonary, and coronary circulation. A large VSD allows oxygen-rich and oxygen-poor blood to mix and circulate throughout the body. Increased pulmonary over-circulation results in signs of congestive heart failure (CHF).

(b) Complete mixing lesion with large VSD present.
(c) Associated with DiGeorge syndrome.
(d) May have associated right-sided aortic arch or interrupted aortic arch.
  (2) Clinical presentation
    (a) Cyanosis may be mild initially
    (b) Increased pulmonary over-circulation as PVR, resulting in signs of congestive heart failure (CHF)
    (c) Single S2 with pansystolic murmur
    (d) Widened pulse pressure and bounding pulses
  (3) Chest x-ray: cardiomegaly, increased pulmonary vascular markings, with or without right-sided aortic arch
  (4) Management of CHF
e. Tricuspid atresia (**Fig. 11-4**)
  (1) Pathophysiology
    (a) Complete absence of tricuspid valve
    (b) Most with VSD; absent or very small VSD leads to poor prognosis due to underdeveloped right ventricle and pulmonary artery
    (c) May be associated with TGA and pulmonary atresia
  (2) Clinical presentation
    (a) Cyanosis at birth

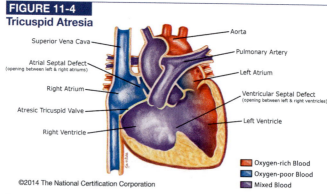

FIGURE 11-4
Tricuspid Atresia

©2014 The National Certification Corporation

Complete absence of tricuspid valve usually combined with a large VSD. If severe, infant will present with significant cyanosis at birth and may have respiratory failure secondary to pulmonary hypoplasia from large right heart *in utero*.

            (b) Holosystolic murmur from VSD
        (3) Chest x-ray
            (a) Variable pulmonary vascular markings
        (4) Management
            (a) Prostaglandins to maintain ductal patency
            (b) May require atrial septostomy
    f. Ebstein's anomaly or tricuspid valve
        (1) Pathophysiology
            (a) Dysplasia of tricuspid valve with downward displacement of septal and posterior leaflets
            (b) Tricuspid regurgitation and resulting right atrial enlargement
            (c) Associated with increased risk of Wolf-Parkinson-White syndrome
        (2) Clinical presentation
            (a) If severe, significant cyanosis at birth
            (b) May have respiratory failure secondary to pulmonary hypoplasia from large right heart *in utero*
            (c) Hepatosplenomegaly
        (3) Chest x-ray
            (a) Characteristic severe cardiomegaly (dilated right atrium)
            (b) Decreased pulmonary vascular markings
        (4) Management
            (a) Prostaglandins may be started to increase pulmonary blood flow.
            (b) Treat CHF.
    g. Total anomalous pulmonary venous return (TAPVR) (**Fig. 11-5**)
        (1) Pathophysiology
            (a) All pulmonary veins do not return to left atrium but return to a systemic vein, right atrium, right ventricle, or pulmonary artery; results in significant pulmonary over-circulation and right heart volume overload
            (b) Types
                i. Supracardiac (most common)
                ii. Cardiac
                iii. Infracardiac
                iv. Mixed
        (2) Clinical presentation: Varies dependent on degree of obstruction

(a) Unobstructed
  i. Minimal symptoms at birth that progress to right heart failure as right ventricular overload worsens
  ii. Typically supracardiac and cardiac
  iii. Wide split S2, systolic murmur
  iv. Mild-moderate cyanosis
(b) Obstructed
  i. Typically infracardiac
  ii. Cyanosis, pulmonary edema
  iii. Decreased systemic perfusion
  iv. No murmur
  v. Loud S2
(3) Chest x-ray
  (a) Unobstructed
    i. May have cardiomegaly
    ii. "Snowman" appearance if supracardiac
    iii. Pulmonary vascular markings increased
  (b) Obstructed: Significant pulmonary vascular markings/pulmonary congestion with similar appearance to interstitial pneumonia
(4) Management
  (a) Treat CHF.
  (b) Prostaglandins may worsen condition in obstructed TAPVR by increasing pulmonary blood flow.

FIGURE 11-5
Total Anomalous Pulmonary Venous Return (TAPVR)

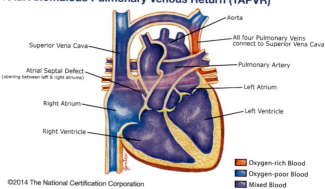

©2014 The National Certification Corporation

Pulmonary veins do not return to left atrium but return to a systemic vein, right atrium, right ventricle, or pulmonary artery. Results in significant pulmonary over-circulation and right heart volume overload.

2. Left-sided obstructive lesions
   a. Coarctation of the aorta (**Fig. 11-6**)
      (1) Pathophysiology
         (a) Narrowing of the aorta in preductal, juxtaductal, or postductal location
         (b) Preductal type presents earlier in neonatal period
         (c) Often associated with bicuspid aortic valve and may have associated hypoplasia of aortic arch and left ventricle
         (d) Increased incidence in patients with Turner syndrome
      (2) Clinical presentation
         (a) Typically asymptomatic until ductal closure; then may develop shock
            i. Hypotension, metabolic acidosis
            ii. Often present after discharge home with septic appearance
         (b) Differential cyanosis typically present
         (c) Decreased femoral pulses
         (d) Systolic murmur typically present; may have diastolic murmur if significant aortic regurgitation present
      (3) Chest x-ray: May have increasing heart size based on degree of coarctation

FIGURE 11-6
Coarctation of the Aorta

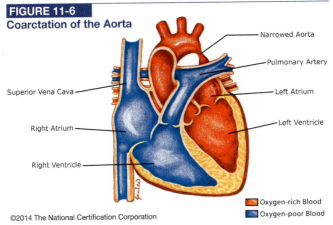

Narrowing of the aorta in the preductal, juxtaductal, or postductal location. Infants may be asymptomatic until ductal closure, but then may develop shock.

(4) Management: Initiate prostaglandins immediately to maintain ductal patency
- b. Aortic valve stenosis
  - (1) Pathophysiology
    - (a) Valvar, subvalvar (idiopathic hypertrophic subaortic stenosis)
    - (b) Supravalvar (associated with Williams syndrome)
  - (2) Clinical presentation
    - (a) Presence and severity of symptoms dependent upon degree of stenosis
    - (b) Acyanotic
    - (c) Systolic ejection murmur present at second right intercostal space and radiates upward, with or without a thrill (palpable vibrations of a loud cardiac murmur on the chest) and systolic ejection click (sound of aortic valve opening that occurs shortly following first heart sound)
    - (d) Severe aortic stenosis (AS); may develop CHF and cardiogenic shock
  - (3) Chest x-ray
    - (a) Normal to slightly increased heart size visualized on x-ray if CHF present
    - (b) May see dilation of aorta post area of stenosis
  - (4) Management
    - (a) Prostaglandins if critical AS
    - (b) Balloon valvuloplasty
- c. Hypoplastic left heart syndrome (**Fig. 11-7**)
  - (1) Pathophysiology
    - (a) Hypoplasia of left ventricle, severe stenosis/atresia of mitral and/or aortic valve, aortic arch hypoplasia (coarctation of aorta is common)
    - (b) Ductal dependent with systemic flow dependent upon L→R atrial flow
  - (2) Clinical presentation
    - (a) May be asymptomatic in immediate neonatal period in presence of PDA
    - (b) If ductus absent or atrial septum intact, immediate decompensation/cyanosis in the delivery room requires emergent intervention
    - (c) Cyanosis, CHF, metabolic acidosis, and shock occur upon closure of ductus arteriosus

(d) Single S2, with or without systolic murmur
   (3) Chest x-ray: Increased pulmonary vascular markings, cardiomegaly
   (4) Management
      (a) Administer prostaglandins immediately to maintain ductal patency.
      (b) Minimize oxygen exposure; oxygen decreases PVR and results in pulmonary over-circulation and decreased systemic blood flow.
      (c) May require atrial septostomy emergently if atrial communication is absent or restrictive.
3. Other lesions
   a. VSD
      (1) Pathophysiology: Most common CHD
      (2) Clinical presentation
         (a) Holosystolic murmur appears after PVR decreases.
         (b) Typically asymptomatic at birth.
         (c) Progression of symptoms depends on size and degree of L→R shunt.
      (3) Chest x-ray: Typically normal but may progress to signs of pulmonary edema
      (4) Management of CHF, if needed
   b. Atrioventricular canal defect
      (1) Pathophysiology

FIGURE 11-7
Hypoplastic Left Heart Syndrome

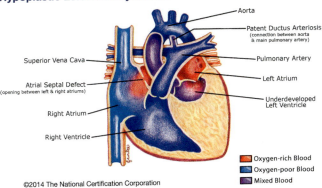

Hypoplasia of left ventricle, severe stenosis/atresia of mitral and/or aortic valve, aortic arch hypoplasia (coarctation of aorta is common).

(a) Abnormality of endocardial cushion that may be complete (common atrioventricular valve, VSD) or partial (intact ventricular septum with separate atrioventricular valves)
(b) If complete, may be balanced or unbalanced (e.g., is there equal development of both ventricles)
(c) Association with Trisomy 21
(2) Clinical presentation
(a) May have some degree of cyanosis
(b) Development of CHF
(c) Systolic murmur
(3) Chest x-ray: Increased pulmonary vascular markings and cardiomegaly
(4) Management of CHF until surgical repair
D. Special considerations
1. VLBW infants are a special population that requires increased awareness and recognition of the signs of a potential severe CHD to ensure timely diagnosis and initiation of necessary therapies.
2. Multidisciplinary care of these infants, including neonatology and pediatric cardiology, is essential.
3. Patient size, immaturity, and comorbid disease processes and complications place VLBW infants with severe CHD at greater risk of mortality (reported up to 44%).

IV. PDA (Fig. 11-8)
A. Pathophysiology
1. *In utero*
a. The ductus connects the pulmonary artery to the descending aorta and provides a pathway for blood to bypass pulmonary circulation.
b. Patency is maintained by high levels of circulating prostaglandins.
c. Increasing muscular wall formation, decreasing sensitivity to prostaglandins, and increased sensitivity to oxygen occurs late in gestation.
2. Normal ductal closure
a. In term infants, the stimulation for ductal closure begins immediately at birth.
b. Increasing arterial PaO_2 results in constriction of ductus after delivery.
c. Closure occurs in two phases:

(1) Functional closure
    (a) Occurs with constriction of the muscular wall in response to increasing oxygen concentration
    (b) Occurs in the majority of healthy term infants by 48 hours
    (c) Can still be medically reopened with prostaglandins or reopen spontaneously, as in preterm infants
(2) Anatomic/structural closure: Constriction of the muscular wall results in area of ischemia and hypoxia, which leads to necrosis

3. PDA in preterm newborns
   a. The ductus in a preterm infant often remains open for a prolonged period after birth.
   b. Decreased muscle content prevents adequate constriction.
   c. Without tight constriction, the hypoxic/ischemic triggers for additional structural closure do not occur.
   d. Delayed closure is greater in lower gestational ages and in infants with significant RDS.

B. Clinical presentation
   1. It is uncommon to have a clinically symptomatic PDA in a VLBW infant in the first three days of life.

FIGURE 11-8
Patent Ductus Arteriosus (PDA)

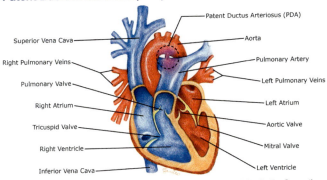

©2014 The National Certification Corporation

The ductus in a preterm infant often remains open for a prolonged period after birth. Delayed closure is greater in lower gestational age and in infants with significant RDS. Clinical findings of a significant PDA often lag 1–2 days behind echocardiographic evidence.

a. Elevated pulmonary pressures may decrease the risk of L→R shunting and pulmonary over-circulation.
b. Clinical findings of a significant PDA often lag 1–2 days behind echocardiographic evidence of significant PDA.
2. Physical examination
   a. Harsh, continuous systolic murmur
   b. Bounding peripheral pulses
   c. Persistent respiratory symptoms/ventilator dependence
3. Chest x-ray: With symptomatic PDA, may see cardiomegaly and pulmonary edema

C. Diagnosis: Echocardiogram to evaluate
   a. Patency, size, and direction of shunt
   b. Left atrial to aortic root ratio
   c. Reversal of flow in descending aorta

D. Management
   1. There is not clear evidence to guide clinicians on when a PDA is symptomatic enough to warrant treatment and there is very limited evidence that treatment has an impact on improving long-term outcomes.
   2. Pharmacologic management
      a. Indomethacin
         (1) Cyclooxygenase inhibitor — blocks prostaglandin synthesis
         (2) Risks of treatment: oliguria, gastrointestinal perforation, hyponatremia, decreased platelet aggregation, decreased intestinal perfusion
         (3) Dosing
            (a) Initial dose of indomethacin IV at 0.2 mg/kg/dose, followed by two doses based on postnatal age (PNA)
            (b) Subsequent two doses
               i. PNA at time of first dose <48 hours: 0.1 mg/kg/dose at 12- to 24-hour intervals
               ii. PNA at time of first dose 2–7 days: 0.2 mg/kg/dose at 12- to 24-hour intervals
               iii. PNA at time of first dose >7 days: 0.25 mg/kg/dose at 12- to 24-hour intervals
            (c) Monitor urine output, potassium, creatinine, platelet counts between doses
               i. Use 12-hour dosing intervals if urine output is >1 mL/kg/hour.

ii. Use 24-hour dosing intervals if urine output is <1 mL/kg/hour but >0.6 mL/kg/hour.
        (d) May repeat one additional 3-dose course if continued presence of PDA
      b. Ibuprofen
        (1) Cyclooxygenase inhibitor
        (2) Decreased effect on intestinal/renal blood flow compared to indomethacin
        (3) Treatment success similar to indomethacin
    3. Surgical ligation
      a. Typically reserved for symptomatic PDA that has failed pharmacologic treatment or treatment is contraindicated
      b. Results in definitive closure of ductus
      c. Significant risks
        (1) Thoracotomy, pneumothorax, unilateral vocal cord paralysis, chylothorax, infection, post-surgical hypotension

V. Cardiac arrhythmias
  A. Fetal arrhythmias
    1. Fetal arrhythmias occur in up to 2% of fetuses
    2. Tachyarrhythmias
      a. Supraventricular tachycardia
        (1) Most common fetal arrhythmia
        (2) HR typically 240–310 beats/min and regular
        (3) At risk for development of hydrops fetalis with prolonged tachycardia; risk of hydrops increases as gestational age decreases
        (4) Treatment
          (a) Maternal digoxin therapy is first-line treatment.
          (b) May require additional antiarrhythmic therapy or delivery preterm, based on complications.
          (c) Following delivery, monitor neonate for complications of antiarrhythmic therapy.
      b. Atrial flutter
        (1) HR typically faster than supraventricular tachycardia (SVT) (425–500 beats/min) and irregular
        (2) Less likely to develop hydrops
        (3) Treatment: Maternal digoxin or sotalol therapy most common

3. Bradycardia
    a. Complete atrioventricular block
        (1) Maternal anti-Ro (SSA) or anti-La (SSB) antibodies (antinuclear autoantibodies)
            (a) Acquired form of heart block
            (b) If complete, can lead to cardiomyopathy and hydrops
B. Neonatal arrhythmias
    1. SVT
        a. Pathophysiology
            (1) Typically a reentrant tachycardia with an accessory pathway allowing conduction to reenter the atrium.
            (2) Most of the accessory pathways will become nonfunctional as the heart matures.
            (3) Most common symptomatic arrhythmia in pediatrics.
            (4) Increased risk with CHD, medications that have cardiac stimulation (caffeine), fever, hyperthyroidism.
            (5) Central line positioning in right atrium may trigger activation of accessory pathway.
        b. Clinical presentation
            (1) Starts and stops abruptly.
            (2) Narrow QRS complex at rate of 220–330 with minimal variation.
            (3) May be stable or unstable; can develop hypotension, poor perfusion.
            (4) If prolonged, can lead to heart failure and cardiogenic shock.
        c. Diagnosis
            (1) Sudden change in heart rate to >220 on telemetry should prompt full bedside evaluation, including blood pressure assessment, capillary refill, and pulses.
            (2) EKG: Narrow QRS complex, P waves not visualized.
            (3) Evaluate central line positioning by x-ray.
        d. Management – acute
            (1) Stable SVT
                (a) Vagal maneuvers
                    i. Endotracheal tube suctioning, deep oral suctioning

ii. Ice to face should be used with caution in extreme preterm infants due to risk of hypothermia and, possibly, intraventricular hemorrhage
 (b) Adenosine
  i. 0.1 mg/kg rapid IV push followed immediately with normal saline flush
  ii. Very short half life; must reach heart to be effective
  iii. May repeat or increase dose to 0.2 mg/kg/dose
  iv. Monitor HR and blood pressure
  v. If possible, it is helpful to capture EKG immediately prior, during, and after therapy
  vi. Always have code cart at bedside and immediately available during adenosine administration
 (2) Unstable SVT
  (a) Synchronized direct-current (DC) cardioversion
  (b) 0.5 joules/kg
 e. Management – chronic
  (1) Propranolol or digoxin is often first-line therapy for chronic management.
  (2) Consultation with pediatric cardiologist should occur for management recommendations.
2. Atrial flutter
 a. Pathophysiology
  (1) Ectopic atrial reentry
  (2) Atrial rate typically 300–500
 b. Clinical presentation
  (1) Typically well tolerated
  (2) May be easily confused with SVT, although P waves typically present
 c. Diagnosis – EKG
   (a) Normal QRS and sawtooth pattern of P waves
   (b) May be difficult to recognize sawtooth pattern
 d. Management
  (1) Adenosine not therapeutic, but may reveal sawtooth pattern on EKG
  (2) Stable: antiarrhythmic therapy

- (3) Unstable: synchronized DC cardioversion or esophageal pacing
- (4) Pediatric cardiology consultation
  e. Prognosis: Unlikely to recur or require long-term medication therapy
3. Ventricular tachycardia
   a. Pathophysiology: Ventricular arrhythmia that occurs secondary to variety of etiologies, including CHD, electrolyte abnormalities (e.g., hyperkalemia), myocarditis, prolonged QT syndrome
   b. Clinical presentation: May be stable or develop signs of CHF or shock
   c. Diagnosis – EKG
      (1) Wide complex QRS
      (2) Premature ventricular beats ≥ 3
      (3) Inverted T waves
   d. Management
      (1) Stable: lidocaine therapy
      (2) Unstable: defibrillation; 1–2 joules/kg
4. Sinus tachycardia
   a. Pathophysiology: Typically secondary to fever, hypovolemia, anemia, shock, medication therapy (caffeine, dopamine)
   b. Clinical presentation
      (1) Narrow complex, rate typically <230 beats/min, P waves present
      (2) Heart rate typically rises and declines slowly (as opposed to rapid, abrupt change with SVT)
   c. Diagnosis
      (1) EKG: narrow complex, P waves present
      (2) Evaluate for potential causes
         (a) Review medication history.
         (b) Consider evaluation for anemia, sepsis, hyperthyroidism.
   d. Management: Treat underlying cause
C. Bradycardia
   1. Complete atrioventricular block
   2. Pathophysiology
      a. Acquired: Secondary to circulating maternal SSA and SSB antibodies that destroy the atrioventricular node
      b. Congenital: Associated with other congenital heart defects; very high mortality rate

c. Results in very slow ventricular rate; heart rate >55 typically well tolerated
3. Clinical presentation
   a. May be asymptomatic if ventricular rate high enough and tolerated.
   b. May present with fetal hydrops or CHF.
4. Diagnosis
   a. EKG
   b. Cardiology consultation
5. Management
   a. Initial delivery room management determined by presence/absence of hydrops
   b. Isoproterenol infusion if hemodynamic compromise
   c. Pacing at direction of cardiologist

D. Premature beats
   1. Premature atrial contractions
      a. Early P waves with altered appearance to normal sinus P waves
      b. Benign and very common in neonatal period
   2. Premature ventricular contraction
      a. Abnormal, prolonged QRS that arises without P wave preceding
      b. If isolated and asymptomatic, treatment not required
      c. Can be associated with electrolyte abnormalities, infections, acidosis, medication therapy

References

Archer JM, Yeager SB, Kenny MJ, Soll RF, Horbar JD. Distribution of and mortality from serious congenital heart disease in very low birth weight infants. *Pediatrics*. 2011;127(2) 293-299.

Brodsky D, Martin C. *Neonatology Review*. 2nd ed. Dara Brodsky; 2010:536.

Gleason CA, Devaskar S, eds. *Avery's Diseases of the Newborn*. 9th ed. Philadelphia, PA: Saunders Elsevier; 2012:1498.

Kilian K. Left sided obstructive congenital heart defects. *Newborn and Infant Nurs Rev*. 2006;6(3):128-136.

Kleinman CS, Seri I, eds. *Hemodynamics and Cardiology: Neonatology Questions and Controversies*. 2nd ed. Philadelphia, PA: Saunders Elsevier; 2012:535.

Polin RA, Fox WW, Abman SH, eds. *Fetal and Neonatal Physiology*. 4th ed. Philadelphia, PA: Saunders Elsevier; 2011.

Polin RA, Yoder MC. *Workbook in Practical Neonatology*. 4th ed. Philadelphia, PA: Saunders Elsevier; 2007:500.

12

Fluids, Electrolytes, and Nutrition

Jan Sherman

I. Introduction
A. Fluid, electrolyte, and acid-base management are essential components in the care of high-risk neonates.
B. Management of fluids and electrolytes, particularly in low birth weight and very low birth weight (VLBW) infants, present significant challenges.
C. Management styles vary from high fluid volumes to fluid restrictions, timing of electrolytes, and proteins and fats.
   1. Base fluid decisions on pathophysiology principles.
      a. Have guidelines for starting volumes and adjust for the clinical and/or environmental situation (such as humidity and incubators).

II. Definitions
A. Total body water (TBW): The total intracellular and extracellular fluids
B. Extracellular fluid: The total intravascular and interstitial fluids
C. Insensible water loss (IWL): The evaporation of water through the skin, respiratory tract, and mucous membranes
   1. The majority of IWL occurs through mucous membranes, but in extremely premature infants, the loss occurs through the skin in large amounts.
   2. IWL increases as gestational age decreases.
   3. May be described as fluid intake + urine output - weight change.

III. General principles
A. Water accounts for 75%–95% of the body weight of the infant, depending upon gestational age.
B. The progressive decrease in TBW with advancing gestational age is primarily due to decreases in the extracellular water compartment.
   1. Premature infants have greater TBW, which is primarily extracellular water. During the first days of life, the physiologic weight loss in term and premature infants represents a contraction of body fluids and is a normal transitional physiologic process.

2. For VLBW infants, weight losses of 10%–15% can be expected within the first 3–5 days of life. Term infants may have up to 10% physiological weight loss.
C. IWL occurs predominantly through evaporation of body water through the skin, mucous membranes, and respiratory tract.
   1. The immature epithelial layer of premature infants allows excessive body water evaporation. Progressive thickening of the stratum corneum and epidermis throughout the third trimester reduces IWL.
   2. Humidifying the infant's environment reduces IWL in premature infants. The heat exchange through evaporation in VLBW infants is twice as high, at 20% vs. 60% ambient humidity.
      a. Studies have demonstrated that 50%–80% humidity in VLBW infants will reduce trans-epidermal water loss (TEWL).
      b. Extremely low birth weight infants at lower gestational ages have the highest TEWL and require the most humidity.
         (1) 80% humidity has been shown to reduce TEWL from 200 g/kg/day to 50 g/kg/day, losing only 5% of birth weight.
      c. It is essential to control TEWL in these infants because it is both a source of heat loss and alters overall water balance. (**Box 12-1** gives one hospital's example of humidity guidelines.)
      d. The stratum corneum will take as long as 4–6 weeks to mature in infants born between 23 and 25 weeks.
   3. Excessive humidity may adversely impact the rate of skin barrier formation.
      a. Skin barrier formation occurs faster in infants nursed in lower relative humidity.
      b. No significant differences occurred between a group of infants nursed at a relative humidity of 75% and those nursed at a relative humidity of 50%.
D. Respiratory rate and humidification of the inspired air oxygen mix alter insensible water loss through the respiratory tract.
   1. Expired air is usually more humid than inspired air and has a higher water vapor pressure. Inspiring warm air with a high humidity will help reduce IWL, as well as promote temperature stability, by gaining heat through the respiratory tract.

BOX 12-1
Example of Humidity Guidelines

1. Have humidified incubator ready on admission.
2. Consider the use of humidified incubator care for infants 32 weeks gestation and/or 1,200 g to decrease TEWL, maintain skin integrity, decrease fluid requirements, and minimize electrolyte imbalance. Strict equipment cleaning protocols should be utilized while providing humidified air.
3. The recommended relative humidity (RH) is 75%–80% for the first seven days, decreasing to 50%–60% RH, **if possible**, during the second week until 30–32 weeks postmenstrual age.
4. The table below shows sample guidelines. Every unit should review the literature and develop guidelines appropriate for their unit.
5. Infants >1,500 g do not require humidity; use should be based on clinical assessment.
6. Continue moderate humidity for infants who remain critically ill until 34 weeks gestation.
7. Change incubator and porthole sleeves every 7 days or if visibly dirty.
8. Porthole sleeves should be used to avoid loss of humidity during patient care.
9. Portholes should be used for all primary access to maintain temperature and humidity. If door access is needed, use a boost-air curtain. Canopies should only be raised during emergencies.

Gestational Age	Initial Humidity	Time Frame	Secondary Humidity	Time Frame	Discontinue Humidity
≤28 weeks	80%	2 weeks	50%	2 weeks	32 weeks
29–30 weeks	80%	1 week	50%	2 weeks	32–33 weeks
31–34 weeks	50%	1 week	0	0	32–35 weeks

Note: Skin maturation occurs after birth; therefore, infants born at 28 weeks of gestation can tolerate removal of humidity at 32 weeks (after 4 weeks of maturation), vs. infants during the first week of life born at 32–34 weeks.

2. Estimated IWL based on birth weight is shown in **Table 12-1**.
   a. Premature infants have almost 15 times higher TEWL then term infants at birth.
3. Methods to reduce IWL are shown in **Box 12-2**.
4. Urine output should be 1–3 mL/kg/hour by the third day of life in infants with normal kidneys.
   a. A urine-specific gravity of 1.005–1.012 is consistent with a balance in TBW.
   b. Oliguria is defined as urine output <1 mL/kg/hour and may be reflective of abnormal renal function based on pre-renal, parenchymal, and post-renal etiologies.
5. Serum electrolytes and creatinine should be routinely monitored to evaluate renal function and fluid balance.
   a. Serum sodium is a useful indicator of hydration in the first few days of life.
      (1) Decreasing sodium from initial baseline (over-hydration)
      (2) Increasing sodium from initial baseline (dehydration)
   b. Serum blood urea nitrogen (BUN) reflects nutrition status and nitrogen balance and has not been found to be as useful in fluid balance.
   c. Creatinine is useful in measuring renal function, understanding that a rise in the first three days of life is normal.

TABLE 12-1

Insensible Water Loss (IWL) in a Thermal-Neutral Environment Based Upon Birth Weight

Birth Weight (g)	IWL (mL/kg/day)
<750	100+
750–1,000	60–70
1,001–1,500	30–65
>1,500	15–30

Note: Numbers are for infants in incubators during the first week of life. Losses can increase by 40% for infants under phototherapy and 50% for infants on radiant warmers. Humidification of environment and respirators will decrease IWL.

(Adapted from Martin RJ, Fanaroff AA, Walsh MC. *Fanaroff and Martin's Neonatal-Perinatal Medicine: Diseases of the Fetus and Infant.* 9th ed. St. Louis, MO: Mosby Elsevier; 2011.)

IV. Fluid and electrolyte needs

A. Careful calculation of fluid volume and electrolyte composition is very important.
   1. Excessive fluid intake may increase the risk of fluid overload and hyponatremia.
      a. Excessive fluid is also associated with patent ductus arteriosus in VLBW infants.
   2. Excessive restriction of fluids may lead to dehydration and/or hypernatremia.
      a. Loss of large volumes of fluid through the skin also leads to hypernatremia and dehydration.
   3. In premature babies, assessing changes in accurate weights best reflects fluid balance.
B. Initial fluid therapy should be aimed at allowing a normal physiologic weight loss while preventing dehydration and electrolyte imbalances.
   1. Normal diuresis occurs after delivery due to a rise in atrial natriuretic peptide and is part of extracellular fluid contraction.
   2. Infants with respiratory distress syndrome have a delay in the diuretic process, which further limits their ability to excrete sodium.
C. Maintenance fluids, deficits, and fluid losses are components of fluid and electrolyte requirements in newborns.
   1. The amount of water required to maintain a newborn in neutral water balance is referred to as maintenance fluid requirement.
   2. The total amount of maintenance fluid required is equal to urine production + insensible losses + fecal water loss (which is usually insignificant).

BOX 12-2
Methods to Reduce Insensible Water Loss (IWL)

Convectively heated, double-walled incubators
Humidified, thermal-neutral environment
Semipermeable skin coverings
Inspiring warm air with a high humidity in respiratory devices

(Adapted from Martin RJ, Fanaroff AA, Walsh MC. *Fanaroff and Martin's Neonatal-Perinatal Medicine: Diseases of the Fetus and Infant.* 9th ed. St. Louis, MO: Mosby Elsevier; 2011.)

D. The maintenance fluids required during the first week of life are displayed in **Table 12-2**. Fluids should be adjusted based upon the infant's clinical condition and any factors that may alter the fluid requirements.
   1. Infants cared for in humidified environments will have lower fluid requirements.
E. The normal glucose requirement is 6–8 mg/kg/min in preterm infants and 3–5 mg/kg/min in term infants.
   1. Preterm infants are at risk for hypoglycemia due to limited glycogen and fat stores.
      a. The human brain relies almost entirely on glucose to provide substrate for metabolism.
      b. Glucose accounts for 95% of cerebral energy supply.
      c. Although the brain can use lactate or ketones, these may not compensate completely for a decrease in glucose availability.
   2. Hypoglycemia
      a. A blood glucose concentration at which cerebral metabolism is irreversibly affected:
         (1) May lead to neuronal cell death and adverse neurodevelopmental outcomes
         (2) Cannot be measured
      b. Careful monitoring to avoid hypoglycemia (plasma glucose level <45 mg/dL is minimal "normal") and hyperglycemia (plasma level >150 mg/dL) is mandatory, with adjustment of dextrose as necessary.
         (1) Some argue that the therapeutic goal should be 60 mg/kL and some believe hypoglycemia is <50 mg/dL.
         (2) Hypoglycemia associated with asphyxia leads to worse neurologic outcomes.

TABLE 12-2
Maintenance Fluid Requirements During the First Week of Life

Birth Weight (g)	Dextrose (g/100 mL)	Day 1–2 (mL/kg/day)	Day 3–7 (mL/kg/day)
<750	5–10	100–200	120–200
750–1,000	10	80–150	100–150
1,001–1,500	10	60–100	80–150
>1,500	10	60–80	100–150

(Adapted from Martin RJ, Fanaroff AA, Walsh MC. *Fanaroff and Martin's Neonatal-Perinatal Medicine: Diseases of the Fetus and Infant.* 9th ed. St. Louis, MO: Mosby Elsevier; 2011.)

c. Potential better practice during the Golden Hours:
   (1) Maintain a "target" blood glucose at 50 mg/dL.
   (2) Respond to blood glucose levels <45 mg/dL (see **Box 12-3**).
   (3) Obtain blood glucose between 30 and 60 min after birth.
      (a) Birth glucose concentration is ~80% of maternal glucose.
      (b) It falls to its lowest nadir between 30 and 90 min after birth.
   (4) Initiate IV fluids within 30 min of birth.
3. Avoid dextrose concentrations of <D5W to minimize osmotic hemolysis.

V. Electrolyte requirements

A. Maintenance sodium and chloride should not be provided in the first 1–2 days of life.
   1. Very premature infants have increased water losses and early administration of sodium supplementation is associated with an increased risk of hypernatremia.
      a. Physiologically, this is often due to delayed diuresis with a restricted ability to excrete sodium.
   2. Sodium supplementation should be based upon serum electrolytes.
      a. Premature infants have a limited ability to excrete or retain sodium, so a fine balance must be maintained.

BOX 12-3
Suggested Response to Blood Glucose <45 mg/dL or Symptomatic Infants

• Bolus: 200 mg/kg (2 mL/kg) D10W if IV fluids have not been initiated yet and start IV fluids.
• Bolus: 200 mg/kg (2 mL/kg) D10W and increase GIR to 6–8 mg/kg/min if IV fluids are already infusing at an adequate rate and GIR.
• Monitor blood glucose every 20–30 min until stable, then every 1–2 hours (if stable), then every 4–6 hours.
• Adjust GIR to maintain blood glucose >50 mg/dL.
• Monitor blood glucose for the first 24–48 hours or until stabilized, especially those infants at risk of hypoglycemia.
• Infants who require high infusion rates or a dextrose concentration >12.5% require placement of a central venous catheter (UVC, PICC).

GIR = glucose infusion rate; PICC = peripherally inserted central catheter; UVC = umbilical venous catheter

B. Potassium should not be routinely provided in parenteral fluid until adequate urine output has been established and normal renal function is attained.

C. From postnatal days 3 to 7, maintenance sodium, potassium, and chloride requirements are ~1–2 mEq/kg/day.

VI. Early nutritional support with parenteral amino acids and intralipids is essential. Approximately 50% of extrauterine growth failure is related to protein and fat deficits.

A. Parenteral nutrition should be provided immediately after birth, if possible.
   1. Protein intakes of 3.0–3.5 g/kg/day in VLBW infants are required and must account for:
      a. Obligate protein loss (1.5–2.0 g/kg/day)
      b. Efficiency of protein retention (~80%)
      c. Achievement of protein accretion
   2. Provision of 1.0–1.5 g/kg/day of intravenous amino acids, even when total caloric intake is low, can help limit catabolism, improve protein balance, and preserve endogenous protein stores. However, these amounts are too low.
   3. Generally, the maximum intake of intravenous amino acids is 3–4 g/kg/day.
   4. The early amino acids provide an antioxidant to critically ill infants, and in addition, provide an anticoagulant function and binder for both bilirubin and free fatty acids.
   5. Urea production is a by-product of amino acid oxidation and acute amino acid. Serum BUN and pH should be monitored since azotemia, hyperammonemia, and metabolic acidosis may be evidence of protein intolerance.
      a. BUN may not be the best marker of amino acid intake because it is also influenced by hydration status, renal function, energy intake, and patient acuity.

B. Intravenous lipids are important to prevent essential fatty acid deficiency (EFAD) and also provide a significant source of non-protein energy.
   1. Failure to provide sufficient non-protein energy leads to increased lipolysis and fatty acid oxidation.
   2. Evidence of EFAD can develop in preterm infants within 72 hours.
      a. This predisposes the infant to hypoglycemia due to disruption in gluconeogenesis.

  b. Failure to provide non-protein energy leads to fatty acids being utilized for energy instead of membrane deposition in the developing brain, leading to abnormal neurodevelopmental outcomes.
3. EFAD can be avoided with a minimum of 0.5–1.0 g/kg/day of intravenous lipid initiated in the first 24 hours of life.
4. Intravenous lipids are available as 10% and 20%.
  a. Currently, the 20% lipid solutions are preferred because they result in lower cholesterol and plasma triglyceride levels.
  b. A 30% lipid solution has recently become available, which may be advantageous, but little data is available.
5. Lipid concentrations can gradually be advanced based on unit policy.
6. Intravenous fat emulsions have been shown to help maintain serum glucose levels.
7. Intravenous lipid is given as a continuous infusion over 24 hours to enhance plasma lipid clearance.
8. Decreases in oxygenation may occur with lipid infusion rates of >0.25 g/kg/hour.
9. Triglyceride concentrations are most often used as an indication of lipid tolerance and should be maintained <200 mg/dL and <150 mg/dL with hyperbilirubinemia.
10. Care should be taken when administering lipids to infants with unconjugated hyperbilirubinemia to avoid bilirubin toxicity as a result of free fatty acids displacing bilirubin from albumin binding sites.
11. Increased risks of sepsis, release of thromboxanes and prostaglandins, and increased pulmonary vascular resistance have been noted when administering lipid emulsions.

C. The appropriate balance of glucose and lipid in parenteral nutrition is critical.
1. A ratio of 60:40 carbohydrate and lipid closely mimics the content of breast milk.
2. Lipid intake should be limited to 40%–50% of total calories to avoid ketosis.

VII. Enteral nutrition

A. Enteral feedings are a controversial subject because of a concern about necrotizing enterocolitis. However, research has shown benefits of enteral intake related to maturation of the intestine, a reduction in liver dysfunction, and improved feeding tolerance without an increase in necrotizing enterocolitis.

B. Breast milk is the ideal choice for feedings, since it provides immunological and antibacterial factors, as well as other components not found in other infant food sources.

C. If mother's breast milk is not available, the American Academy of Pediatrics (AAP) recommends pasteurized donor milk. If neither mother's nor donor milk is available, premature formula is acceptable.

D. Low-volume hypo-caloric feedings, called minimal enteral or trophic feedings, do not contain sufficient calories to sustain growth, but are meant to prime the gut and to help prevent intestinal atrophy.

E. While there is not a universal definition, a typical trophic feeding volume would be 1–2 mL/kg every 2–3 hours.

F. Once the infant has stabilized clinically, feedings can be advanced based upon unit guidelines.
   1. A common strategy is to advance feedings by 10–20 mL/kg/day as tolerated.
   2. Advancement typically results in full enteral feeding (150 mL/kg/day) in 7–10 days.
   3. A slow rate of advancement is thought to decrease the risk of necrotizing enterocolitis.

G. Follow hospital policies for the implementation of parenteral and enteral nutrition.

References

Agren J, Sjörs G, Sedin G. Ambient humidity influences the rate of skin barrier maturation in extremely preterm infants. *J Pediatr*. 2006;148(5):613-617.

American Academy of Pediatrics. Breastfeeding and the use of human milk. *Pediatrics*. 2012;129(3):e827-e841. http://pediatrics.aappublications.org/content/early/2012/02/22/peds.2011-3552.full.pdf+html. February 27, 2012.

Cloherty JP, Eichenwald EC, Hansen AR, Stark AR. *Manual of Neonatal Care*. 7th ed. Philadelphia, PA: Wolters Kluwer Health/Lippincott Williams & Wilkins; 2012.

Dell KM. Fluid, electrolytes, and acid-base homeostasis. In: Martin RJ, Fanaroff AA, Walsh MC. *Fanaroff and Martin's Neonatal-Perinatal Medicine: Diseases of the Fetus and Infant*. 9th ed. St. Louis, MO: Mosby Elsevier; 2011.

Dinerstein A, Nieto RM, Solana CL, Perez GP, Otheguy LE, Larguia AM. Early and aggressive nutritional strategy (parenteral and enteral) decreases postnatal growth failure in very low birth weight infants. *J Perinatol.* 2006;26(7):436-442.

Ehrenkranz RA. Early, aggressive nutritional management for very low birth weight infants: what is the evidence? *Semin Perinatol.* 2007;31(2):48-55.

Gleason CA, Devaskar S, eds. *Avery's Diseases of the Newborn.* 9th ed. Philadelphia, PA: Saunders Elsevier; 2012.

Gomella TL, Cunningham MD, Eyal FG, eds. *Neonatology: Management, Procedures, On-Call Problems, Diseases, and Drugs.* 7th ed. New York, NY: McGraw Hill/Lange; 2013.

Hammarlund K, Sedin G. Transepidermal water loss in newborn infants. VI. Heat exchange with the environment in relation to gestational age. *Acta Paediatr Scand.* 1982;71(2):191-196.

Hartnoll G. Basic principles and practical steps in the management of fluid balance in the newborn. *Semin Neonatol.* 2003;8(4):307-313.

Martin RJ, Fanaroff AA, Walsh MC. *Fanaroff and Martin's Neonatal-Perinatal Medicine: Diseases of the Fetus and Infant.* 9th ed. St. Louis, MO: Mosby Elsevier; 2011.

Poindexter BB, Denne S. Nutrition and metabolism in the high-risk neonate. In: Martin RJ, Fanaroff AA, Walsh MC. *Fanaroff and Martin's Neonatal-Perinatal Medicine: Diseases of the Fetus and Infant.* 9th ed. St. Louis, MO: Mosby Elsevier; 2011.

Poindexter BB, Langer JC, Dusick AM, Ehrenkranz RA. Early provision of parenteral amino acids in extremely low birth weight infants: relation to growth and development outcome. *J Pediatr.* 2006;148(3):300-305.

Polin RA, Fox WW, Abman SH, eds. *Fetal and Neonatal Physiology.* 4th ed. Philadelphia, PA: Saunders Elsevier; 2011.

Rutter N. Clinical consequences of an immature barrier. *Semin Neonatol.* 2000;5(4):281-287.

Simmer K, Rao S. Early introduction of lipids to parenterally-fed preterm infants. *Cochrane Database of Systematic Reviews* 2005, Issue 2. Art. No. CD005256. DOI:10.1002/14651858.CD005256.

te Braake FW, van den Akker CH, Wattimena DJ, Huijmans JG, van Goudoever JB. Amino acid administration to premature infants directly after birth. *J Pediatr.* 2005;147(4):457-461.

13

Hypoglycemia

Jan Sherman

I. Definitions
  A. Glycogenolysis: Hydrolysis of glycogen to glucose
  B. Gluconeogenesis: Synthesis of glucose from molecules that are not carbohydrates, such as amino and fatty acids
  C. Hypoglycemia: Typically defined as a serum glucose of <45

II. Pathophysiology of glucose homeostasis
  A. *In utero*
   1. The fetus depends on the mother for a continuous supply of glucose for both energy metabolism and the synthesis of other metabolic substrates.
   2. Glucose is the primary substrate for the fetus, with lactate and amino acids providing ~20% of fetal energy.
   3. Fetal glucose level is ~80% of the maternal level.
  B. Hepatic glycogen content
   1. Low levels early in gestation
   2. Begins to increase at 15 and 20 weeks
   3. Rapid accumulation noted late in gestation
   4. Key hepatic enzymes necessary for gluconeogenesis present in fetus, though at lower levels than in adults
  C. At birth
   1. Newborn must have glucose and other nutrients to meet energy requirements.
   2. Glucose is the primary metabolic fuel for the brain and is supplied by the blood via diffusion.
   3. Levels of circulating epinephrine, norepinephrine, and glucagon rise.
   4. Levels of insulin fall.
   5. These hormonal changes stimulate hepatic glycogen utilization and stimulate gluconeogenesis.
   6. The result is a steady rate of glucose production and maintenance of the plasma glucose concentration.
   7. On average, the neonate produces glucose at rates between 4 and 6 mg/kg/min.
   8. Venous plasma glucose concentration at birth is ~60%–80% of maternal venous glucose concentration.

9. Glucose is initially maintained after birth by glycogenolysis and gluconeogenesis until either IV fluids or feeds are established.
10. Premature infants have limited stores of glycogen and fat.
11. Plasma glucose concentration falls, reaching its lowest value 30–90 min after birth.
12. In full-term, healthy neonates, plasma glucose concentration rises to 40–80 mg/dL.

D. Definition of hypoglycemia: The exact definition of hypoglycemia remains controversial. Most guidelines suggest it is defined as a serum glucose level of <45–50 mg/dL. Follow your institutional guidelines. If an infant is diagnosed with hyperinsulinemia, serum glucose levels should not be <60. It is critical for providers to understand that lower limits are unknown and probably need to be higher in patients who have higher cerebral demands for glucose, such as in hypoxemia, asphyxia, and seizures.

1. **Symptomatic infants should be treated, regardless of the degree of hypoglycemia.**
2. Severe hypoglycemia may cause neuronal cell death, glial cell injury, and subsequent adverse neurodevelopmental outcomes.
   a. The exact glucose level when damage starts is unknown.
   b. Sequelae may occur without acute signs of hypoglycemia.
   c. Hypoglycemia is thought to potentiate brain injury in sick newborns, which describes most extremely low birth weight (ELBW) infants.
3. Clinicians should maintain "target" glucose that is considered acceptable in their unit and have a standard of care for treatment. Less than 45 mg/dL seems to be the consensus in the first two days of life in premature infants.

III. Incidence
A. Hypoglycemia has been estimated to occur in 16% of large for gestational age (LGA) infants and 15% for small for gestational age (SGA) infants.

IV. Clinical presentation
A. Treatment should be started in the presence of signs of hypoglycemia, even with marginal glucose levels.
B. Clinical symptoms of hypoglycemia are nonspecific and similar to those of many neonatal disorders (**Box 13-1**).

C. Clinical symptoms should improve with correction of low glucose concentration.
D. Careful attention should be given to ensure that other associated disorders (e.g., sepsis, asphyxia) are not missed.
E. Seizures are seen more often in infants with delayed diagnosis and treatment and poor control.

V. Etiologies of hypoglycemia
A. Glucose metabolism after birth is a common metabolic problem seen in the NICU.
B. Transitional hypoglycemia can occur in the first 6–12 hours of life from the loss of maternal substrate at birth and/or failure to adapt after delivery.
   1. In premature infants, this is often due to lack of glycogen stores.
   2. This may also occur in hypothermic or hypoxic infants.
   3. Premature infants are at higher risk due to low glycogen stores.
   4. In these situations, hypoglycemia occurs early and is very responsive to treatment.
   5. Symptoms, if any, are usually stupor (lethargy) and jitteriness; respiratory disturbances and hypotonia may be seen.
C. Most cases of hypoglycemia are transient and respond readily to treatment (**Box 13-2**).

BOX 13-1
Clinical Presentation of Hypoglycemia

Irritability
Apnea, cyanotic spells
Seizures, jitteriness, tremors
Lethargy
Grunting, tachypnea
Hypothermia
Sweating
Hypotonia, limpness
Tachycardia
Changes in level of consciousness

(Adapted from Martin RJ, Fanaroff AA, Walsh MC. *Fanaroff and Martin's Neonatal-Perinatal Medicine: Diseases of the Fetus and Infant.* 9th ed. St. Louis, MO: Mosby Elsevier; 2011.)

D. Persistent or recurrent hypoglycemia may occur and is usually related to hyperinsulinism, endocrine abnormalities, or inborn errors of metabolism (**Box 13-3**).
  1. Onset varies but hypoglycemia is usually severe.
  2. Outcomes will depend on rapid and adequate treatment.

VI. Screening neonatal hypoglycemia
A. Anticipation of the group at high risk with goal of prevention
B. Correction of acute hypoglycemia
C. Prevention of subsequent hypoglycemia
D. Investigation and treatment of cause of hypoglycemia
E. Obtain blood glucose between 30 and 90 min of life
F. Steady state usually achieved by 2–4 hours of age

VII. Infants at high risk of hypoglycemia include:
A. LGA >90th percentile
B. SGA <10th percentile
C. Infants of diabetic mothers
D. Acutely ill infants
E. Infants born to mothers who received beta-adrenergic blockers (propranolol), oral hypoglycemic agents, or glucose infusions during the intrapartum period

VIII. Management of hypoglycemia
A. If infant is symptomatic or if there is a need to rapidly increase the plasma glucose level, administer a bolus of 2 mL/kg of 10% dextrose solution over 1 min.

BOX 13-2
Possible Etiologies of Transient Neonatal Hypoglycemia

Intrapartum administration of glucose
Intrapartum administration of terbutaline, ritodrine, propranolol, oral hypoglycemic agents
Intrauterine growth restriction
Birth depression
Infection
Hypothermia
Hyperviscosity
Congenital cardiac malformations

(Adapted from Martin RJ, Fanaroff AA, Walsh MC. *Fanaroff and Martin's Neonatal-Perinatal Medicine: Diseases of the Fetus and Infant.* 9th ed. St. Louis, MO: Mosby Elsevier; 2011.)

B. Administer parenteral glucose at a rate of 6–8 mg/kg/min, corresponding to 3.6–4.8 mL/kg/hour of 10% dextrose solution by 30 min of age.
C. Goal for peripheral intravenous catheter (PIV) or umbilical venous catheter (UVC) should be within 30 min of delivery in very low birth weight (VLBW) infants.
D. Any infant with persistent hypoglycemia requiring high rates of glucose infusions should have a central line.

IX. Monitoring

A. Goal of parenteral glucose therapy is to maintain the plasma glucose concentration at a level >45–150 mg/dL.
B. Monitor plasma glucose levels every 1–2 hours stable and then every 4–6 hours, depending on diagnosis. Follow your institutional guidelines.
C. If glucose concentrations do not increase to normal levels, increase rate of infusion by 1–2 mg/kg/min while monitoring the glucose response.
D. A UVC or central line should be considered in infants with severe hypoglycemia and those who require high rates of glucose.

X. American Academy of Pediatrics (AAP) guidelines

A. A report titled "Postnatal Glucose Homeostasis in Late-Preterm and Term Infants" provides guidelines for screening and detection in late-preterm and term infants. There is currently no AAP guideline for the premature infant.

BOX 13-3
Possible Etiologies of Persistent or Recurrent Hypoglycemia

Hyperinsulinism
β-cell hyperplasia
Beckwith-Wiedemann syndrome
Genetic causes: glutamate dehydrogenase HI, SCHADD-III

Endocrine disorders
Cortisol (adrenal) deficiency
Congenital hypopituitarism
Growth hormone deficiency

Inborn errors of metabolism
Galactosemia
Hepatic glycogen storage diseases
Hereditary tyrosinemia
Maple syrup urine disease

(Adapted from Martin RJ, Fanaroff AA, Walsh MC. *Fanaroff and Martin's Neonatal-Perinatal Medicine: Diseases of the Fetus and Infant.* 9th ed. St. Louis, MO: Mosby Elsevier; 2011.)

XI. Persistent hypoglycemia
   A. Assess the ratio of glucose to insulin by drawing both simultaneously.
      1. The insulin-to-glucose (I/G) ratio should be <0.30.
      2. If the ratio is higher, consider hyperinsulinemia.
   B. Assess serum ketones, lactate, ammonia, and cortisol.
      1. If ketones are low to absent, consider hyperinsulinemia.
      2. High ketones and/or low cortisol may indicate cortisol deficiency.
      3. Abnormal lactate levels may indicate metabolic defects.
      4. Further evaluation should be considered with endocrinology.

XII. Weaning the glucose infusion
   A. When plasma glucose concentration has been stable at ~70–100 mg/dL for 2–3 days, the infant may be weaned from glucose infusion if no longer needed for nutrition.
   B. Glucose infusions can be decreased every 6–12 hours, as long as the blood glucose concentration remains stable (>50 mg/dL) and the goal is to discontinue IV fluids.
   C. At each concentration change, monitor serum glucose.

XIII. Adjunct therapies
   A. Hydrocortisone
      1. Should only be used if there is evidence of adrenal insufficiency
      2. Should be considered in infants who require 12–15 mg/kg/min with ongoing episodes of hypoglycemia
      3. A cortisol level should be sent prior to starting therapy
      4. Increases gluconeogenesis and the effects of glucagon
      5. Can be weaned over several days once blood glucose is stabilized
   B. Diazoxide
      1. Diazoxide is a benzothiadiazine derivative that is similar to the thiazide diuretics, yet has none of the diuretic effects of thiazides.
      2. Initially used as a antihypertensive agent, now it is more often used for the treatment of hypoglycemia due to hyperinsulinism.
      3. Diazoxide has been shown to cause decreased insulin and catecholamine release.
      4. The drug is eliminated primarily by glomerular filtration.
      5. 90% of circulating diazoxide is bound to albumin.

6. Side effects are uncommon, except for hypertrichosis lanuginosa and fluid retention. Others may include sodium and water retention, expansion of plasma volume, edema, thrombocytopenia, anorexia, vomiting, and sometimes, extrapyramidal symptoms.

C. Somatostatin
1. When administered exogenously, somatostatin inhibits the secretion of glucagon, insulin, growth hormone, and thyrotropin.
2. It suppresses the secretion of both insulin and glucagon, causing a fall in plasma glucose followed by a transient increase.
3. In the neonate, somatostatin has been used to treat nesidioblastosis (hyperinsulinemic hypoglycemia) as an emergency measure — with variable success — and evaluate the usefulness of pancreatectomy.
4. Octreotide, the first somatostatin analogue introduced for clinical use, is significantly more potent in its hormone-suppressive effect.
    a. After subcutaneous injection, its elimination half-life is reported to be 2 hours.
    b. It has been used with some success in the management of islet cell tumors, insulinomas, and nesidioblastosis.

D. Glucagon
1. Glucagon should only be given in infants with adequate glycogen stores and should not be used in SGA or ELBW infants.
2. Glucagon is a peptide hormone produced in the pancreas and used most often for the diagnosis of hepatic glycogen storage disease.
3. A minimum increase in plasma glucose concentration is seen in response to glucagon with hepatic glycogen storage disease.
4. Glucagon increases the blood glucose concentration by stimulating glycogenolysis and gluconeogenesis.
5. Acute administration of glucagon increases blood glucose by >50% in most normal infants. However, the effect is transient.
6. To maintain increased serum glucose levels following glucagon, administer IV glucose.

XIV. Potential outcomes

A. Disturbances of neurological development and intellectual function
   1. Deficits reflect cerebral cortical neuronal and white matter injury.
   2. Seizures as a symptom in hypoglycemic infants are associated with abnormal outcomes 50% of the time.
   3. Asymptomatic infants have abnormal neurological outcomes ~6% of the time. Symptomatic infants without seizures do almost as well.
   4. There has been a study of premature infants showing that even moderate hypoglycemia (a plasma glucose of less than ~47 mg/dL) increases the incidence of neurodevelopmental sequelae (29%) if it is present for 3 or more days, and this incidence increases to 40% if the duration is 5 or more days.
   5. Early treatment of hypoglycemia is essential.
B. Visual and motor disturbances (spasticity and ataxia)
C. Seizure disorders
D. Microcephaly

References

American Academy of Pediatrics. Postnatal glucose homeostasis in late-preterm and term infants. *Pediatrics*. 2011:127(3):575-579. doi: 10.1542/peds.2010-3851.

Briggs J. Management of asymptomatic hypoglycaemia in neonates. *Nurs Stand*; 2007;22(8):35-38.

Chan SW. Neonatal hypoglycemia. UptoDate Web site. http://www.uptodate.com/contents/neonatal-hypoglycemia. Accessed September 9, 2008.

Cloherty JP, Eichenwald EC, Hansen AR, Stark AR. *Manual of Neonatal Care*. 7th ed. Philadelphia, PA: Wolters Kluwer Health/Lippincott Williams & Wilkins; 2012.

Deshpande S, Ward Platt M. The investigation and management of neonatal hypoglycaemia. *Semin Fetal Neonatal Med*. 2005;10(4):351-361.

Garg M, Devaskar SU. Glucose metabolism in the late preterm infant. *Clin Perinatol*. 2006;33(4):853-870.

Gleason CA, Devaskar S, eds. *Avery's Diseases of the Newborn*. 9th ed. Philadelphia, PA: Saunders Elsevier; 2012.

Gomella TL, Cunningham MD, Eyal FG, eds. *Neonatology: Management, Procedures, On-Call Problems, Diseases, and Drugs*. 7th ed. New York, NY: McGraw Hill/Lange; 2013.

Kalhan S, Peter-Wohl S. Hypoglycemia: what is it for the neonate? *Am J Perinatol*. 2000;17(1):11-18.

Martin RJ, Fanaroff AA, Walsh MC. *Fanaroff and Martin's Neonatal-Perinatal Medicine: Diseases of the Fetus and Infant*. 9th ed. St. Louis, MO: Mosby Elsevier; 2011.

Mitanchez D. Glucose regulation in preterm newborn infants. *Horm Res*. 2007;68(6):265-271.

Polin RA, Fox WW, Abman SH, eds. *Fetal and Neonatal Physiology*. 4th ed. Philadelphia, PA: Saunders Elsevier; 2011.

Rozance PJ, Hay WW. Hypoglycemia in newborn infants: features associated with adverse outcomes. *Biol Neonate*. 2006;90(2):74-86.

Volpe JJ. *Neurology of the Newborn*. 5th ed. Philadelphia, PA: Saunders Elsevier; 2008.

Ward Platt M, Deshpande S. Metabolic adaptation at birth. *Semin Fetal Neonatal Med*. 2005;10(4):341-350.

14

Neonatal Sepsis

Jan Sherman

I. Definitions

A. Early-onset sepsis (EOS): Defined by the NICHD and the Vermont Oxford Networks (VON) as sepsis with onset at ≤3 days of age

B. Hospital acquired infection (HAI): A blood or cerebrospinal fluid (CSF) infection in a newborn >3 days (72 hours) after birth, proven by culture

C. Bacterial infections and meningitis are a major cause of morbidity and mortality in very low birth weight (VLBW) infants
   1. Bacteremia: positive blood culture
   2. Meningitis: positive CSF culture

D. Clinical sepsis: Clinically ill but with a negative blood culture

E. Sensitivity: Percentage of patients with infection who have an abnormal test result

F. Specificity: Percentage of patients without infection who have a normal test result

G. Positive predictive value: If test result is abnormal, percentage of patients with infection

H. Negative predictive value: If test result is normal, percentage of patients with no infection

II. Early-onset bacterial sepsis

A. The incidence of neonatal sepsis ranges from 1–2 cases per 1,000 live births; the case fatality rate is 5%–10%.
   1. This is 10-fold higher in VLBW infants.

B. EOS is generally acquired vertically from bacteria colonizing the mother's lower genital tract, or from infected amniotic fluid. The exception is transplacental transmission of *Treponema pallidum* and *Listeria monocytogenes*.

C. Risk factors for EOS: Although risk factors are often used, they have not been shown to have any specificity or sensitivity.
   1. Maternal factors
      a. Intrapartum fever >37.5°C (99.5°F)
      b. Chorioamnionitis (intramnionic)
         (1) Complicates as many as 40%–70% of premature births

(2) Diagnosis of clinical chorioamnionitis
   (a) Maternal fever >38 °C (100.4 °F) and at least two of the following:
      i. Maternal leukocytosis (>15,000 cells/mm^3)
      ii. Maternal tachycardia (>100 beats/min)
      iii. Fetal tachycardia (>160 beats/min)
      iv. Uterine tenderness
      v. Foul odor of amniotic fluid
   (b) Can be masked by medications and epidurals
  c. Prolonged rupture of membranes (ROM), >18 hours
  d. Presence of meconium-stained amniotic fluid
  e. Maternal colonization with group B *Streptococcus* (GBS)
     (1) GBS is not a risk factor if the mother has received penicillin, ampicillin, or cefazolin at least 4 hours before the delivery.
     (2) GBS is not a risk factor if the mother had a cesarean delivery with intact membranes and did not labor.
  f. Colonization with genital mycoplasmas
2. Neonatal factors
  a. Less than 37 weeks gestation (prematurity)
  b. Birth weight <2,500 g
     (1) Incidence is 10 times higher in infants with a birth weight of <1,000 g.
  c. Higher risk in African-American infants

III. Predominant organisms

A. GBS is the most common cause of EOS in term newborns (**Table 14-1**).
  1. This has significantly decreased with the use of intrapartum prophylaxis antibiotics in GBS-positive mothers (0.34 cases per 1,000 live births).
     a. Penicillin or ampicillin is the recommended treatment by the Centers for Disease Control and Prevention (CDC), unless the mother is allergic.
  2. There is a higher risk of death for culture-positive VLBW infants.
B. Gram-negative enteric bacteria (*Escherichia coli*) are the most common cause of EOS in VLBW infants.
  1. *E. coli*: anaerobic Gram-negative rods

a. In critically ill newborns with suspected sepsis, third-generation cephalosporins are recommended secondary to the risk of ampicillin-resistant, Gram-negative sepsis.
   2. Other organisms frequently seen are *Klebsiella*, *Pseudomonas*, *Haemophilus*, and *Enterobacter*.
   C. Coagulase-negative *Staphylococci* (CoNS), *Candida* species; and *Staphylococci aureus*, which is often methicillin resistant (MRSA); are more common causes of HAIs (**Table 14-2**).
   D. HAIs due to Gram-negative organisms are associated with higher mortality.

IV. Clinical presentation of sepsis
A. The signs and symptoms of neonatal sepsis are often nonspecific.
B. It is important to note that EOS can be present in a healthy appearing newborn.
C. The infant with sepsis may have a normal temperature, or may be hyperthermic or hypothermic.
   1. Hyperthermia or fever — temperature 38.0°C–38.3°C (100.4°F–100.9°F) — is rare, and iatrogenic causes should be ruled out.
D. Respiratory distress is frequently seen.
   1. Tachypnea
   2. Apnea
E. Feeding difficulties or lethargy may be present.
F. Gastrointestinal symptoms may include hepatomegaly, abdominal distention, vomiting, diarrhea, guaiac-positive stools, and jaundice.

TABLE 14-1
Percentage of Organisms Associated with Early-Onset Sepsis (EOS)

EOS		VLBW EOS	
Organism	%	Organism	%
GBS	46%	E. coli	49%
Other *Streptococci*	26%	CoNS	17%
E. coli	20%	GBS	14%
Enterococcus	4%	Other *Streptococci*	11%
S. aureus	4%	Other Gram positive	9%

CoNS = coagulase-negative *Staphylococci*; GBS = group B *Streptococcus*
(Adapted from Falciglia G, Hageman JR, Schreiber M, Alexander K. Antibiotic therapy and early onset sepsis. *Neoreviews*. 2012;13(2):e86-e93. doi:10.1542/neo.13-2-e86.)

G. Focal infections may be present and can present with cellulitis, soft tissue abscesses, omphalitis, and conjunctivitis. Causative agents associated with focal infections may include:
   1. *Streptococci* with cellulitis
   2. *Staphylococci* with abscesses
   3. *Pseudomonas aeruginosa* with necrotic skin lesions

V. Diagnosis of sepsis: Diagnostic tests used to diagnose sepsis have poor positive predictive value.

A. Microbiologic tests
   1. Blood culture: A blood culture should be obtained from all infants with suspected sepsis.
      a. Obtaining more than one blood culture can be helpful in distinguishing blood culture contaminants from true pathogens; however, one culture at birth is adequate.
      b. A minimum of 1.0 mL of blood per bottle is recommended.
      c. Umbilical arterial blood culture is preferred with a newly placed line, if available.
      d. Both aerobic and anaerobic cultures can be sent if 2 cc of blood is available.
         (1) *Bacteroides fragilis* only grows in anaerobic media.
      e. Blood culture bacterial growth time to positivity:
         (1) 90% by 36 hours
         (2) 93% by 48 hours
         (3) 98.5% by 60 hours

TABLE 14-2
Percentage of Organisms Associated with Hospital Acquired Infection (HAI)

Gram-Positive Organisms (70.2%)		Gram-Negative Organisms (17.6%)		Fungal (12.2%)	
Organism	%	Organism	%	Organism	%
CoNS	47.9%	*E. coli*	4.9%	*C. albicans*	5.8%
S. aureus	7.8%	Klebsiella	4.0	*C. parapilosis*	4.1%
Enterococcus	3.3%	Pseudomonas	2.7	Other	2.3%
GBS	2.3%	Enterobacter	2.5		
Other	8.9%	Serratia	2.2		

CoNS = coagulase-negative *Staphylococci*; GBS = group B *Streptococcus*
(Adapted from Chu A, Hageman JR, Schreiber M, Alexander K. Antimicrobial therapy and late onset sepsis. *Neoreviews*. 2012;13(2):e94-e102. doi:10.1542/neo.13-2-e94.)

(4) After 72 hours, generally classified as contaminant
2. Urine culture:
   a. A urine culture should not be obtained during the workup for EOS.
   b. A positive urine culture is rarely seen in EOS and most often reflects a spread to the bladder in the setting of bacteremia.
3. CSF cultures: Remain controversial in EOS
   a. Meningitis, while rare, may be seen in ~10% of infants with EOS.
      (1) Meningitis cannot be diagnosed or excluded solely on the basis of symptoms.
      (2) Blood cultures can be sterile in 10%–15% of infants with early-onset meningitis and in one-third of VLBW infants with late-onset meningitis.
   b. A lumbar puncture (L/P) should be performed if:
      (1) Blood cultures are positive
      (2) Clinical or laboratory course suggests bacterial sepsis
      (3) Infant worsens despite antimicrobial therapy
   c. The L/P should be delayed in unstable infants with cardiovascular or respiratory instability.
4. Tracheal aspirate: If pneumonia is suspected, a tracheal-aspirate Gram stain and culture should be obtained immediately after intubation.
5. Drainage from skin and soft tissue lesions should be sent for Gram stain and culture.

B. Laboratory evaluation: It is important to note that normal tests usually give more assurance that infection is absent than diagnose the presence of infection.
   1. Complete blood count (CBC)
      a. A white blood cell count of $<5.0 \times 10^3$/mcL is a risk factor for infection.
      b. Serial CBC should be sent, since a single leukocyte count obtained shortly after birth is not adequately sensitive for diagnosing sepsis.
      c. The immature-to-total ratio (I:T ratio) has a good negative predictive value and the best sensitivity. There is a high likelihood that infection is absent if the I:T ratio is normal (≤ 0.2).

(1) Calculation: The number of immature polymorphonuclear (PMN) lymphocytes (e.g., bands, metas, myelos, etc.) divided by the total number of PMN lymphocytes (mature and immature)
2. Acute phase reactants (APRs)
   a. The acute-phase response is an inflammatory response of the body to infection or trauma.
   b. C-reactive protein (CRP) is the most commonly measured APR.
   c. The peak CRP is seen at 6–8 hours after onset of an infection and peaks at 24 hours.
   d. Sensitivity is low at birth since it requires an inflammatory response, but improves within 6–12 hours of birth.
   e. Two normal CRP determinations between 8 and 12 hours, and then again 24 hours later, has been shown to have a high negative predictive value in which antimicrobial therapy can safely be discontinued (by 48 hours of age).
   f. Infants with elevated CRP (≥ 1.0 mg/dL) do not benefit from serial CRPs.
3. Future biomarkers
   a. Proinflammatory cytokines: Interleukin-6 and interleukin-8
      (1) Initially thought to be excellent markers for detecting infection.
      (2) Very short half-life of circulating cytokines significantly increases the rate of false negative results.
   b. Calprotectin: Major product of innate immune cells
      (1) Have higher sensitivity and specificity (89% and 96%, respectively) for HAIs than CRP. Levels are not influenced by postnatal age.
      (2) Advances in flow cytometry have allowed the investigation of cell surface antigens as potential markers.
   c. Molecular microbiology: Identifies bacteria on the basis of genotypic analysis
      (1) Whole-cell mass spectrophotometry (WC-MS)
      (2) Amplification and sequencing of 16S ribosomal nucleic acid

d. Broad-range polymerase chain reaction (PCR): Uses amplification of nonspecific 16S ribosomal DNA primers on DNA extracted directly from blood or spinal fluid without previous culturing
   e. Granulocyte colony stimulating factor (G-CSF): Mediator produced by bone marrow that facilitates neutrophil proliferation and differentiation
      (1) Investigated as a marker of neonatal infection
      (2) Shows high sensitivity (95%) and a predictive negative value of 99% in initial studies
C. Decisions to treat
   1. Utilize your specific hospital guidelines.
      a. Should be based on American Academy of Pediatrics (AAP) guidelines and algorithms
   2. Normal diagnostic tests with high negative predictive values give some assurance that infection is not present.
   3. As risk factors increase, so should the decision to treat, especially in VLBW infants.
D. Antimicrobial therapy
   1. Antibiotic therapy can alter the neonatal microbiome, potentially making the infant more susceptible to opportunistic infection and increasing the incidence of antibiotic-resistant organisms.
   2. Antibiotic coverage should initially be directed against the most likely pathogenic bacteria, which are GBS and *E. coli* in the United States.
   3. Antibiotics should be discontinued after 48 hours if negative cultures, unless there is compelling clinical evidence against stopping.
   4. Empiric antibiotics should target the **likely bacteria** until the infecting organism is identified and antimicrobial susceptibilities are determined (**Table 14-3**).
      a. **Ampicillin and gentamicin** (aminoglycoside) are the most widely used empirical antibiotics.
      b. The combination of ampicillin and gentamicin is synergistic and effective against all strains of GBS, most strains of *E. coli*, and *Listeria*.
      c. Cefotaxime, a third-generation cephalosporin, has been used as a replacement for gentamicin in empiric therapy.
         (1) At least one report links the drug to a higher mortality in neonates.

TABLE 14-3
Common Antibacterials

Type	General Information	Spectrum of Activity	Comments
Natural Penicillins Aminopenicillins Ampicillin	Bactericidal; Interfere with cell wall synthesis Acts synergistically with gentamicin.	Gram-positive *cocci* Gram-positive *bacilli* *Neisseria* *Clostridia*	Allergic reactions, hematologic toxicity
Antistaphylococcal penicillins Nafcillin Methicillin	Semisynthetic penicillin derivatives Nafcillin has the greatest CSF penetration of the anti-staphylococcal penicillins	*S. aureus* CoNS	Nafcillin is excreted through the biliary system, accumulation can occur with jaundice
Cephalosporins	Classified into four generations based on spectrum of activity		IV site pain, phlebitis, fever, increased liver enzymes, cholelithiasis
1st generation cefazolin	1st generation used to treat skin and soft tissue infections 2nd generation — limited use in infants		Serious adverse effects include seizure, hemolytic anemia, thrombocytopenia, leukopenia
3rd generation cefotaxime	3rd generation — cefotaxime has enhanced Gram-negative coverage with excellent CNS penetration; **new reports demonstrate increased mortality with use of this drug in neonates**		
4th generation cefepime	4th generation — reserved for multidrug-resistant organisms		
Carbapenems Imipenem Meropenem	Ideal for polymicrobial infections	Imipenem used to treat cephalosporin-resistant citrobacter and enterobacter species Meropenem is more active against Gram-negative bacteria	Thrombophlebitis and seizures Risk of seizure is lower with meropenem
Aminoglycides Gentamicin	Synergistic with penicillins and cephalosporins Used with vancomycin to treat *S. aureus*	Used with Gram-negative infections	Nephrotoxicity, ototoxicity
Glycopeptides Vancomycin	Concern for vancomycin-resistant *Enterococcus*	Bactericidal for aerobic and anaerobic Gram-positive bacteria Used to treat *S. aureus*, *Staphylococcus epidermis*, *Enterococcal* species	Red man syndrome — histamine-mediated rash Nephrotoxicity, ototoxicity

CNS = central nervous system; CoNS = coagulase-negative *Staphylococci*; CSF = cerebrospinal fluid

(Table 14-3 adapted from Chu A, Hageman JR, Schreiber M, Alexander K. Antimicrobial therapy and late onset sepsis. *Neoreviews*. 2012;13(2):e94-e102. doi:10.1542/neo.13-2-e94; Falciglia G, Hageman JR, Schreiber M, Alexander K. Antibiotic therapy and early onset sepsis. *Neoreviews*. 2012;13(2):e86-e93. doi:10.1542/neo.13-2-e86; Martin RJ, Fanaroff AA, Walsh, MC. *Fanaroff and Martin's Neonatal-Perinatal Medicine: Diseases of the Fetus and Infant*. 9th ed. St. Louis, MO: Mosby Elsevier; 2011; Yaffe SJ, Aranda JV, eds. *Neonatal and Pediatric Pharmacology: Therapeutic Principles in Practice*. 4th ed. Philadelphia, PA: Wolters Kluwer Heath/Lippincott Williams & Wilkins; 2011.)

            (2) Studies report a rapid development of organism resistances.
            (3) **Cefotaxime should be used judiciously to avoid resistance**.
            (4) Consider only if meningitis is suspected.
    5. The best way to ensure that ampicillin and gentamicin remain effective is responsible antibiotic stewardship.
        a. Antibiotic therapy should be narrowed as much as possible once an organism is identified and susceptibility is known.
            (1) Consider 10 days of treatment if there is bacteremia without an identifiable focus.
                (a) Treat focal infections longer.
            (2) Uncomplicated GBS meningitis: Treat 14 days.
            (3) Gram-negative meningitis: Treat a minimum of 21 days or 14 days after the first negative culture (use the longest treatment).
                (a) Treat with cefotaxime and an aminoglycoside until susceptibility is known.
        b. Empirical antibiotic therapy should be limited to 48 hours if cultures are negative.

VI. Viral infections
    A. Herpes virus family
        1. Epidemiology and transmission
            a. Eight viruses in the family infect infants: Herpes simplex (HSV) types 1 and 2; cytomegalovirus (CMV); varicella-zoster (VZV); Epstein-Barr (EBV); and human herpes viruses (HHV) 6, 7, and 8.
            b. The incidence of neonatal herpes simplex infections is 1 in every 3,200 live births per year.
            c. Labial and oropharyngeal infections are predominantly caused by HSV-1 and may be transmitted by respiratory droplet spread or by direct contact with infected secretions.

- d. Genital infections are usually transmitted by direct sexual contact with HSV-2.
- e. Transmission from mother to infant may occur by a transplacental route (5%), or may be acquired during the intrapartum (85%) and postnatal periods (10%).

B. Presentation and classification
1. Two-thirds of term newborns have a normal neonatal course and are discharged before the onset of disease.
2. Vesicles may not be present, particularly with disseminated and encephalitis infections.
3. Neonatal infections are classified as:
   - a. Disseminated (25% of cases): Involve multiple organs, which may or may not include the central nervous system (CNS). Infants will generally present within 10–12 days of birth with signs of bacterial sepsis or shock, thrombocytopenia, hepatosplenomegaly, and purpura.
   - b. Encephalitis (30% of cases): Present with lethargy, poor feeding, irritability, and localized or generalized seizures. EEGs will have nonspecific abnormalities.
   - c. Localized (45% of cases): Usually present with lesions on the skin, eyes, or mouth within 10–11 days of birth.

C. Diagnosis
1. Cultures (scrapings of mucocutaneous lesions, CSF, stool, urine, nasopharynx, and conjunctivae) should be delayed 24–48 hours after birth to differentiate viral replication in the newborn from transient colonization of the newborn at birth.
2. Serologic testing is not useful in neonatal disease because of transplacentally transferred maternal antibody.
3. PCR testing of the CSF, blood, scrapings of lesions, conjunctivae, or nasopharynx should be done. There is a very low recovery rate for HSV cultures, particularly in the CSF.

D. Treatment
1. IV acyclovir remains the drug of choice for neonatal HSV disease and HSV encephalitis.
2. Oral acyclovir is the first choice for skin recurrences after HSV disease.
3. If parenteral acyclovir is unavailable, IV ganciclovir may be used as a second-line therapy, and IV foscarnet as third-line therapy for neonatal HSV disease or HSV encephalitis.
4. Skin recurrences may be treated with oral valacyclovir.

5. Infants with CNS disease need to have a repeat L/P at the end of the course of treatment. Treatment should be continued until the CSF is PCR negative.

E. Potential outcomes
1. Mortality is 29% for disseminated disease; 4% for CNS disease; and 0% for skin, eye, or mouth disease.
2. The percentage of survivors with normal development (31%) has not changed for CNS disease: Normal development among survivors of disseminated disease is now 83%; and >98% for skin, eye, or mouth disease.

VII. Fungal infections

A. Microbiology
1. *Candida albicans* is usually acquired maternally.
2. *Candida parapsilosis* accounts for one quarter of all cases of invasive fungal infection in VLBW infants.

B. Clinical presentation
1. Pseudomembranous candidiasis (thrush): Manifests with white patches that cover the buccal mucosa, gingiva, and tongue.
2. Candida diaper dermatitis: Begins with an erythematous vesiculopapular eruption that coalesces, producing large areas with satellite lesions that are surrounded by a fine, white, scaly area.
3. Congenital cutaneous candidiasis: Presents with erythematous maculopapular lesions on the trunk and extremities that rapidly become pustular and rupture, leaving denuded skin with well-defined, raised, scaling borders.
4. Catheter-associated and systemic candidiasis: Generally occur at a mean of 30 days of age. Presentation may be similar to bacterial infections.
5. Meningitis: Occurs in ~40% of affected infants. Therefore, an L/P should be part of the workup.
6. Renal involvement: May manifest as candiduria, multiple renal abscesses, or fungus balls that can obstruct flow of urine. Renal ultrasound should be performed if renal involvement is suspected.
7. Endophthalmitis: May manifest as retinitis. A retinal examination should be part of the diagnostic evaluation for all infants.
8. Microabscesses of the liver or spleen may be seen.
9. Endocarditis and extension of infection to the lungs, bones, or joints may also occur.

C. Diagnosis: Established by growth of *Candida* species in cultures
D. Treatment
   1. Thrush usually responds to nystatin suspension.
   2. Candida diaper dermatitis may be treated with nystatin cream or ointment.
   3. Systemic candidiasis is mainly treated with amphotericin B.
      a. Consider additional therapies when treating meningitis, since CSF concentrations are only 2%–4% of serum concentrations.
      b. Approximately 80% of cases develop either infusion-related toxicity or nephrotoxicity, especially with other nephrotoxic drugs.
      c. Fever, shaking chills, hypotension, vomiting, and tachypnea may be seen 1–3 hours after starting the infusion.
      d. Rapid IV infusion has been associated with hypotension, hypokalemia, arrhythmias, and shock.
   4. Lipid formulations were approved in the 1990s and are marketed under the trade names Abelcet and AmBisome. The lipid formations have reduced toxicity but provide slower onset of action and are not as potent as amphotericin B.
   5. 5-fluorocytosine (5-FC) enhances the activity of amphotericin B. Toxic effects include azotemia, leukopenia, and thrombocytopenia.
   6. Fluconazole is a synthetic compound, which can be used in conjunction with amphotericin B to enhance CSF penetration. Side effects are rare and may include rash, vomiting, and diarrhea.
   7. Echinocandins such as caspofungin are a new class of antifungals, which interfere with cell wall biosynthesis and target the CNS. They are particularly useful for refractory cases of disseminated candidiasis and for aspergillosis. Side effects are usually minimal; hepatotoxicity may be seen.

VIII. Infection control practices in the NICU
   A. Hand hygiene practices
      1. Hand hygiene is the single most important intervention to prevent nosocomial infection.
         a. Routine, meticulous hand hygiene should occur before and after every patient contact.

     b. Fingernails should be natural, trimmed short, and free of artificial nails or wraps.
     c. Sinks and alcohol-based hand sanitizer dispensers should be numerous and conveniently located throughout the unit.
  B. Standard precautions to follow during every patient encounter
     1. Gloves: Use to prevent contamination of health care workers' hands during:
        a. Direct contact with mucous membranes, blood, body fluids, or non-intact skin
        b. Direct contact with infants who are infected or colonized with pathogens transmitted by contact route
        c. Direct contact with visibly soiled or potentially contaminated surfaces or equipment
     2. Droplet precautions, such as masks: Consider with pathogens spread via close contact (≤ 3 feet) with respiratory secretions, such as pertussis.
     3. Airborne precautions, such as fit-tested respirators: Use to prevent transmission of pathogens that are capable of traveling long distances when suspended in air, such as measles, varicella, and tuberculosis.
     4. Combination of gloves and gown: Use to prevent transmission of pathogens that are spread by direct or indirect contact with the patient or his/her environment. Such precautions should be used with multidrug-resistant organisms.
     5. Combination of gloves, gown, and mask: Consider when direct and droplet contact may be encountered, such as with adenovirus bronchiolitis.

IX. **Implementation of care bundles**
  A. A care bundle is a group of best practices that, when implemented together, show proven success in improving patient outcomes.
  B. Care bundles are valuable tools for ensuring that evidence-based medicine is delivered reliably and consistently.
  C. Implementation of bundles, such as a central-line insertion and maintenance bundle, with a checklist to monitor adherence to the bundle elements, will standardize insertion and care, which should reduce nosocomial infections.

1. Sterile procedures
    a. Sterile gloves, sterile gowns, hats, and masks are required.
        (1) In small delivery areas or areas that cannot prevent traffic, everyone should wear hats and masks.
        (2) Anyone at the sterile field or assisting should wear sterile gloves, sterile gowns, hats, and masks.
    b. Sterile drapes for procedures should be clear and cover the entire surface of the bed.
    c. A nontransparent drape may be used to continue the sterile field from the bed surface down to the front of the provider.

References

Chu A, Hageman JR, Schreiber M, Alexander K. Antimicrobial therapy and late onset sepsis. *Neoreviews*. 2012;13(2):e94-e102. doi:10.1542/neo.13-2-e94.

Cloherty JP, Eicherwald EC, Hansen AR, Stark AR. *Manual of Neonatal Care*. 7th ed. Philadelphia, PA: Lippincott Williams & Wilkins; 2012.

Falciglia G, Hageman JR, Schreiber M, Alexander K. Antibiotic therapy and early onset sepsis. *Neoreviews*. 2012;13(2):e86-e93. doi:10.1542/neo.13-2-e86.

Gleason CA, Devaskar S, eds. *Avery's Diseases of the Newborn*. 9th ed. Philadelphia, PA: Saunders Elsevier; 2012.

Gomella TL, Cunningham MD, Eyal FG, eds. *Neonatology: Management, Procedures, On-Call Problems, Diseases, and Drugs*. 7th ed. New York, NY: McGraw Hill/Lange; 2013.

Guzman-Cottrill JA. Infection control practices in the NICU: what is evidence-based? *Neoreviews*. 2010;11(8):e419-e425. doi:10.1542/neo.11-8-e419.

Lachman P, Yuen S. Using care bundles to prevent infection in neonatal and paediatric ICUs. *Curr Opin Infect Dis*. 2009;22(3):224-228.

Martin RJ, Fanaroff AA, Walsh, MC. *Fanaroff and Martin's Neonatal-Perinatal Medicine: Diseases of the Fetus and Infant*. 9th ed. St. Louis, MO: Mosby Elsevier; 2011.

Polin RA, Committee on Fetus and Newborn. Management of neonates with suspected or proven early-onset bacterial sepsis. *Pediatrics*. 2012;129(5):1006-1015.

Polin RA, Fox WW, Abman SH, eds. *Fetal and Neonatal Physiology*. 4th ed. Philadelphia, PA: Saunders Elsevier; 2011.

Puopolo K. Epidemiology of neonatal early-onset sepsis. *NeoReviews*. 2008;9(12):e571-e579.

Schulman J, Stricof R, Stevens TP, et al. Statewide NICU central-line-associated bloodstream infection rates decline after bundles and checklists. *Pediatrics*. 2011; 127(3):436-44. doi:10.1542/peds.2010-2873.

Yaffe SJ, Aranda JV, eds. *Neonatal and Pediatric Pharmacology: Therapeutic Principles in Practice*. 4th ed. Philadelphia, PA: Wolters Kluwer Heath/Lippincott Williams & Wilkins; 2011.

15

Intraventricular Hemorrhage

Bresney Crowell and David J. Annibale

I. Overview

A. An intraventricular hemorrhage (IVH) is an intracranial hemorrhage that begins in the subependymal germinal matrix with subsequent entrance of blood into the ventricular system. (See **Fig. 15-1**.)

B. Predominately found in preterm infants, IVH is associated with an increased risk of adverse neurodevelopmental outcomes. The associated risks increase with severity.

II. Pathophysiology

A. Pathogenesis of grades I–III IVH (see Section IV.D.) is multifactorial and the reasons for the preterm infant's vulnerability to IVH are both anatomical and pathophysiologic.

B. IVH largely originates in the germinal matrix located in the subependymal region around the lateral ventricles. Origination of IVH in this region is related to the fragility of the germinal matrix vasculature, the disturbance of cerebral blood flow (CBF), and coagulation and platelet disorders.
   1. Intrinsic vascular fragility of the germinal matrix
      a. The germinal matrix produces new glial cells early in gestation, requiring a rich blood supply due to increased quantities of substrate and energy. Glial fibers develop with increasing maturation.

FIGURE 15-1
Intraventricular Hemorrhage (IVH)

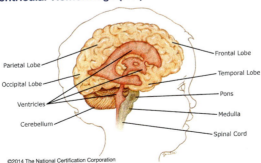

An IVH begins in the subependymal germinal matrix with subsequent entrance of blood into the ventricular system. Predominately found in preterm infants, IVH is associated with increased risk of adverse neurodevelopmental outcomes.

    b. This area lacks muscular layers or supporting structures, leaving the small, fragile, immature vessels susceptible to rupture.

    c. The vessels in this capillary bed do not resemble arterioles or venules and are sometimes called channels. They do not become real capillary beds until the germinal matrix disappears.

    d. The region's microvasculature and poor connective tissue results in a poor blood-brain barrier due to an abundance of blood vessels that have paucity of pericytes, immature basal lamina, and a deficiency of tight junctions, as well as glial fibrillary acidic protein in the astrocyte endfeet.

    e. It is thought that the venous system that drains the fragile capillary network is prone to venous congestion and stasis, which contributes to germinal matrix IVH.

    f. The greatest risk period for IVH is the first three days of life, after which the germinal matrix vessels are believed to become less fragile.

2. Increased risk of the germinal matrix to hypoperfusion injury

    a. The cellular elements of the germinal matrix are rich in mitochondria and metabolically active, making them more susceptible to hypoxic insult.

    b. The vulnerability of the germinal matrix in the first three days is compounded by the physiological instability after birth of a preterm infant.

    c. In the preterm brain, autoregulatory and cerebral vasoreactivity mechanisms are poorly developed. Infants have limited control of cerebral perfusion pressure and CBF during periods of low systemic pressure, and limited protection to cerebral circulation during periods of elevated systemic pressure.

    d. The range of arterial pressures over which a premature infant can maintain autoregulation is narrow and abrupt changes in blood pressure can overwhelm the neonate's ability to protect cerebral circulation.

    e. Poor autoregulatory mechanisms result in a pressure-passive cerebral circulation in which CBF is determined by moment-to-moment changes in systemic blood pressure.

f. Pressure-passiveness is directly correlated with lower gestational age and birth weight and most often identified in medically unstable, ventilated infants.
   g. Physiologic and non-physiologic states, such as sleep cycles, spontaneous movements, positive-pressure ventilation, noxious stimuli, rapid volume infusion, and others may result in rapid fluctuations in CBF and IVH, secondary to alterations in arterial blood pressure.
   h. Alterations in carbon dioxide also disrupt cerebral autoregulation:
      (1) Hypercarbia: vasodilatation
      (2) Hypocarbia: vasoconstriction
3. Exposure to biochemical and mechanical disturbances
   a. Fluctuations in CBF can be related to hypotension, hypoxemia, hypercapnia, acidosis, patent ductus arteriosus, and restlessness. Increases in CBF can cause IVH as well as reperfusion injury after periods of decreased CBF.
   b. Elevations in cerebral venous pressure (CVP) during mechanical ventilation, pneumothorax, and positive-pressure ventilation can cause decreases in cerebral perfusion.
4. Intrinsic disturbance in coagulation
   a. Multiple studies have shown that thrombocytopenia is a risk factor for IVH, but the role of coagulopathy in the pathogenesis of IVH has not been completely elucidated.
   b. Drugs that affect coagulation may also contribute to increased risk for IVH.
5. Genetic predisposition: Conflicting data regarding mutations of hemostasis genes and predisposition to IVH in preterm infants
6. Prenatal hemorrhage
   a. Relatively rare
   b. Maternal risk factors
      (1) Von Willebrand disease
      (2) Anticoagulation therapy
      (3) Cocaine abuse
      (4) Seizures
      (5) Abdominal trauma
      (6) Amniocentesis
      (7) Febrile illness

(8) Chorioamnionitis
  c. Fetal risk factors
    (1) Immune thrombocytopenia
    (2) Congenital tumors
    (3) Clotting factor deficiencies
    (4) Fetomaternal hemorrhage
    (5) Twin-twin transfusion
    (6) Co-twin death
C. Pathogenesis of grade I, II, and III hemorrhages appears to be related to a disruption in autoregulation that leads to a pressure-passive CBF that is determined entirely by blood pressure.
  1. Fluctuation in blood flow results in disruption of the capillary rete in the germinal matrix, resulting in a local hemorrhage.
  2. A germinal matrix hemorrhage can result in local edema and vascular congestion in the region, leading to increasing venous pressure in the terminal vein.
  3. The veins take a very sharp turn where the terminal vein in the germinal matrix and the internal cerebral vein meet. This narrow area is sensitive to high pressure.
  4. Bleeding can extend into the ventricles.
D. Pathogenesis of grade IV hemorrhage appears to be related to anatomical characteristics of the cerebral venous circulation and increased cerebral pressure that results from lower-grade hemorrhage.
  1. Increased cerebral pressure in the region of a germinal matrix hemorrhage results in increased venous pressure within the germinal matrix.
  2. Blood flow is impaired in the medullary veins, which drain the cerebral white matter into the terminal vein.
  3. The increased venous pressure is transmitted in a retrograde direction along the venous drainage of the periventricular white matter.
  4. Increased venous pressure results in a periventricular hemorrhagic infarction (also known as grade IV IVH) with destruction of periventricular white matter.
  5. The hemorrhagic venous infarction tends to be most concentrated near the ventricular angle where the medullary veins drain the cerebral white matter.

III. Incidence

A. Although incidence of IVH in very low birth weight (VLBW) infants (<1,500 g) has declined to 20%–25% from ~40%–50% in the early 1980s, it remains a major complication.

B. In extremely low birth weight (ELBW) infants (<1,000 g), the incidence of IVH increases to ~45%.

C. There are ~12,000 new cases of IVH diagnosed in preterm infants each year in the United States.

D. 10%–15% of VLBW infants suffer from more severe grades of hemorrhage and about three-fourths of these infants suffer from mental retardation and/or cerebral palsy.

E. Overall incidence is inversely related to gestational age.

IV. Diagnosis

A. Timing
   1. Approximately 90% of IVH occurs within the first five postnatal days.
   2. 50% occur within the first day, 25% in the second, and 15% in the third.
   3. Most extensions of a lesion occur 3–5 days after the initial hemorrhage.

B. Clinical presentation
   1. Silent syndrome occurs in 25%–50% of cases and is diagnosed by routine brain sonography.
   2. Saltatory syndrome can evolve over hours or days and is characterized by an altered level of consciousness, hypotonia, and subtle changes in eye movement and positioning.
   3. Catastrophic presentation is the least common and can develop within minutes or hours of injury.
      a. This presentation includes coma or stupor, irregular respirations (apnea/hypoventilation), seizures, or posturing.
      b. Other features include bulging fontanel, hypotension, bradycardia, and anemia. Metabolic acidosis, as well as inappropriate antidiuretic hormone secretion, can occur.

C. Screening
   1. Cranial sonography
      a. Procedure of choice for diagnosis
         (1) High resolution
         (2) Portable
         (3) Non-radiating

- b. Screening guidelines from the American Academy of Neurology and the Practice Committee of Child Neurology Society
  - (1) Routine cranial ultrasound on infants <30 weeks gestational age or <1,500 g
  - (2) Should be performed at 7–14 days and repeated at 36–40 weeks postmenstrual age
 2. Lumbar puncture
    - a. Used if cranial ultrasonography is not available.
    - b. Cerebrospinal fluid (CSF) with IVH typically includes numerous red blood cells and elevated protein levels.
- D. Grading system
  1. Described by Papile
     - a. Grade I IVH: Hemorrhage subependymal and confined to germinal matrix (**Figs. 15-2A** and **15-2B**)
     - b. Grade II IVH: Hemorrhage in lumen of lateral ventricle(s) without ventricular distention (**Fig. 15-3**)
     - c. Grade III IVH: Hemorrhage within lumen of lateral ventricle(s) with dilation of ventricle (**Figs. 15-4A** and **15-4B**)

FIGURE 15-2A
Neonatal Cranial Sonogram

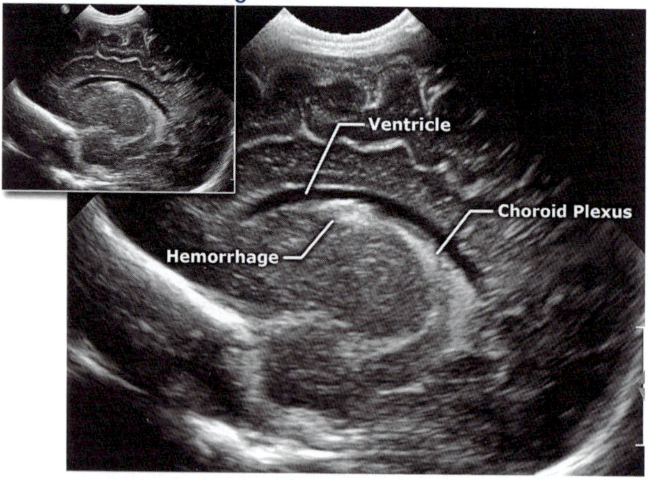

Images courtesy of J. Hill, MD, Department of Radiology and Radiological Science at the Medical University of South Carolina.

Grade I IVH, left sagittal view. Note the hemorrhage is subependymal and confined to the germinal matrix.

d. Grade IV IVH: Combination of blood within lateral ventricle(s) and an echogenic area in periventricular tissue (**Fig. 15-5**)
 2. Modified by Volpe
    a. Grade I IVH: Germinal matrix hemorrhage with no or minimal intraventricular blood (**Figs. 15-2A** and **15-2B**)
    b. Grade II IVH: Hemorrhage with intraventricular blood occupying 10%–50% of ventricular volume (**Fig. 15-3**)
    c. Grade III IVH: Hemorrhage with intraventricular blood occupying >50% of ventricular volume (**Figs. 15-4A** and **15-4B**)
    d. Grade IV IVH: Periventricular hemorrhagic infarction (**Fig. 15-5** and Section VI.A.)

V. Management

A. Treatment of IVH is mostly supportive. Care should be aimed toward preventing further injury, preserving cerebral perfusion, and detecting associated complications.
 1. Maintain blood pressure to preserve cerebral perfusion.

FIGURE 15-2B
Neonatal Cranial Sonogram

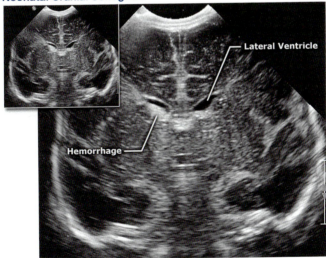

Images courtesy of J. Hill, MD, Department of Radiology and Radiological Science at the Medical University of South Carolina.

Coronal view of grade I IVH.

2. Ensure adequate oxygenation and ventilation.
3. Provide efficient nutritional and fluid support.
4. If seizures present, initiate treatment to avoid impairments of cerebral oxygenation or perfusion.
5. Detect and manage associated complications.

B. Follow-up care is important for outcomes and developmental intervention programs are indicated for patients with IVH.

VI. Associated lesions and complications

A. Periventricular hemorrhagic infarction (PHI)
1. PHI was initially described as an extension of a germinal matrix hemorrhage (GMH). It is now known that PHI is a direct complication, affecting 10%–15% of preterm infants with GMH.
2. PHI is a large region of hemorrhagic necrosis in the periventricular white matter.
3. It is usually unilateral (asymmetrical).
4. PHI occurs when pressure is exerted on the periventricular terminal drain, leading to venous congestion and subsequently causing ischemia and further hemorrhage.

FIGURE 15-3
Neonatal Cranial Sonogram

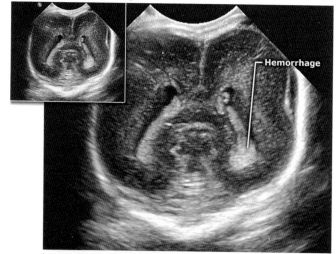

Images courtesy of J. Hill, MD, Department of Radiology and Radiological Science at the Medical University of South Carolina.

Coronal view of grade II IVH. Note the intraventricular blood can occupy 10%–50% of the ventricle (Volpe), but the ventricle is not distended (Papile).

FIGURE 15-4A
Neonatal Cranial Sonogram

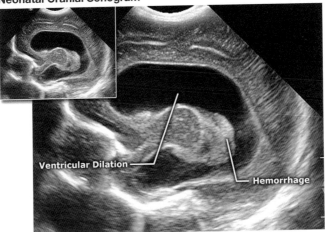

Images courtesy of J. Hill, MD, Department of Radiology and Radiological Science at the Medical University of South Carolina.

Grade III IVH, sagittal view. Note the hemorrhage within the lumen of the lateral ventricle(s) with dilation of the ventricle (Papile).

FIGURE 15-4B
Neonatal Cranial Sonogram

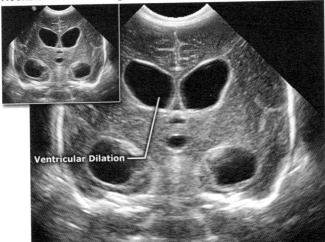

Images courtesy of J. Hill, MD, Department of Radiology and Radiological Science at the Medical University of South Carolina.

Coronal view of grade III IVH, which shows ventricular dilation.

B. Periventricular leukomalacia (PVL)
   1. PVL refers to the necrosis of the white matter in the brain. It has a characteristic distribution and consists of periventricular focal necrosis with cystic formation and more diffuse gliotic cerebral white matter injury. (See **Figs. 15-6, 15-7A, and 15-7B**.)
      a. Non-hemorrhagic
      b. Usually symmetrical (bilateral)
      c. Necrosis of all cellular elements
      d. Watershed injury due to vascular insults

FIGURE 15-5
Neonatal Cranial Sonogram

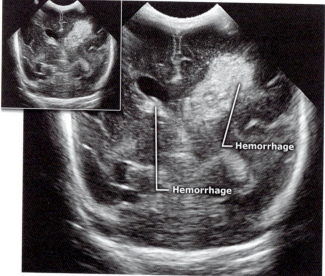

Images courtesy of J. Hill, MD, Department of Radiology and Radiological Science at the Medical University of South Carolina.

Grade IV IVH, coronal view. Note the combination of blood within the lateral ventricle(s) and the echogenic area in the periventricular tissue (Papile). PHI (Volpe) is a large region of hemorrhagic necrosis in the periventricular white matter.

2. While PVL and IVH may occur independently, they can be associated and are often found in the same patients. The association might be related to similarities in pathogenesis and/or the initiation of pathological mechanisms such as perfusion abnormalities and reperfusion injury.
3. PVL has been associated with maternal chorioamnionitis, possibly due to cytokines, inflammatory damage, and perfusion.
4. PVL is associated with increased development of cerebral palsy, intellectual impairment, and visual disturbances.

C. Posthemorrhagic hydrocephalus (PHH)

FIGURE 15-6
Neonatal Cranial Sonogram

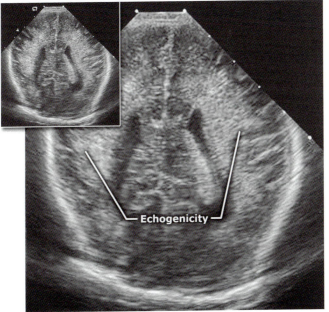

Images courtesy of J. Hill, MD, Department of Radiology and Radiological Science at the Medical University of South Carolina.

Early PVL, which refers to necrosis of the white matter. PVL is usually non-hemorrhagic and symmetrical. Although PVL and IVH may occur independently, they may be associated and found in the same patients.

1. PHH occurs in ~50% of infants with IVH and can present within 1–3 weeks after the initial hemorrhage. It appears to be most common in neonates with severe-grade IVH, found in as many as 75% of infants with grades III or IV IVH.
2. Infants with PHH usually present with rapidly increasing head circumference, ventricular dilatation on ultrasound, and signs of increased intracranial pressure (ICP). Symptoms of PHH may not be evident for weeks after the initial hemorrhage due to brain compliance in the neonate.
3. Effects of PHH are believed to be caused by injury to the periventricular white matter.
4. Communicating PHH is the most common form and is caused by the inability to reabsorb CSF due to inflammation of the subarachnoid villi.
5. Some patients may develop non-communicating hydrocephalus due to an obstruction from a clot or subependymal scarring within the ventricular system.
6. PHH may be non-progressive or resolve spontaneously without intervention.

FIGURE 15-7A
Neonatal Cranial Sonogram

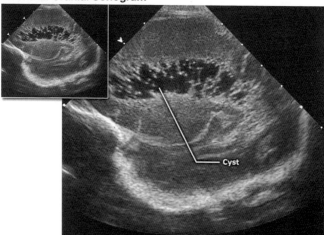

Images courtesy of J. Hill, MD, Department of Radiology and Radiological Science at the Medical University of South Carolina.

Cystic PVL, sagittal view. Periventricular focal necrosis with extensive cyst formation.

7. Some treatment options have significant drawbacks, especially in VLBW infants.
   a. Close surveillance
      (1) Monitor head growth (>2 cm/week).
      (2) Monitor for signs of increasing ICP (agitation, decreased responsiveness, coma).
      (3) Consider neurosurgery consult for infants with rapidly increasing head growth or changes on head ultrasound.
   b. Lumbar and ventricular taps
      (1) Most common short-term therapeutic approach for early stages of slowly progressing, communicating hydrocephalus.
      (2) Drawbacks include procedure failure, which may enhance the risk for clot formations and lead to non-communicating hydrocephalus. There is also a significant rate of infection associated with taps (7%–27%).

FIGURE 15-7B
Neonatal Cranial Sonogram

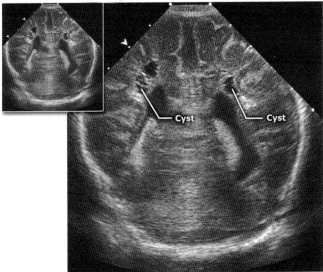

Images courtesy of J. Hill, MD, Department of Radiology and Radiological Science at the Medical University of South Carolina.

Coronal view of cystic PVL with bilateral cyst formation.

(3) Hyponatremia may also occur with the removal of CSF.
c. External ventricular drainage (EVD)
   (1) This involves placement of an intraventricular catheter that is connected to an external drainage system. CSF drainage is adjusted by the level of the external system.
   (2) Associated problems include over-drainage and the possible development of subdural hygromas. EVDs have low infection rates.
   (3) The rate of needing a permanent shunt after an EVD is ~64%–68%.
d. Subcutaneous reservoir (SC)
   (1) This is a temporary treatment. Taps are performed through an SC, thereby preventing the need for ventricular taps with needle tracking and possible further brain injury.
   (2) These reservoirs are accessed as many as 2–3 times per day, depending on the ICP. Drawbacks include the rise of the ICP in between taps. Infection and skin necrosis are ongoing problems.
   (3) Permanent shunting is required in 75%–88% of patients with SC.
e. Ventriculoperitoneal (VP) shunting
   (1) This is the most common long-term treatment of PHH, usually for infants >2 kg.
   (2) There are multiple problems associated with this method of treatment.
      (a) The surgery is complicated and has a high revision rate. Shunts may need to be adjusted or replaced to account for changes in pressures as the child ages.
      (b) Due poor immune systems in preterm infants, the infection rate is ~5%–15%.
      (c) Shunt failure is common due to obstructions caused by increased CSF protein levels.

VII. Outcomes
A. Each year, there are >3,600 new cases of mental retardation related to IVH in the United States, according to data from the U.S. Census Bureau, the NICHD Neonatal Network, and the Centers for Disease Control.
B. Lifetime care costs exceed $3.6 billion for these children.

C. Long-term outcomes are inversely associated with birth weight and gestational age and are correlated with the location, extent, and laterality of the lesion. For example, in IVH associated with PVI, bilateral lesions spanning frontal-temporal-occipital regions carry the worst prognosis. Small, unilateral, frontal, white matter lesions have the best prognosis.
  1. Severe IVH is associated with an increased mortality rate (~20%). Approximately 75% of survivors develop PHH, which increases the mortality rate to 55%.
  2. With mild IVH, mortality rates drop to 5%, with only 7% of infants developing PHH.
  3. 45%–85% of preterm infants with moderate to severe IVH have major cognitive deficits.
  4. 90% of infants with severe IVH and PHI develop neurological sequalae.
  5. Studies have shown an increase in cerebral palsy to 24% in ELBW infants with grade II IVH, vs. 6% in infants who had grade I IVH or no IVH.
D. Major predictors of poor outcome include PVI, cystic PVL, need for VP shunt placement, and shunt infections and revisions.
  1. The mortality rate for infants with PHH requiring VP shunt placement is ~25%. Of these infants, 20% have severe neurological abnormalities, with only ~30% having a normal outcome.
  2. 87% of infants with severe PVL or PVI have major deficits and 75% have impaired cognitive function.
  3. Epilepsy develops in 50% of infants with PVL.

VIII. Prevention
A. Prenatal and delivery-room intervention: Prevention of preterm delivery most effective
  1. Antenatal corticosteroids are known to reduce risk of respiratory distress syndrome (RDS) associated with increased risk for IVH.
     a. Most beneficial with completed course
     b. Protective effect in regard to IVH
  2. Recent studies suggest that administration of magnesium sulfate may have a protective effect against IVH.
  3. Delayed cord clamping increases hematocrit at birth, decreasing the need for transfusions and thereby decreasing the risk for IVH.

B. Postnatal management
 1. Promptly and appropriately resuscitate, avoiding hemodynamic instability or conditions that impair cerebrovascular autoregulation.
    a. Synchronize ventilation.
    b. Limit suctioning.
    c. Prevent pneumothorax.
    d. Maintain neutral head position (midline).
 2. Avoid hypotension or hypertension; if present, correct while avoiding large bolus infusions. Manage fluid carefully.
 3. Avoid metabolic abnormalities.
    a. Hyperosmolality
    b. Hyper/hypoglycemia
    c. Acidosis or alkalosis-bicarbonate therapy associated with increased risk
 4. Correct coagulopathies.
 5. Studies have looked at the use of prophylactic indomethacin to reduce the incidence of IVH. These studies resulted in clear short-term benefits with a decrease in IVH in preterm infants. Although research supports indomethacin for the reduction of IVH, this is not the current standard of care. More research is indicated to identify optimal dosing regimen as well as optimal patient population in regard to gestational age, birth weight, and illness severity.

IX. Conclusion
A. Despite research and developments in medicine, prevention of IVH remains an unsolved problem affecting preterm infants.
B. Careful assessment and observation with timely and appropriate treatment may reduce the long-term effects of IVH.
C. More research is needed to implement therapies that may reduce the incidence of IVH.
D. Infant follow-up clinics and early referrals to intervention programs may also improve neurological and developmental outcomes.

References

Adcock LM. Clinical manifestations and diagnosis of intraventricular hemorrhage in the newborn. UpToDate Web site. http://www.uptodate.com/contents/clinical-manifestations-and-diagnosis-of-intraventricular-hemorrhage-in-the-newborn?source=search_result&search=head+ultrasounds+screening+for+ivh&selectedtitle=2%7E150. Accessed June 1, 2012.

Adcock LM. Management and complications of intraventricular hemorrhage in the newborn. UpToDate Web site. http://www.uptodate.com/contents/management-and-complications-of-intraventricular-hemorrhage-in-the-newborn. Accessed June 1, 2012.

Alcohol's damaging effects on the brain. National Institute on Alcohol Abuse and Alcoholism Web site. http://pubs.niaaa.nih.gov/publications/aa63/aa63.htm. October 2004.

Annibale DJ. Periventricular hemorrhage-intraventricular hemorrhage. Medscape Web site. http://emedicine.medscape.com/article/976654-overview. Accessed June 2012.

Ballabh P. Intraventricular hemorrhage in preterm infants: mechanism of disease. *Pediatr Res.* 2010;67(1):1-8.

Fowlie PW, Davis PG, McGuire W. Prophylactic intravenous indomethacin for preventing mortality and morbidity in preterm infants. *Cochrane Database of Systematic Reviews* 2010, Issue 7. Art. No.: CD000174. DOI: 10.1002/14651858.CD000174.pub2.

Horinek D, Cihar M, Tichy M. Current methods in the treatment of posthemorrhagic hydrocephalus in infants. *Bratisl Lek Listy.* 2003;104(11):347-351.

Lazzara A, Ahmann P, Dykes F, Brann AW Jr, Schwartz J. Clinical predictability of intraventricular hemorrhage in preterm infants. *Pediatrics.* 1980;65(1):30-34.

McCrea HJ, Ment LR. The diagnosis, management and postnatal prevention of intraventricular hemorrhage in the preterm neonate. *Clin Perinatol.* 2008;35(4):777-792.

Robinson S. Neonatal posthemorrhagic hydrocephalus from prematurity: pathophysiology and current treatment concepts. *J Neurosurg Pediatr.* 2012;9(3):242-258.

Roland EH, Hill A. Germinal matrix-intraventricular hemorrhage in the premature newborn: management and outcome. *Neurol Clin.* 2003;21(4):833-851.

Roze E, Kerstjens JM, Maathuis CG, ter Horst HJ, Bos AF. Risk factors for adverse outcome in preterm infants with periventricular hemorrhagic infarction. *Pediatrics.* 2008;122(1):e46-e52.

Shooman D, Portess H, Sparrow O. A review of the current treatment methods for posthemorrhagic hydrocephalus of infants. *Cerebrospinal Fluid Res.* 2009;6(1). http://www.ncbi.nlm.nih.gov/pmc/articles/PMC2642759/#!po=2.17391. January 30, 2009.

Volpe JJ. *Neurology of the Newborn.* 5th ed. Philadelphia, PA: Saunders Elsevier; 2008.

Whitelaw A. Core concepts: intraventricular hemorrhage. *NeoReviews.* 2011;12(2):e94-e101.

16

Hematologic Emergencies

James R. Kiger

I. Red blood cells (RBCs)

A. Normal values
1. Average hematocrit (Hct) varies between 40% and 50%, depending on estimated gestational age.
   a. Average hemoglobin (Hgb) is between 14 and 20 g/dL.
2. Preterm infants have a lower average Hct vs. term infants, with infants <28 weeks having an average Hct ~10% lower than term infants.

B. Anemia
1. Signs
   a. Infants who are born or become severely anemic shortly after birth develop signs of distress, including pallor, hypotension, tachycardia, and tachypnea. In the most severe cases, infants are in florid hypovolemic shock.
   b. Normal neonatal respiratory resuscitation will not correct the above signs.
   c. Cyanosis is not observed from anemia alone.
2. Causes
   a. Hemorrhage
      (1) Placental abruption (**Fig. 16-1**)
         (a) Blood loss from premature placental separation is usually from the maternal side of the placenta.
         (b) Incidence is ~1% of births.
         (c) Vaginal bleeding is a poor predictor of blood loss or potential for fetal compromise.
      (2) Vasa previa, placenta previa, or surgical incision of the placenta may cause fetal blood loss (FBL) with placental abruption.
      (3) Fetomaternal hemorrhage (FMH)
         (a) Large-volume blood loss from the fetal to maternal circulation through defects in the placental trophoblast.

(b) Usually, the etiology of the placental defect that leads to passage of fetal blood is unclear. Specific placental pathology, such as intraplacental choriocarcinoma, has been reported in association with massive FMH.
(c) FBL of 30 mL is considered significant FMH; massive FMH may have blood loss of ≥150 mL.
(d) The incidence of significant FMH is ~3 in 1,000 live births, with massive FMH occurring in ~0.2 in 1,000 live births.
(e) The Kleihauer-Betke (KB) test may be performed on the mother following delivery.
  i. The KB test is an assessment of the percentage of erythrocytes in maternal circulation that carry hemoglobin F.
  ii. Approximate FBL may be calculated from the KB value for the percentage of fetal blood cells in maternal circulation, the maternal blood volume (MBV), and the maternal and fetal Hcts:
  $$FBL = (Hct_{mat}/Hct_{fet}) \times (MBV) \times (\% \text{ fetal cells})$$

FIGURE 16-1
Placental Abruption

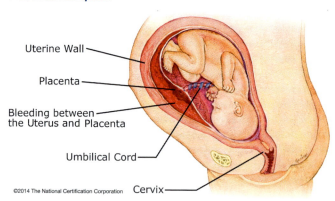

Blood loss from premature placental separation is usually from the maternal side of the placenta. Vasa previa, placenta previa, or surgical incision of the placenta may cause FBL with placental abruption.

(4) Umbilical cord hemorrhage
   (a) Umbilical cord rupture can cause significant acute FBL.
(5) Penetrating trauma to placenta

b. Twin-twin transfusion syndrome (**Fig. 16-2**)
   (1) May occur in monochorionic twin pregnancies (either diamniotic or monoamniotic).
   (2) Unbalanced blood flow through placental anastomoses between the infants' circulations results in one twin receiving less umbilical blood flow (the donor twin) and the other receiving increased umbilical blood flow (the recipient twin).
   (3) Prevalent in 10%–15% of monochorionic pregnancies.
   (4) Treatment options include fetoscopic laser ablation of placental anastomoses to reduce unbalanced blood flow.
   (5) Fetal/neonatal consequences:
      (a) Extremely high mortality, especially for cases with onset in the first trimester

FIGURE 16-2
Twin-Twin Transfusion Syndrome

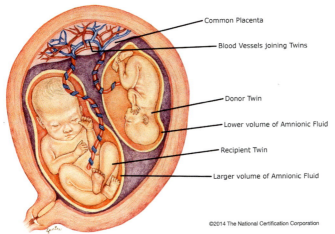

©2014 The National Certification Corporation

Twin-twin transfusion syndrome may occur in monochorionic twin pregnancies, either diamniotic or monoamniotic. Unbalanced blood flow through placental anastomoses between the infants' circulations results in the donor twin receiving less umbilical blood flow and the recipient twin receiving increased blood flow.

- (b) Growth discordance
- (c) Polyhdramnios in recipient fetus, oligohydramnios in donor fetus
- (d) Polycythemia in recipient fetus (see Section I.C.2.)
- (e) Anemia in donor fetus
    - i. Suggested prenatally by increased middle cerebral artery Doppler flow velocities on ultrasound
    - ii. Donor twin may be profoundly anemic (Hgb level as low as 4.5 g/dL)
- c. Hemolysis
    - (1) Immune mediated hemolysis
        - (a) Maternal antibodies to antigens on fetal RBCs transported across the placenta
        - (b) Requires maternal sensitization to fetal antigens the mother does not possess (e.g., the antigens are paternally derived) due to FMH during the current pregnancy or a prior pregnancy or abortion
        - (c) Rh incompatibility
            - i. Two genes encode Rh antigens.
                1) One encodes RhC/c and RhE/e, which are isoforms of specific RBC membrane proteins.
                2) The other encodes the RhD protein. RhD and Rhd indicate the presence or absence of the D antigen protein, respectively. This is the most important protein for immune mediated hemolysis.
                3) Rh-negative status signifies the absence of the RhD protein, resulting from a deletion of the encoding gene on both chromosomes. Rh-positive status signifies the presence of this protein on the RBC membrane.
                4) Rh-negative status varies across populations; ~15% of Caucasians and 5% of African Americans are Rh negative.

ii. Mothers are given Rh immunoglobulin following delivery, spontaneous or therapeutic abortion, or after significant hemorrhage during pregnancy to reduce risk of maternal sensitization to Rh antigen.
iii. Percutaneous umbilical cord blood sampling may be used when hydrops develops during the pregnancy to determine the degree of fetal anemia and to administer blood transfusions.
iv. Clinical presentation of hemolysis in a newborn due to Rh alloimmunization:
1) Positive direct Coombs test (direct antiglobulin test) indicating presence of maternal antibody attached to infant RBCs
2) Mild to severe anemia
3) Stillbirth or hydrops fetalis (due to high-output cardiac failure), in severe cases
4) Hyperbilirubinemia, which may require phototherapy or double-volume exchange transfusion
5) Liver dysfunction
6) Occasionally, leukemoid reaction or thrombocytopenia of unknown etiology

(d) ABO incompatibility
  i. Mediated by maternal antibodies against fetal A or B antigens
   1) Hemolytic disease is mostly limited to type O mothers, as the anti-A and anti-B antibody types produced are mostly immunoglobulin G (IgG), which may cross the placenta.
   2) In contrast, mothers who are type A or type B produce immunoglobulin M (IgM) anti-B antibodies, which will not cross the placenta.
  ii. This may occur during the first pregnancy, e.g., it does not require sensitization as Rh-mediated disease does.

iii. This is usually a milder degree of hemolysis than Rh-mediated disease, but may still be severe enough to cause hydrops.
iv. Clinical presentation
1) Direct Coombs test often negative, as fetal RBCs express fewer type-specific A and B antigens
2) Indirect Coombs test sometimes positive, indicating presence of type-specific antibodies in the serum
3) Spherocytes seen on peripheral blood smear, due to removal of parts of the RBC membrane in the spleen
4) Mild to moderate anemia
5) Hyperbilirubinemia

(e) Minor blood group incompatibility
  i. Kell and Rhc antibodies may cause severe hemolytic disease.
  ii. Kidd and Duffy antibodies have been associated with mild hemolytic disease.
  iii. Positive direct Coombs test in the absence of ABO or Rh incompatibility is suggestive of minor blood group incompatibility.

(f) Treatment of hyperbilirubinemia due to hemolysis
  i. Phototherapy
     1) The American Academy of Pediatrics (AAP) has published guidelines for the level of hyperbilirubinemia that requires phototherapy.
     2) Expose as much skin as possible with diaper off.
     3) Irradiate at least 30 microWatts/cm^2/nm.
  ii. Double-volume exchange transfusion
     1) The AAP has published guidelines for the level of hyperbilirubinemia that requires double-volume exchange transfusion.
     2) Preterm infant (100 mL/kg x 2, or 200 mL/kg)

iii. Intravenous immunoglobulin (IVIG)
 1) The utility of IVIG for Rh-mediated disease is controversial; studies have shown conflicting results.
 2) IVIG has been associated with increased incidence of necrotizing enterocolitis.
(2) RBC defects
 (a) Membrane defects
  i. Spherocytosis and elliptocytosis
   1) Defects in the RBC cytoskeleton increase fragility and risk for hemolysis.
   2) Both defects are usually inherited in an autosomal dominant fashion.
   3) Diagnosis is by blood smear.
   4) 50% of cases will manifest hemolysis with the presence of anemia, splenomegaly, and hyperbilirubinemia in the newborn period.
   5) Spherocytosis is the most common hereditary hemolytic anemia.
  ii. Glucose-6-phosphate dehydrogenase (G6PD) deficiency
   1) X-linked enzyme defect
   2) Common in populations from the Mediterranean, Asia, and Africa
   3) Reduced ability of RBC to neutralize oxidative stress
   4) Hemolysis provoked by exposure to certain drugs or infection
   5) Diagnosis made by RBC G6PD activity or by G6PD gene test
   6) Bilirubin should be monitored closely and infant should be treated with phototherapy or exchange transfusion as required
(3) Infection
 (a) Certain viral or bacterial infections may increase the risk for hemolysis.
  i. Sepsis (bacterial)
  ii. Cytomegalovirus
  iii. Toxoplasmosis
(4) Disseminated intravascular coagulation (DIC)

- (a) Anemia associated with coagulopathy and thrombocytopenia
- (b) Treat symptomatic anemia and underlying condition
  d. Hypoplastic anemia
   (1) Suggested by anemia with low reticulocyte count
   (2) Infection
   - (a) Parvovirus infection in a fetus can lead to aplastic anemia.
   - (b) Severe cases can cause hydrops.
   (3) Congenital hypoplastic anemia (Diamond-Blackfan)
   - (a) Mostly sporadic cases
   - (b) Congenital absence of erythroblast stem cells in bone marrow
   - (c) May present as profound anemia at birth

C. Polycythemia
  1. Definition
     a. Hct ≥65% from a freely flowing venous sample
     b. Capillary Hct often overestimates central venous Hct
     c. Hct the most important factor affecting viscosity of blood in a neonate
  2. Clinical presentation
     a. Plethora
     b. Hypoglycemia
     c. Hypocalcemia
     d. Irritability or lethargy
     e. Poor feeding
     f. Decreased urine output
     g. Respiratory distress, tachypnea
     h. Stroke, in rare cases
  3. Causes
     a. Twin-twin transfusion
        (1) See Section I.B.2.b.
        (2) Recipient twin may have significantly elevated Hct.
     b. Chronic fetal hypoxia
        (1) Increased erythropoietin in fetus
        (2) Maternal diabetes
        (3) Maternal tobacco use
        (4) Placental insufficiency
           (a) Preeclampsia

(b) Chronic abruption
- (5) Intrauterine growth restriction or small for gestational age infant
  c. Cord stripping or delayed cord clamping
     (1) Extra bolus of blood delivered to infant prior to clamping
  d. Syndromes
     (1) Trisomy 13, 18, 21
     (2) Beckwith-Wiedemann syndrome
  e. Neonatal thyrotoxicosis
4. Management
   a. Indicated if venous Hct is >70% or ≥65% with symptoms attributable to polycythemia (see Section I.C.3.b).
   b. Partial exchange transfusion
      (1) Goal is to reduce Hct to 50%–55%.
      (2) Isotonic crystalloid solution replacement (normal saline) is as effective as fresh frozen plasma or other colloid solution.
      (3) Replacement volume is calculated by:

      $$[(\text{Current Hct} - \text{Goal Hct})/\text{Current Hct}] \times \text{Weight} \times (80 \text{ mL/kg})$$

      (4) Volume is replaced in aliquots of 5–10 mL, preferably through umbilical venous/arterial access.

II. White blood cells

A. Normal values
1. Term infants have higher neutrophil counts than preterm infants.
2. In term infants at birth, the 5th–95th percentiles for neutrophil count are ~4,000–17,000/µL.
3. For preterm infants (28–36 weeks estimated gestational age at birth), the 5th–95th percentiles are ~1,000–10,000/µL.
4. Neutrophil counts rise over the first seven days of life, then gradually fall off again.

B. Neutropenia
1. Neutropenia occurs in 6%–8% of hospitalized patients in the NICU.
2. Neutropenia in the absence of signs of sepsis has not been shown to predispose the infant to an infection.
3. Causes

a. Maternal hypertension or preeclampsia
   (1) Thought to be due to a released inhibitory factor from the placenta.
b. Anemia
   (1) Bone marrow is pushed to make erythroid line cells.
c. Congenital conditions
   (1) Kostmann syndrome
      (a) Autosomal recessive disorder with very low absolute neutrophil counts (<500/μL)
   (2) Schwachman-Diamond syndrome
      (a) Dwarfism, pancreatic insufficiency, and neutropenia
   (3) Severe combined immunodeficiency
d. Alloimmune neonatal neutropenia
   (1) Maternal IgG antibodies to a fetal neutrophil antigen
   (2) Most common antigens NA1 and NA2
e. Infection
   (1) Bacterial sepsis
   (2) Fungal sepsis
   (3) Cytomegalovirus infection
4. Therapy
   a. Significant neutropenia may indicate sepsis; evaluate infants according to clinical presentation
   b. Granulocyte-colony stimulating factor (G-CSF) and granulocyte-macrophage colony-stimulating factor (GM-CSF)
      (1) Administration of G-CSF or GM-CSF will cause a significant increase in absolute neutrophil count (ANC).
      (2) Human studies have not conclusively shown that either G-CSF or GM-CSF reduce the chance of infection when given prophylactically, or increase odds of survival when given to infants with presumed infection.
C. Leukocytosis/neutrophilia
   1. Increased neutrophil production
      a. Bacterial or fungal sepsis
      b. Leukemoid reaction (with increased blast and immature forms)
         (1) Trisomy 21
      c. Neonatal leukemia

(1) Acute myelocytic leukemia (AML)
(2) Associated with trisomy 21
(3) Leukemia associated with trisomy 21 may be self-limited and self-resolving, or may be lethal
2. Increased release from bone marrow
   a. Corticosteroid therapies
3. Therapies
   a. Leukocytosis may be a harbinger of infection; evaluate for sepsis if appropriate to the clinical presentation.
   b. Significant leukocytosis (>100,000/μL) may increase blood viscosity.
      (1) Partial exchange transfusion has been suggested, but is not of proven benefit.
      (2) Consultation with hematology specialist is warranted.

III. Platelets

A. Normal values
   1. Infants have lower mean platelet counts than adults. The adult standard of 150,000 platelets/μL is not accurate to indicate thrombocytopenia in neonates.
   2. The 5th–95th percentiles for platelet count for newborns is between ~100,000/μL and 350,000/μL.
   3. Term infants have slightly higher average platelet counts than preterm infants.
   4. Average platelet count at birth ranges from 200,000/μL for 23- to 24-week infants to 250,000/μL for term infants.

B. Thrombocytopenia
   1. Definition
      a. Mild: 100–150 x 10^9/L
      b. Moderate: 50–99 x 10^9/L
      c. Severe: <50 x 10^9/L
   2. Causes
      a. Bacterial or fungal sepsis
         (1) Should always be considered when etiology unknown
      b. Necrotizing enterocolitis
      c. Asphyxia with total body cooling
      d. Thrombosis
      e. Maternal hypertension or preeclampsia
         (1) Frequently with neutropenia
      f. Placental insufficiency
         (1) Often a transient, mild thrombocytopenia

(2) Consider infectious causes if thrombocytopenia does not resolve
g. Consumptive
   (1) Disseminated intravascular coagulation
   (2) Giant hemangioma (Kasabach-Merritt syndrome)
      (a) Platelets and fibrinogen are consumed in coagulation occurring in hemangiomas.
h. Syndromes
   (1) Trisomy 13, 18, 21
i. Immune mediated
   (1) Neonatal alloimmune thrombocytopenia (NAIT)
      (a) Isolated, early onset, profound thrombocytopenia in an otherwise healthy infant
         i. May see diffuse petechiae, bruising, hemorrhage, and jaundice
         ii. Platelet count of 20,000–50,000/μL in the first day of life.
      (b) Maternal IgG antibodies directed against paternally derived antigen on fetal platelets
      (c) HPA-1a most common targeted antigen
      (d) Diagnosis
         i. DNA platelet typing to determine paternal inheritance of antigen
         ii. Blood from the mother and father for confirmatory testing
         iii. Testing for anti-platelet antibody in maternal serum
      (e) Management
         i. IVIG should be given
         ii. Platelet transfusion if infant platelet count <30,000/μL or there is active bleeding
         iii. Initial treatment with 10mL/kg transfusion of platelets if diagnosis unknown (marked platelet response seen in 1 hour in absence of disease)
         iv. Maternal platelets preferable if diagnosis made before delivery, will not react with maternal antibody in infant's blood
      (f) Requires communication with mother and obstetrician about risk of recurrence/fetal morbidity in future pregnancies
   (2) Autoimmune neonatal thrombocytopenia

                (a) Maternal autoantibodies due to a maternal history of idiopathic thrombocytopenic purpura (ITP)
                (b) Milder course than NAIT
                (c) Presents in first 72 hours of life
                (d) Platelet transfusions of limited effectiveness
    3. Management
        a. Laboratory evaluation for thrombocytopenia of unknown origin
            (1) Sepsis evaluation
            (2) Evaluation for disseminated intravascular coagulation
            (3) Evaluation for other blood cell lines
            (4) Inborn errors of metabolism
            (5) Thrombosis
        b. Therapies
            (1) Platelet transfusion
                (a) Leukocyte depleted, cytomegalovirus negative
                (b) Usually 15–20 mL/kg of body weight per transfusion
                (c) Have been associated with transfusion-associated lung injury (TRALI)
                    i. Bilateral pulmonary infiltrates and hypoxemia occurring within 6 hours of transfusion

IV. Bleeding disorders seen in neonates
   A. Inherited coagulation disorders
      1. Factor VIII deficiency (hemophilia A) and factor IX deficiency (hemophilia B)
         a. X-linked diseases
         b. May present with bleeding
      2. Bleeding from umbilicus and after circumcision common presentations
      3. Factor V, VII, X, and von Willebrand factor deficiencies
   B. Acquired coagulation disorders
      1. Hemorrhagic disease of the newborn (vitamin K deficiency)
         a. Early presentation
            (1) First 24 hours of life
            (2) Presents with significant bleeding: intracranial hemorrhage, intra-abdominal bleeding, bleeding at venipuncture or intramuscular injection sites

(3) Linked to maternal use of anti-vitamin K drugs (warfarin, anti-epileptics, etc.)
  b. Classic presentation
    (1) First 2–7 days of life
    (2) More common in breast-fed infants (greater vitamin K concentration in formula than in breast milk)
    (3) Bleeding from umbilical stump, gastrointestinal tract, and venipuncture sites common presentations
    (4) Intracranial hemorrhage rare
  c. Late presentation
    (1) Weeks 2–8 of life
    (2) May present with bruising, gastrointestinal bleeding, intracranial hemorrhage
    (3) Associated with liver disease
    (4) More common in breast-fed infants
  d. Prophylaxis
    (1) Vitamin K given shortly after birth:
      (a) 1 mg intramuscular dose
      (b) 2–4 mg oral dose
    (2) Intramuscular administration prevents nearly all cases of hemorrhagic disease.
    (3) Oral dose is effective at preventing classic hemorrhagic disease, but is of unknown efficacy in preventing late-onset hemorrhagic disease.
C. Secondary coagulopathy
  1. Consumptive
    a. Disseminated intravascular coagulation
    b. Kasabach-Merritt syndrome
    c. Intracranial hemorrhage
  2. Sepsis
  3. Acidosis
  4. Liver dysfunction or injury
  5. Hypothermia (therapeutic or accidental)
  6. Thrombocytopenia (see Section III.B.)
  7. Hypoxic–ischemic injury

References

American Academy of Pediatrics Subcommittee on Hyperbilirubinemia. Management of hyperbilirubinemia in the newborn infant 35 or more weeks of gestation. *Pediatrics*. 2004;114(1):297-316.

Bhutani VK, Committee on Fetus and Newborn, American Academy of Pediatrics. Phototherapy to prevent severe neonatal hyperbilirubinemia in the newborn infant 35 or more weeks of gestation. *Pediatrics*. 2011;128(4):e1046-e1052.

Christensen RD, Henry E, Jopling J, Wiedmeier SE. The CBC: reference ranges for neonates. *Semin Perinatol*. 2009;33(1):3-11.

de Alarcon PA, Werner EJ, Christensen RD, eds. *Neonatal Hematology: Pathogenesis, Diagnosis, and Management of Hematologic Problems*. 2nd ed. Cambridge, England: Cambridge University Press; 2013.

Figueras-Aloy J, Rodriguez-Miguelez JM, Iriondo-Sanz M, Salvia-Roiges MD, Botet-Mussons F, Carbonell-Estrany X. Intravenous immunoglobulin and necrotizing enterocolitis in newborns with hemolytic disease. *Pediatrics*. 2010;125(1):139-144.

Gabbe SG, Niebyl JR, Simpson JL, et al. *Obstetrics: Normal and Problem Pregnancies*. 6th ed. Philadelphia, PA: Saunders Elsevier; 2012.

Gleason CA, Devaskar S, eds. *Avery's Diseases of the Newborn*. 9th ed. Philadelphia, PA: Saunders Elsevier; 2012.

Gottstein R, Cooke RW. Systematic review of intravenous immunoglobulin in haemolytic disease of the newborn. *Arch Dis Child Fetal Neonatal Ed*. 2003;88(1):F6-10.

Isaacs H, Jr. Fetal and neonatal leukemia. *J Pediatr Hematol Oncol*. 2003;25(5):348-361.

Koike Y, Wakamatsu H, Kuroki Y, Isozaki A, Ishii S, Fujitsuka S. Fetomaternal hemorrhage caused by intraplacental choriocarcinoma: a case report and review of literature in Japan. *Am J Perinatol*. 2006;23(1):49-52.

Lopriore E, Slaghekke F, Oepkes D, Middeldorp JM, Vandenbussche FP, Walther FJ. Hematological characteristics in neonates with twin anemia-polycythemia sequence (TAPS). *Prenat Diagn*. 2010;30(3):251-255.

Nittala S, Subbarao GC, Maheshwari A. Evaluation of neutropenia and neutrophilia in preterm infants. *J Matern Fetal Neonatal Med*. 2012;25(suppl 5):100-103.

Pappas A, Delaney-Black V. Differential diagnosis and management of polycythemia. *Pediatr Clin North Am*. 2004;51(4):1063-1086, x-xi.

Sarkar S, Rosenkrantz TS. Neonatal polycythemia and hyperviscosity. *Semin Fetal Neonatal Med*. 2008;13(4):248-255.

Smits-Wintjens VE, Walther FJ, Rath ME, et al. Intravenous immunoglobulin in neonates with rhesus hemolytic disease: a randomized controlled trial. *Pediatrics*. 2011;127(4):680-686.

WAPM Consensus Group on Twin-to-Twin Transfusion, Baschat A, Chmait RH, Deprest J, et al. Twin-to-twin transfusion syndrome (TTTS). *J Perinat Med*. 2011;39(2):107-112.

Wylie BJ, D'Alton ME. Fetomaternal hemorrhage. *Obstet Gynecol*. 2010;115(5):1039-1051.

17

Surgical Emergencies: Abdominal Wall Defects

Robin L. Bissinger and Ellen Tappero

I. Introduction
A. The most common defects in very low birth weight (VLBW) infants are abdominal wall defects.
B. Diagnosis is often made by fetal ultrasound, otherwise at birth.

II. Omphalocele (Fig. 17-1)
A. Overview
1. Embryologic defect caused by failure of the intestine to return to the abdominal cavity during the eleventh week of gestation
2. Translucent membrane covers the herniated sac, which is part of the umbilical cord
B. Incidence
1. Approximately 1 in 5,000 to 1 in 7,000 live births
2. 30%–50% have associated chromosomal anomalies or other structural defects
   a. Trisomy 12, 13, 18, or Turner syndrome

FIGURE 17-1
Omphalocele

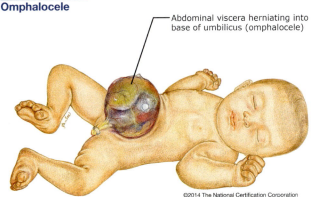

©2014 The National Certification Corporation

Omphalocele is an embryologic defect caused by failure of the intestine to return to the abdominal cavity. If the omphalocele is intact, the infant is not usually in distress, unless associated pulmonary hypoplasia is present. Infants with giant omphaloceles (>5 cm in size with liver involvement) are at higher risk for respiratory distress due to lung hypoplasia. If omphalocele is ruptured, treat the same way as gastroschisis.

- b. Beckwith-Wiedemann syndrome
- c. Congenital heart disease
- d. Malrotation and/or intestinal atresia
- e. Genitourinary anomalies: bladder exstrophy
- f. Pentalogy of Cantrell
3. Most common in males
4. 33% will be born premature
5. Mortality depends on size and severity of defects
6. Approximately 30% of cases isolated without heart disease

C. Physical characteristics
1. Prenatal ultrasounds often identify omphaloceles before birth.
2. Defects appear at birth as a herniation into the base of the umbilical cord.
3. Omphaloceles differ in size; large defects may contain stomach, liver, spleen, and intestines.
4. Small defects may not be readily apparent and appear as a fat umbilical cord.
5. If umbilical cord is unusual or any question of a small herniation exists, clamp cord well away from the base and the suspected defect.
6. The defect is usually covered with a transparent sac.
   a. At birth, the appearance of a herniated bowel is normal unless the sac is ruptured.
   b. Sac may rupture before or at the time of delivery, exposing the contents to amniotic fluid and causing the bowel to appear edematous.
   c. Even if ruptured, the remnants of the sac will usually be visible.

D. Immediate management
1. Neonates with intact omphaloceles are usually not in distress unless associated pulmonary hypoplasia is present.
   a. Infants with giant omphaloceles (>5 cm in size with the liver) are at higher risk for respiratory distress due to lung hypoplasia.
   b. Consider intubation since bag mask ventilation can cause distention of the intestines.
2. At birth, carefully examine the infant to detect any associated problems, such as Beckwith-Wiedemann syndrome, chromosomal abnormalities, congenital heart disease, or other malformations.
3. Immediately after delivery, cover defect with a waterproof barrier, such as a bowel bag or plastic wrap.

    a. Avoid moist gauze dressings; they quickly become cold and can lead to hypothermia.
    b. If moist dressings are used, place loosely around defect and ensure warmth is maintained.
 4. These infants often have latex allergies, so ensure all products are latex-free.
 5. Observe for vascular compromise of the bowel.
 6. Position infant on side or support defect with a small roll to avoid positional-related pressure or trauma to the defect.
 7. Handle bowel minimally.
 8. Place a large-caliber suction catheter to decompress the intestines; decompression facilitates bowel reduction.
 9. Obtain genetics consult to examine infant for other defects and signs of chromosomal abnormalities.
 10. In nursery, use echocardiogram to rule out congenital heart disease.
 11. Immediate surgical evaluation is necessary for decisions about primary or staged repair.
 12. Neonatologists and pediatric surgeons share responsibility for management.
 13. Consultation with cardiologist, pulmonologist, and gastroenterologist may be indicated.
 14. Fluid management is a challenge due to insensible water losses; may need 2–3 times maintenance fluids.
 15. Administer prophylactic, broad-spectrum antibiotics.
 16. Repair can be primary or staged if the defect is large.
 17. Treat ruptured omphalocele the same way as gastroschisis.

III. Gastroschisis (Fig. 17-2)
 A. Overview
   1. Herniation of abdominal contents through a defect in the abdominal wall; lateral and usually to the right of the umbilical cord insertion
   2. Thought to occur by 6–10 weeks after gestation
   3. Theories of causes
      a. Failure of embryonic-disk infolding during third week of development
      b. No herniation of umbilical cord; intestines rupture through the abdominal cavity
      c. Vascular accident leaves cord necrotic at base, allowing an opening for intestinal evisceration

4. Isolated structural anomaly; no single definitive genetic or environmental cause identified

B. Incidence
1. Occurs in 1 in 2,000 to 1 in 5,000 live births, with increasing incidence.
2. 50%–60% are associated with prematurity and low birth weights, secondary to *in utero* growth restriction.
3. Young maternal age, primigravida status, and low socioeconomic level are associated with increasing prevalence.
4. Alcohol, recreational drugs, and smoking may increase risk.
5. Isolated defect without associated chromosomal abnormalities.
6. 10%–15% may have associated anomalies such as intestinal malrotation and atresia.
7. Mortality rate is <5%.

C. Physical characteristics
1. Easily identified at birth; diagnosed prenatally using ultrasonography
2. Full thickness defect of the abdominal wall
   a. Usually includes the small and large intestines, rarely the liver
   b. Abdominal cavity small and underdeveloped
3. Umbilical cord intact, not part of defect
   a. Inserted normally

FIGURE 17-2
Gastroschisis

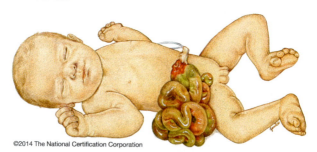

©2014 The National Certification Corporation

Gastroschisis, herniation of abdominal contents through a defect in the abdominal wall, is an isolated structural anomaly. Manage respiratory distress first. Minimize losses of fluids, electrolytes, and heat. Place the infant in a right side-lying position or support defect with a small roll. Handle bowel minimally. Immediate surgical evaluation is necessary.

b. Defect usually a 2- to 4-cm opening to the right of the umbilicus
4. No protective sac
   a. Defect is uncovered.
   b. Amniotic fluid exposure may cause peritonitis.
   c. Bowel may appear edematous, thickened, and inflamed at birth, rather than as distinguishable loops, from prolonged exposure to amniotic fluid.
   d. Intestinal stenosis or atresia, matted bowel, and decreased or no bowel sounds may be found.

D. Delivery
   1. Timing should be based on fetal well-being.
   2. Mode of delivery remains controversial.

E. Immediate management
   1. Respiratory distress must be managed first.
      a. Intubation may be indicated; prevent abdominal distention caused by bag mask ventilation.
      b. Place a large-caliber suction catheter to suction for gastric decompression.
   2. Fluid, electrolyte, and heat losses must be minimized and corrected to prevent hypotension, hypovolemia, hypothermia, and hypoglycemia.
      a. Neutral thermal environment is critical.
      b. Establish vascular access.
   3. Because of significant fluid losses with open abdominal wall defect, IV fluids should be administered as soon as possible.
      a. May take 2–3 times maintenance due to large insensible water losses through the defect, third-spacing of fluid into the exposed bowel, and water loss through the premature skin.
         (1) Maintenance fluids at birth are usually 80–100 mL/kg/day, based on environment.
         (2) These infants can require 160–240 mL/kg/day or higher if water loss is not controlled.
   4. The defect should be covered with a waterproof barrier, such as a bowel bag or plastic wrap, immediately following delivery.
      a. Moist gauze dressings should be avoided since they quickly become cold and can lead to hypothermia.
      b. If utilized, place loosely around the lower abdomen and ensure warmth is maintained.

c. Clear plastic allows for ongoing visualization of the bowel to assess blood supply and perfusion.
5. Observe for vascular compromise of the bowel and place the infant in a right side-lying position or support defect with a small roll to avoid positional-related pressure or trauma to the defect.
   a. Prevent mesenteric artery kinking.
   b. When the bowel drapes to the side in a supine position, there is risk of bowel necrosis.
6. Handle bowel minimally.
7. Examine infant for other defects.
8. Monitor urine output closely to assess fluid balance; consider insertion of urinary catheter per unit guidelines.
9. Administer broad-spectrum antibiotics to prevent contamination of the peritoneal cavity.
10. Immediate surgical evaluation is necessary for a decision on the need for primary or staged repair; in staged repairs, a silo will be placed, allowing for serial reduction over 7–10 days.
11. Neonatologists and pediatric surgeons share responsibility for management.
12. Consultation with a pulmonologist and gastroenterologist may be indicated.

IV. Bladder exstrophy
A. Overview
   1. Malformation of the urinary, genital, and musculoskeletal system
   2. Bladder comes through an abdominal defect; pubis symphysis is widely spaced
      a. Growth failure in lower abdominal wall
      b. Umbilicus in a lower position
   3. Pathophysiology unknown
   4. Timing of rupture leads to the type of defect
      a. Early defect: cloacal exstrophy
         (1) Bladder and large intestines exposed
         (2) Anal, genital, and colon abnormalities
         (3) 88%–100% have omphaloceles
         (4) Widely spaced pubic bones
         (5) Usually involves hip dislocation
      b. Late defect: epispadias, abnormal dorsal urethral location

B. Incidence
   1. Increased risk in males, Caucasians, and with maternal smoking, use of alcohol and drugs, and lower maternal age.
   2. Rare: 1 in 40,000 live births
   3. Cloacal exstrophy the least common; occurs in 0.5 in 200,000 to 1 in 200,000 live births.
C. Physical characteristics
   1. Bladder is outside the abdomen as well as the posterior urethra
   2. Widened pubis symphysis
   3. Umbilicus always below the iliac crest
   4. Hip dislocation associated with cloacal exstrophy
   5. Assess for neural tube defects, omphaloceles, imperforate anus, and limb anomalies; can be part of a syndrome
   6. Inguinal hernias common, 81% in males
   7. Assess further for horseshoe kidneys, ureteral ectopy, ureteroceles, megaureters, and ureteropelvic obstruction
   8. Vesicoureteral reflux found in all patients
   9. Epispadias often seen
   10. Short, dorsally curved penis
   11. In females, vaginal orifice is stenotic and clitoris is bifid
D. Immediate management
   1. Do not clamp the umbilical cord; utilize umbilical tape to prevent bladder trauma and tie off high.
   2. Keep bladder moist, covered, and in plastic wrap or bowel bag.
   3. Ultrasound of both kidneys is needed.
   4. Abdominal x-ray and measurement of the pubis is needed.
   5. Start antibiotic therapy after delivery and continue through the early postoperative period.
   6. Surgical consult is necessary for staged or complete repair based on the extent of the defect.
   7. Monitor renal function closely.
      a. Strict intake and output
      b. Electrolytes
   8. Examine infant for other defects.
   9. Reconstructive surgery will be required.

References

Baradaran N, Gearhart JP. Bladder exstrophy-epispadias-cloacal exstrophy complex: a contemporary overview. *NeoReviews*. 2010;11(12):705-713.

Barksdake EM, Chwals WJ, Magnuson DK, Parry RL. Selected gastrointestinal anomalies. In: Martin RJ, Fanaroff AA, Walsh MC. *Fanaroff and Martin's Neonatal-Perinatal Medicine: Diseases of the Fetus and Infant.* 9th ed. St. Louis, MO: Mosby Elsevier; 2011:1408-1412.

Chabra S. Management of gastroschisis: prenatal, perinatal, and neonatal. *NeoReviews*. 2006;7(8):419-427.

Chabra S, Gleason CA. Gastroschisis: embryology, pathogenesis, epidemiology. *NeoReviews*. 2005;6(11):e493-e499.

Colby CE, Carey WA, Blumenfeld YJ, Hintz SR. Infants with prenatally diagnosed anomalies: special approaches to preparation and resuscitation. *Clin Perinatol*. 2012;39(4):871-887.

Glasser JG. Pediatric omphalocele and gastroschisis. Medscape Reference Web site. http://emedicine.medscape.com/article/975583-overview. Updated May 8, 2013. Accessed June 2013.

Ledbetter DJ. Gastroschisis and omphalocele. *Surg Clin North Am*. 2006;86(2):249-260.

Lund CH, Bauer K, Berrios M. Gastroschisis: incidence, complications, and clinical management in the neonatal intensive care unit. *J Perinat Neonatal Nurs*. 2007;21(1):63-68.

18

Congenital Anomalies

Ellen Tappero

I. Overview
A. Congenital anomalies are common causes for medical intervention in the first few hours of life. They may lead to long-term illness or neonatal death.
B. The identification of congenital anomalies has important diagnostic and prognostic implications for neonates.
C. Because many infants with congenital anomalies are identified in the delivery room or shortly after birth in the nursery, the neonatal health care provider is often the first person families turn to for information about the significance of an anomaly.
D. It is important that the neonatal provider is familiar with physical characteristics of minor anomalies; certain minor anomalies may suggest the need for further diagnostic studies and the search for related conditions.
E. In recent years, improvements in prenatal care have led to increased prenatal detection of anomalies.
F. Early detection facilitates frank discussions with families and helps the neonatal provider anticipate challenges that may occur in the delivery-room resuscitation of the neonate.

II. Definitions
A. Congenital: A finding present at birth; does not denote the cause of the defect and should not be confused with the term genetic
B. Genetic: Determined by genes or gene regulation
   1. Translocation: A chromosome breaks and a portion of the original attaches to a different chromosome.
   2. Mosaicism: A person has two or more cell populations with different genetic or chromosomal constitutions.
C. Anomalies: Structural defects that deviate from the norm; classified as minor, major, or multiple
   1. Minor congenital anomalies
      a. Unusual visible features or alterations of normal form that have no serious medical or surgical consequences
      b. Of cosmetic concern and may indicate altered and/or abnormal developmental process or morphogenesis
      c. Most commonly seen on the hands, feet, face, or ears
   2. Major congenital anomalies

a. Unusual visible features or alterations of normal form that are present at birth
   b. Require significant surgical or cosmetic treatment
3. Major and minor congenital anomalies usually fall into one of four categories:
   a. Malformation: Structural defect of an organ, tissue, or part of the body resulting from an intrinsically abnormal developmental process due to genetic or teratogenic reasons (e.g., neural tube defect or congenital heart defect); recurrence risk 1%–5%
   b. Deformation: Altered form or position of a body part caused by abnormal extrinsic mechanical forces acting on (otherwise) normally developing tissue (e.g., altered head shape, clubfoot); good prognosis and low recurrence rate
   c. Disruption: Defect of a body part resulting from breakdown of (previously) normally developed tissue (e.g., amniotic banding); usually sporadic with low recurrence risks
   d. Dysplasia: Tissue anomaly due to abnormal organization of cells in that tissue; may be localized (e.g., hemangioma) or generalized (e.g., achondroplasia); usually not correctable
4. Multiple congenital anomalies
   a. Two or more major malformations, such as a neural tube defect, cardiac defect, missing limb
   b. Three or more minor malformations, such as syndactyly, clubfoot, abnormally formed pinna
   c. If more than one anomaly is present, the neonatal provider should consider whether it is part of a sequence, association, or syndrome, which have different prognostic implications
      (1) Sequence: Single defect as the cause for other anomalies; sometimes called the snowball effect
      (2) Association: Multiple defects without specific or common cause; occur together more frequently than normal by chance, but less than the pattern seen in a syndrome
      (3) Syndrome: Recognizable pattern of anomalies, often of more than one system, with a single specific cause

III. Incidence

A. Birth defects affect 3%–5% of all newborns in the United States.
B. Multiple defects or syndromes occur in 1% of newborns.
C. Approximately 40%–60% of congenital anomalies have no known cause/origin.
D. 20% of birth defects are most likely the result of combined genetic and environmental factors.

IV. Sequence anomalies

A. Potter's sequence (**Fig. 18-1**)
  1. May result from a variety of events, including absent kidneys, cystic kidneys, obstruction of the urinary tract, autosomal recessive polycystic kidney disease, autosomal dominant polycystic kidney disease (rare), renal hypoplasia, and chronic leakage of amniotic fluid, which result in oligohydramnios or absent amniotic fluid
  2. Decreased volume of amniotic fluid causes fetus to become compressed by mother's uterus with resulting physical deformities, most commonly Potter's facies
  3. Incidence
     a. Ranges from 1 in 4,000 to 1 in 10,000 live births
     b. Male predominance
  4. Physical characteristics
     a. Small for gestational age
     b. Pulmonary hypoplasia

FIGURE 18-1
Potter's Sequence

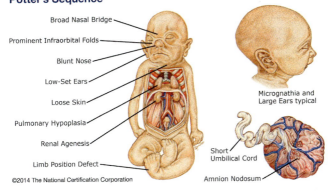

Potter's sequence is the result of decreased or absent amniotic fluid, which causes the fetus to become compressed in the uterus. Physical characteristics include parrot-beaked nose, low-set ears, and recessed chin.

c. Potter's facies
      (1) Parrot-beaked nose
      (2) Low-set ears
      (3) Recessed chin
      (4) Wide-spaced eyes
      (5) Depressed nasal bridge
      (6) Prominent skin fold extending from the medial canthus across the cheek and below the eye
   d. Anuria
5. Management
   a. If respiratory support is needed in the delivery room, avoid using high pressures during resuscitation to prevent complications such as pneumothoraces.
   b. Once a clearly lethal prognosis with severe pulmonary hypoplasia is determined, redirection of care needs to be planned with families.
   c. Include palliative care consult, if available.
   d. Maximize the time the baby can spend with the family before dying, while causing no harm and ensuring that the baby is comfortable and free of pain.
   e. Provide grief support for the family.
B. Robin sequence/complex (**Fig. 18-2**)
   1. Incidence

FIGURE 18-2
Robin Sequence

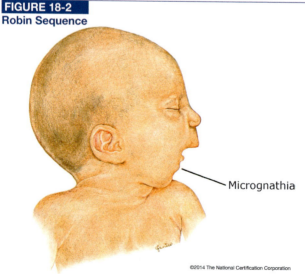

Infant with Robin sequence; note smaller than normal lower jaw (micrognathia).

a. Robin sequence/complex is rather uncommon.
b. Frequency estimates range from 1 in 2,000 to 1 in 30,000 births, based on how strictly the condition is defined.
c. Up to 80% of cases are associated with other syndromes.
2. Physical characteristics
   a. Smaller than normal lower jaw (micrognathia)
   b. Posterior displacement of the tongue causing partial or complete airway obstruction (relative hyperglossia)
   c. U-shaped cleft soft palate, a high-arched or complete cleft palate
3. Management
   a. Initial airway management
      (1) Prone positioning to prevent tongue from falling back into airway and to facilitate anterior displacement of tongue
      (2) Nasopharyngeal airway with or without use of nasal continuous positive airway pressure to avoid airway blockage in some infants
      (3) Endotracheal tube for temporary treatment of obstructive apnea in infants with persistent respiratory distress
   b. Non-emergent surgical airway management
      (1) Tongue-lip adhesion, where tongue is sutured to the lower lip
      (2) Mandibular distraction
      (3) Tracheostomy
C. Amniotic banding (**Fig. 18-3**)
   1. Believed to be caused by the early rupture of the amnion during pregnancy, which results in amniotic bands (constricting bands of fibrous tissue) that encircle fetal body parts.
   2. Most often affects the extremities, but complications can range from ring constrictions to amputations to major organ defects.
   3. Incidence
      a. Approximately 1 in 1,200 to 1 in 15,000 live births
      b. Sporadic occurrence not associated with genetic disorders
      c. Hand malformations twice as common as those of feet
   4. Physical characteristics

a. Constricting bands of fibrous tissue encircle developing structures, usually the limbs, and result in constriction deformities, amputations and/or umbilical cord constriction.
b. Features seen on external examination are usually the only abnormalities. There is no one feature that consistently occurs.
c. Deformation defects seen on examination are secondary to decreased fetal movement or constraint.
   (1) Foot abnormalities
   (2) Scoliosis
   (3) Edema
   (4) Necrosis
5. Management
   a. Condition should be identified at delivery.
   b. Treatment depends on the severity of the defect.
   c. Initially, evaluate vascular supply/perfusion.
   d. Evaluate for evidence of neurologic compromise.

FIGURE 18-3
Amniotic Banding

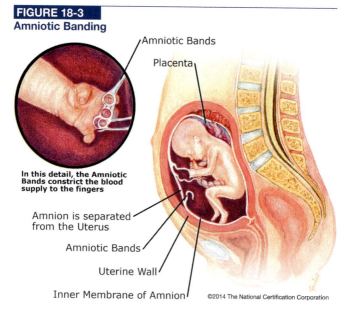

In this detail, the Amniotic Bands constrict the blood supply to the fingers

- Amniotic Bands
- Placenta
- Amnion is separated from the Uterus
- Amniotic Bands
- Uterine Wall
- Inner Membrane of Amnion

©2014 The National Certification Corporation

Believed to be caused by the early rupture of the amnion, amniotic banding is characterized by constricting bands of fibrous tissue that usually encircle fetal extremities. Complications may range from amputations to major organ defects.

e. Ongoing assessment of the affected extremity includes monitoring circulation, edema, movement, and function.
   f. Surgical intervention is geared toward functional improvement and is rarely an urgent need.
D. Arthrogryposis (**Figs. 18-4A and 18-4B**)
   1. Overview
      a. A heterogeneous group of disorders that include the common feature of multiple congenital joint contractures
      b. Thought to be due to fetal akinesia (decreased fetal movements) related to fetal abnormalities; such as neurogenic, muscle, or connective tissue abnormalities; or mechanical limitations to fetal movement
      c. Akinesia attributed to maternal disorders such as drugs or trauma
      d. No genetic disorder known
   2. Incidence: ~1 in 3,000 live births
   3. Physical characteristics vary but may include:

FIGURE 18-4A AND 18-4B
Arthrogryposis

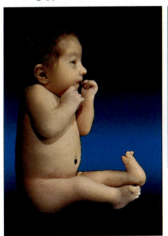
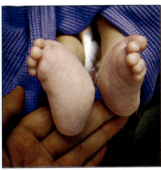

©2014 The National Certification Corporation

Arthrogryposis is a heterogeneous group of disorders that include the common factor of multiple congenital joint contractures. Physical characteristics may include symmetric joint contractures, flexion, and internal rotation of the shoulder, as well as vascular and respiratory issues.

    a. Symmetric joint contractures with marked limitations of movement of the involved joint (rigidity). Severity increases distally, with the hands and feet typically the most deformed. If only two extremities are affected, the lower extremities are affected more often.
    b. Flexion and, sometimes, joint dislocation occurs at the hips or knees.
    c. Internal rotation of the shoulder, extension at the elbow, and flexion of the wrist and fingers may also occur.
    d. Intrinsically derived contractures are frequently associated with oligohydramnios; contractures are accompanied by a wax-like appearance of the skin across joints and a lack of flexion creases.
    e. Deformities of the face include asymmetry, flat nasal bridge, hemangioma, and micrognathia.
    f. Respiratory problems include tracheal stenosis and laryngeal clefts; weak muscles or hypoplastic diaphragm may affect lung function.
    g. Vascular abnormalities may cause hemangiomas and cutis marmorata; distal limbs may be blue and cold.
    h. Other deformities include scoliosis and hernia (inguinal, umbilical).
  4. Management
    a. Assess for respiratory compromise in the delivery room.
    b. Assess range of motion and other anomalies.
  5. Ongoing care
    a. Maximize the infant's potential and prevent further deformity.
    b. X-rays usually confirm the diagnosis when evaluating stiff or dislocated joints.
    c. Additional tests include blood tests, muscle biopsies, and other imaging studies to help confirm the diagnosis.
  6. Support the family, highlighting the infant's normal intelligence and favorable functional prognosis.
E. VATER/VACTERL association anomalies
  1. Overview
    a. VACTERL is an acronym for a disorder that affects multiple body systems: **v**ertebral defects, **a**nal atresia, **c**ardiac defects, **t**racheo-**e**sophageal (TE) fistula, **r**enal anomalies, and **l**imb abnormalities.

b. Infants diagnosed with VACTERL association typically have at least three of the characteristic features.
c. Additional abnormalities may occur that are not among the characteristic features.
d. Anomalies may or may not be identified in the delivery room.
e. Infants with VACTERL association tend to have normal development and normal intelligence.

2. Incidence
   a. Approximately 1 in 5,000 to 1 in 40,000 newborns; wide range of manifestation makes exact incidence within the population uncertain
   b. Seen more frequently in infants of diabetic mothers
   c. Rarely seen more than once in one family

3. Physical characteristics
   a. Vertebral anomalies
      (1) Defects of the spinal column; usually consist of small (hypoplastic) vertebrae or hemivertebra
      (2) Rarely cause any difficulties in infancy
      (3) Usually discovered on a chest x-ray
      (4) Later in life, may put child at risk for developing scoliosis
   b. Anal anomalies
      (1) Narrowing or atresia of anus seen in ~55% of patients
      (2) May be accompanied by abnormalities of the genitalia and urinary tract (genitourinary anomalies)
      (3) Usually noted at birth and often require surgery in the first days of life
   c. Cardiac defects
      (1) May range in severity from a life-threatening problem to a subtle defect that does not cause health problems
      (2) Ventricular septal defect (VSD), atrial septal defects, and tetralogy of Fallot most commonly seen
   d. Esophageal atresia with TE fistula
      (1) Seen in ~70% of patients with VACTERL association
      (2) May be a cause of respiratory distress at delivery
   e. Renal anomalies

- (1) Missing (one or both), abnormally developed, and/or misshapen kidneys
- (2) May affect kidney function
- (3) Many have a single umbilical artery, which can often be associated with kidney or urologic problems
  f. Limb anomalies
  - (1) Most commonly include poorly developed or missing thumbs or underdeveloped forearms and hands
  - (2) Radial agenesis
4. Management
   a. Assessment and observation to maintain airway and resuscitate as needed
   b. Initial care in the delivery room and nursery influenced by:
      (1) Severity of identified defects
      (2) Presence of complicating factors
   c. Identification of functional deficits
   d. Prompt surgical consultation and treatment for anal atresia or stenosis, esophageal atresia, tracheoesophageal fistula
   e. Appropriate consultation with subspecialists as needed
5. Recognition and diagnosis
   a. Usually do not have dysmorphic facial features, abnormalities of growth, or mental deficiency
   b. Diagnosis through exclusion; may not be immediately evident to the health care provider

F. CHARGE syndrome (**Fig. 18-5**)
   1. Overview
      a. CHARGE is an acronym for a disorder that affects multiple body systems: **c**oloboma, **h**eart disease, choanal **a**tresia, **r**etarded growth and development, **g**enital hypoplasia, and **e**ar anomalies with deafness.
      b. Not all features must be present and the extent of involvement of each system is widely variable.
      c. Because mutations in at least one gene (CHD7) are attributed to causing CHARGE, the association is now referred to as CHARGE syndrome.
   2. Incidence
      a. 1 in 10,000 to 1 in 15,000 births
      b. Autosomal dominant disorder; most cases represent the first in a family

c. Risk of recurrence in family ~1%–2%
3. Physical characteristics
   a. Colobomas
      (1) Present in 80%–90% of cases
      (2) More common in retina than iris
   b. Heart defects
      (1) Frequency is ~75% of cases.
      (2) Types of defects vary widely.
      (3) Most frequent types include tetralogy of Fallot, double-outlet right ventricle, truncus arteriosus, and perimembranous VSD.
      (4) Aortic arch anomalies like interrupted aortic arch, vascular ring, or aberrant subclavian artery make up 38%–40%.
   c. Choanal atresia
      (1) Present in 50% of cases
      (2) May be unilateral (one-sided) or bilateral (both sides), bony or membranous
   d. Growth deficiency
      (1) Frequency is ~15% of cases.
      (2) Growth parameters are normal at birth.

FIGURE 18-5
CHARGE Syndrome

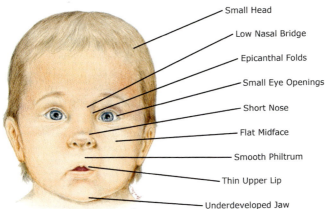

©2014 The National Certification Corporation

CHARGE is an acronym for a disorder that affects multiple systems: coloboma (C), heart disease (H), choanal atresia (A), retarded growth and development (R), genital hypoplasia (G), and ear abnormalities (E). Not all features need to be present. Because the sequence is associated with mutation in at least one gene, it is called CHARGE syndrome.

(3) Linear growth declines by infancy.
    e. Genital hypoplasia
        (1) Present in ~50%–60% of male cases; may manifest as microphallus, hypospadias, chordee, or undescended testes
        (2) Present in ~25% of female cases, more difficult to recognize externally; includes hypoplastic labia and clitoris and small or missing uterus
    f. Ear anomalies
        (1) Occur in ~90% of cases
        (2) May involve the outer, middle, or inner ear
4. Management: CHARGE syndrome often presents as a medical emergency due to:
    a. Choanal atresia leading to respiratory distress and/or failure; requires ongoing respiratory assessment
    b. Serious heart defects; require assessment of cardiovascular status
    c. Swallowing difficulties; require monitoring for possible aspiration and initial feeding assessment
G. Differentiating VACTERL and CHARGE associations
    1. Infants who have VACTERL association are not dysmorphic and have an excellent prognosis for normal growth and development.
    2. Infants who have CHARGE syndrome are dysmorphic and usually have significant feeding and developmental issues.
    3. A careful eye evaluation for retinal coloboma may help differentiate between these two associations.

V. Syndromes

A. Trisomy 21 (Down syndrome) **(Fig. 18-6)**
    1. Overview
        a. Genetic disorder in which infant has 47 chromosomes rather than the normal 46
        b. Three copies of genetic material on chromosome No. 21
        c. No visible abnormalities if chromosomes are balanced; parent passes on a translocated chromosome, along with the chromosome No. 21 that lost a section due to translocation; child is balanced translocation carrier
    2. Incidence
        a. 1 in 800 live births
        b. Spans all ethnicities and economic levels
        c. Risk increases with maternal age (35 years or older)

d. Maternal age not primary predictor; 80% born to women <35
3. Physical characteristics
   a. 20% premature
   b. Muscular hypotonia
   c. Poor Moro reflex
   d. Hyperflexibility of joints
   e. Slanted palpebral fissures
   f. Flat facial profile
   g. Prominent epicanthal fold
   h. Brushfield's spots
   i. Hand
      (1) Single palmar crease: unilateral or bilateral
      (2) Low-set thumb
      (3) Fifth finger short and curves inward
   j. Feet
      (1) Wide space between great toe and second toe
      (2) Deep crease that starts between great toe and second toe and curves toward medial edge of the sole
   k. Congenital heart defects

FIGURE 18-6
Trisomy 21 (Down Syndrome)

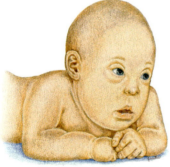

Flattened Nose and Face and Upward Slanting Eyes

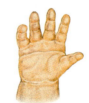

Single Palmer Crease and Short 5th Finger that Curves Inward

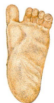

Widely Separated 1st and 2nd Toes with a Deep Crease in Between

©2014 The National Certification Corporation

Down syndrome is a genetic disorder in which the infant has 47 chromosomes rather than the normal 46. The disorder is not related to ethnicity or economic levels.

l. Duodenal atresia
m. Hematologic abnormalities, e.g., transient neonatal leukemia
4. Management
   a. Most infants with Down syndrome have a normal transition period at birth and need little, if any, intervention.
   b. If infant is premature, monitor for respiratory distress and support as necessary.
   c. Assess for congenital heart defects and support as necessary. A cardiology consult is needed soon after admission into the nursery.
   d. Monitor feeding pattern and for changes in abdominal assessment. Surgical consult if infant develops symptoms of duodenal atresia.
   e. Consult appropriate subspecialists as needed.
   f. Support the family. Provide information about Down syndrome and support groups to the parents.
B. Trisomy 18 (Edwards syndrome) (**Fig. 18-7**)
   1. Overview
      a. Genetic disorder caused by the presence of all or part of an extra chromosome No. 18

FIGURE 18-7
Trisomy 18 (Edwards Syndrome)

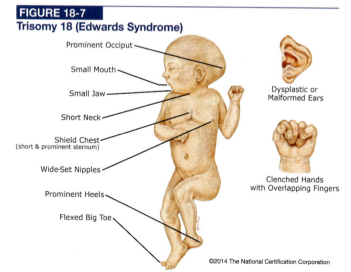

©2014 The National Certification Corporation

Edwards Syndrome, a genetic disorder, is caused by the presence of all or part of an extra chromosome No. 18. Most infants with the disorder die before birth; few survive longer than a year.

b. Second most common autosomal trisomy, after Down syndrome, that carries to term
c. Very low rate of survival; 50% mortality within the first week of life
d. 5%–10% survive first year

2. Incidence
   a. Approximately 1 in 6,000 live births
   b. Approximately 80% female
   c. Majority of cases die before birth
   d. Incidence increases as mother's age increases

3. Physical characteristics: Some or all may be present
   a. Prenatal and postnatal growth deficiency in infants carried to term
   b. Head: Microcephaly, prominent occiput
   c. Eyes: Ptosis of one or both eyelids
   d. Micrognathia and microstomia (small jaw and mouth)
   e. Ears: Low set and/or malformed
   f. Hands: Clenched fist, with index finger overlapping the third and fifth finger overlapping the fourth; undeveloped or altered thumbs
   g. Feet: Rocker bottom and/or clubfeet
   h. Redundant skin at back of neck
   i. Short sternum

4. Management
   a. If available, palliative care prenatally or post birth
   b. Usually no treatment beyond supportive care
   c. Gavage feeds as needed for feeding difficulties
   d. Oxygen as needed for respiratory support
   e. Maximize time with family, while ensuring that infant is comfortable and free of pain
   f. Family support

C. Trisomy 13 (Patau syndrome) **(Fig. 18-8)**
   1. Overview
      a. Genetic disorder in which infant has three copies of genetic material on chromosome No. 13, instead of the usual two copies
      b. Extra material may be attached to another chromosome (translocation, rare)
      c. Highly lethal; >80% die in the first year
   2. Incidence
      a. Occurs in ~1 in 10,000 newborns.
      b. Most cases are not inherited.

    c. Unless one of the parents is a carrier of a translocation, the chances of a couple having another child affected with trisomy 13 is <1% (less than that of Down syndrome).
3. Physical characteristics: Often identifiable at birth
    a. Microcephaly
    b. Cleft lip or palate
    c. Ears: Malformed or low set
    d. Eyes: Microphthalmia, colobomas of the iris, cataracts, close-set eyes where the eyes may fuse into one
    e. Heart: Usually ventricular septal defect, patent ductus arteriosus, or positional anomalies such as dextrocardia
    f. Hands: Clenched hands with outer fingers on top of the inner fingers; flexion deformities of the hand, fingers, and wrist; postaxial polydactyly; single palmar crease
    g. Feet: Polydactyly, rocker bottom
    h. Umbilicus: Hernia, omphalocele

FIGURE 18-8
Trisomy 13 (Patau Syndrome)

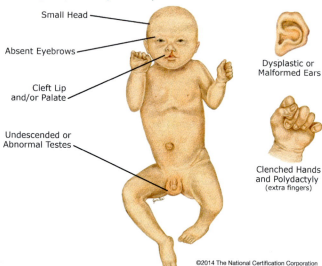

Patau syndrome indicates the infant has three copies of the genetic material on chromosome No. 13. Many infants do not survive because of complex heart defects or severe neurological problems. Management should focus on specific physical problems.

i. Cutis aplasia
j. Genitalia (male): Small scrotum with anterior placement, undescended testes
k. Holoprosencephaly: Failure of the forebrain to divide properly

4. Management
   a. Should be planned on a case-by-case basis, focusing on specific physical problems.
   b. Many infants have difficulty surviving the first few days or weeks due to severe neurological problems or complex heart defects.
   c. Surgery may be necessary to repair heart defects or cleft lip/palate anomalies.
   d. If diagnosed prenatally, involve families in direction of care in the delivery room and nursery.
   e. If available, include palliative care prenatally or post birth.
   f. Provide routine newborn care/anticipatory guidance for parents.
   g. Cardiac evaluation may be necessary.
   h. Neurology evaluation is required, as seizures are relatively common.
   i. If comfort care is offered, maximize the infant's time spent with family, while causing no harm and ensuring that the infant is comfortable and free of pain.
   j. Support the family.

D. Beckwith-Wiedemann syndrome
   1. Overview
      a. An overgrowth disorder, usually present at birth, thought to be caused by a deletion or abnormality on chromosome No. 11.
      b. Features include macroglossia, macrosomia, midline abdominal wall defects, ear creases or ear pits, and neonatal hypoglycemia.
      c. Most cases do not have all five features and no two infants are the same.
      d. Some premature newborns do not have macroglossia until closer to their anticipated delivery date.
   2. Incidence
      a. Estimated 1 in 12,000 to 1 in 14,000 live births
         (1) Variability in presentation and difficulties with diagnosis make exact incidence unknown.

(2) Reported incidence is likely low because of clinical features that are less prominent and therefore missed.
  b. Documented in a variety of ethnic groups; occurs equally in males and females
  c. Most cases (>85%) sporadic; usually has not occurred in other family members; parents not at increased risk of having another child with Beckwith-Wiedemann syndrome
  d. Up to 15% may be familial, with autosomal dominant transmission but variable phenotypes
  e. Infant mortality rate ~20%, mainly caused by complications of prematurity
3. Physical characteristics
  a. Prenatal history of polyhydramnios and prematurity
  b. Macrosomia: Birth weight and length >90th percentile
  c. Head: Prominent occiput, large fontanel
  d. Macroglossia: Presents in >90%
  e. Anterior abdominal wall defects, including omphalocele or other umbilical anomaly
  f. Linear fissures in the lobe of the external ear, ear pits
  g. Other significant clinical findings
    (1) Hypoglycemia: Usually after the first day of life
    (2) Accelerated osseous maturation
    (3) Large kidneys
    (4) Polycythemia
  h. Port wine stain (nevus flammeus) often found on forehead or back of neck (benign, usually does not require treatment)
4. Management
  a. Support airway as indicated.
  b. Place infant on side to facilitate breathing; may need oral airway.
  c. Monitor glucose closely; treat hypoglycemia.
  d. Facilitate feeding with a large soft nipple.
  e. Follow hemoglobin/hematocrit; many are polycythemic, may need partial exchange transfusion.
  f. Provide information about web sites and support groups to parents.

VI. Cleft lip with or without cleft palate (Fig. 18-9)

A. Overview
1. Craniofacial defect; among the most common of all birth defects
2. Due to defective embryonic development of the primary and secondary palate; both genetic and environmental factors contribute
3. May be isolated defect or component of inherited disease or syndrome

B. Incidence
1. 1 in 14,000 births
2. Cleft lip more common than cleft palate
3. The Centers for Disease Control and Prevention (CDC) estimates:
   a. Cleft palate occurs in 2,651 babies born in the United States.
   b. Cleft lip with or without a cleft palate occurs in 4,437 babies born in the United States.
      (1) In Caucasians, occurs in ~1 in 4,000 live births
      (2) In Asian population, occurs twice as often as Caucasians

FIGURE 18-9
Cleft Lip with Cleft Palate

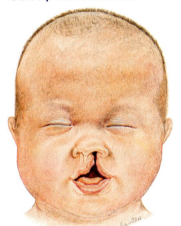
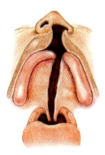

Unilateral Cleft Lip and Palate
©2014 The National Certification Corporation

Cleft lip may present with or without cleft palate. This craniofacial defect is among the most common of all birth defects. Genetic and environmental factors may contribute to incidence. Outcomes are usually good with surgical correction.

(3) In African Americans, occurs in ~0.4 in 10,000 births
C. Physical characteristics
1. Condition is apparent at birth.
2. Cleft lip may be unilateral or bilateral.
3. Bilateral cleft lip is commonly accompanied by a cleft palate.
4. Varying degrees of nasal deformities may be noted.
D. Management
1. Obstruction of the airway may present shortly after birth.
2. Intubation may be difficult; have laryngeal mask airway (LMA) available in the delivery room in case respiratory support is needed.
3. Aerophagia (swallowing of air) and nasopharyngeal reflux are commonly seen.
4. Infants may experience feeding difficulties because of the inability to form an airtight seal around the nipple.
5. Infants have increased risk of aspiration.
6. Include speech therapy evaluation, if available.
7. Surgical consult is needed; initiate treatment soon after birth, depending on the severity of the defect.
8. Outcomes are good with surgical correction and influence facial aesthetics, psychological impact, maxillary growth, dental development, and speech therapy.

VII. Ambiguous genitalia (Fig. 18-10)

A. Overview
1. Rare condition in which external genitals are neither clearly male nor female.
2. Genitals may be poorly formed or characteristic of both sexes.
3. External and internal sex organs may not match.
4. Not a disease; a sign of a condition affecting sexual development, for example:
   a. Congenital adrenal hyperplasia
   b. 5-alpha reductase deficiency
B. Incidence
1. Approximately 1 in 5,000
2. Etiologies vary, not well-documented
3. Incidence varies by source and ethnic group
   a. Estimate for Switzerland is 1 in 5,000 live births.
   b. Estimate for Maryland is 1 in 67,000 live births.

4. Congenital adrenal hyperplasia considered most common cause of ambiguous genitalia, occurring in 1 in 14,000 to 1 in 28,000 live births
5. Associated malformations common, affecting 37.5% of all infants

C. Physical characteristics
1. Suspect problems in a phenotypic male with:
   a. Bilateral nonpalpable testes
   b. Perineal hypospadias
   c. Unilateral undescended testis with hypospadias
   d. Slight phallic enlargement
   e. Unusually small genitalia
2. Suspect problems in a phenotypic female with:
   a. Clitoral hypertrophy
   b. Palpable gonad, inguinal masses
   c. Fused labia of varying degrees
   d. Abnormal opening or dimpling on the perineum (urogenital sinus)
3. Excessive genital pigmentation, signs of dehydration (may indicate congenital adrenal hyperplasia)

FIGURE 18-10
Ambiguous Genitalia

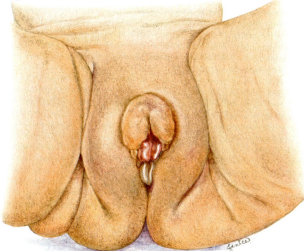

©2014 The National Certification Corporation

This rare condition may involve poorly formed genitals or external and internal sex organs that do not match. Evident at birth, chromosomal testing may be necessary to identify the infant's gender.

4. Dysmorphic features suggestive of Turner syndrome (may indicate gonadal dysgenesis)
5. Multiple congenital anomalies (may indicate a variety of syndromes associated with ambiguous genitalia)

D. Management
1. Disorders of sex development are evident at birth and are considered a psychosocial emergency.
2. In the delivery room, it is recommended to tell the parents that the genitalia are incompletely developed and further testing is needed.
3. During counseling, use gender-neutral terms (e.g. "your baby"); avoid gender-specific pronouns.
4. Review prenatal history to determine if an amniocentesis was performed using chromosomes to identify the infant's gender.
5. Further investigation is imperative before gender assignment can be made.
6. Laboratory studies:
   a. Chromosome analysis: High resolution and fluorescence in situ hybridization (FISH)
   b. Basic biochemical studies and tests for underlying endocrine disorders, including 17-hydroxyprogesterone (17-OHP), testosterone, dihydrotestosterone, sodium, and potassium
7. Radiographic studies:
   a. Pelvic ultrasonography to look for the presence and localization of internal gonadal structures
   b. Adrenal ultrasonography to identify abnormalities related to adrenal hyperplasia
   c. In complex cases, contrast studies to outline the internal anatomy
8. Early referral to a specialist familiar with disorders of sex differentiation, such as a pediatric endocrinologist, geneticist, pediatric urologic surgeon, psychiatrist, or social worker.
9. Genetic consultation, particularly if features or constellation of findings suggest a possible syndrome disorder.
10. State newborn screening tests for congenital adrenal hyperplasia (CAH).
11. Assess the newborn for signs and symptoms of CAH, including lethargy, poor feeding, vomiting, diarrhea, dehydration, failure to thrive, apnea, and seizures.

VIII. Summary

A. Identification of congenital anomalies has important diagnostic and prognostic implications for neonates.

B. The neonatal health care provider's expertise in identifying abnormal findings on physical examination is very useful.

C. Families look to the neonatal health care provider for initial information about the significance of an anomaly.

D. The Internet helps health care professionals and families find more information about specific birth defects and support groups.

E. Online, an enormous amount of up-to-date information from experts can be assessed in a short period of time.

F. Reputable web sites are good places to refer families for a general search about their infant's condition, including:
   1. March of Dimes Birth Defects Foundation: http://www.marchofdimes.com/
   2. Centers for Disease Control and Prevention: http://www.cdc.gov/ncbddd/birthdefects/index.html
   3. Online Mendelian Inheritance in Man: http://www.ncbi.nlm.nih.gov/omim
   4. National Institute of Child Health and Human Development: http://www.nichd.nih.gov/health/topics/birthdefects/Pages/default.aspx
   5. National Organization of Rare Diseases: www.rarediseases.org

References

Arthrogryposis page. Boston Children's Hospital Web site. http://www.childrenshospital.org/health-topics/conditions/a/arthrogryposis. Accessed April 12, 2012.

Beckwith-Wiedemann syndrome. Genetics Home Reference Web site. http://ghr.nlm.nih.gov/condition/beckwith-wiedemann-syndrome. Accessed May 3, 2012.

Bishara N, Clericuzio CL. Common dysmorphic syndromes in the NICU. *NeoReviews*. 2008;9(1):e29-e38.

Burstein FD, Williams JK. Mandibular distraction osteogenesis in Pierre Robin sequence: application of a new internal single-stage resorbable device. *Plast Reconstr Surg*. 2005;115(1):61-67.

Chi C, Lee HC, Neely EK. Ambiguous genitalia in the newborn. *NeoReviews*. 2008;9(2):e78-e84.

Cohen JN, Ringer SA. Congenital kidney abnormalities: diagnosis, management, and palliative care. *NeoReviews*. 2010;11(5):e226-235.

Cooperman DR, Thompson GH. Congenital abnormalities of the upper and lower extremities and spine. In: Martin RJ, Fanaroff AA, Walsh MC. *Fanaroff and Martin's Neonatal-Perinatal Medicine: Diseases of the Fetus and Infant*. 9th ed. St. Louis, MO: Mosby Elsevier; 2011:1797.

Crotwell PL, Hoyme HE. Core concepts: chromosome aneuploidies. *NeoReviews*. 2012;13(1):e30-e39.

Facts about cleft lip and cleft palate. Centers for Disease Control and Prevention Web site. http://www.cdc.gov/ncbddd/birthdefects/CleftLip.html. Accessed April 12, 2012.

Gomella TL. Common multiple congenital anomaly syndromes. In: Gomella TK, Cunningham MD, Eyal FG, eds. *Neonatology: Management, Procedures, On-Call Problems, Diseases, and Drugs*. 7th ed. New York, NY: McGraw-Hill/Lange; 2013:599-606.

Gomella TL. Disorders of sex development. Gomella TK, Cunningham MD, Eyal FG, eds. *Neonatology: Management, Procedures, On-Call Problems, Diseases, and Drugs*. 7th ed. New York, NY: McGraw-Hill/Lange; 2013:619-627.

Kalhan SC, Devaskar SU. Metabolic and endocrine disorders. In: Martin RJ, Fanaroff AA, Walsh MC. *Fanaroff and Martin's Neonatal-Perinatal Medicine: Diseases of the Fetus and Infant*. 9th ed. St. Louis, MO: Mosby Elsevier; 2011:1511-1512.

Kaplan J, Hudgins L. Neonatal presentations of CHARGE syndrome and VATER/VACTERL association. *NeoReviews*. 2008;9(7):e299-e304.

Lakovschek IC, Streubel B, Ulm B. Natural outcome of trisomy 13, trisomy 18, triploidy after prenatal diagnosis. *Am J Med Genetics A*. 2011;155A(11):2626–2633.

Lin-Su K, New MI. Ambiguous genitalia in the newborn. In: Gleason CA, Devaskar S, eds. *Avery's Diseases of the Newborn*. 9th ed. Philadelphia, PA: Saunders Elsevier; 2012:1286-1306.

Merritt TA, Catlin A, Wool C, Peverini R, Goldstein, M. Trisomy 18 and trisomy 13: treatment and management decisions. *NeoReviews*. 2012;13(1):e40-e48.

Purandare SM, Zackai EH. Amniotic band sequence. *NeoReviews*. 2005;6(12):e567-e571.

Support Organization for Trisomy 18, 13 and Related Disorders Web site. http://www.trisomy.org/. Accessed April 21, 2012.

Thimmappa B, Hopkins E, Schendel SA. Management of micrognathia. *NeoReviews*. 2009;10(10):e488-e493.

Thyen U, Lanz K, Holterhus PM, Hiort O. Epidemiology and initial management of ambiguous genitalia at birth in Germany. *Horm Res*. 2006;66(4):195-203.

Tighe D, Petrick L, Cobourne MT, Rabe H. Cleft lip and palate: effects on neonatal care. *NeoReviews*. 2011;12(6):e315-e324.

Tonge A. Perioperative care of the pediatric patient with Down syndrome. *AORN J*. 2011;94(6):606-617.

Trisomies and monosomies page. Boston Children's Hospital Web site. http://childrenshospital.org/az/Site1789/mainpageS1789P0.html. Accessed April 12, 2012.

19

Developmentally Supportive and Family-Centered Care

Jacqueline M. McGrath, Ana Francisca Diallo, Rebecca J. Paquette, and Haifa (Abou) Samra

I. Introduction
A. For best outcomes, developmentally supportive care of the infant and family must begin before birth and continue through delivery and into early infancy.
B. Bundling interventions that are already evidenced to support best outcomes increases the potential for positive results.
   1. Family-centered, developmentally supportive interventions are essential elements of any bundle in the NICU, especially during the Golden Hours.
   2. It is the authors' belief that if these supportive interventions are missing from among the other bundled interventions, the care is incomplete.

II. Developmentally supportive strategies
A. Developmental care in the prenatal period just prior to birth
   1. Neuroprotective strategies in the prenatal period support the long-term development of the child; the *in utero* environment is most often the best place for the infant to grow and develop.
   2. The family unit requires support during this time; decision making about the infant must be collaborative and take into account the family's needs and beliefs.
B. Developmental strategies in the delivery room
   1. Consider the environment; decrease chaos whenever possible.
   2. Provide warmth and consider positioning with warm nesting on the warming table.
   3. Support the needs of the parents and any other family members who are present.
   4. Provide open communication.
C. Developmental care during admission to the NICU
   1. Consider the environment during admission; reduce chaos and unnecessary staff, activity, and noise.
   2. Use light sparingly when needed; protect the infant as quickly as possible.
   3. Admit the smallest and sickest of infants to a quiet area or single room that is out of the main traffic aisle.

4. Based on the stability or instability of the infant, consider avoiding certain routine tasks and whether the benefits outweigh the costs during this time of transition.
    a. Work as a health care team to assess the infant and eliminate the need for individual assessments by nursing, medicine, or others.
5. Regularly assess the infant's behavioral cues in response to caregiving and procedures; use these assessments to choose strategies that best support the infant and decrease stress.
    a. During the Golden Hours, the infant often has reduced energy reserves; every effort must be made to conserve energy and reduce stress.
    b. Stress can be heightened in the Golden Hours and can lead to fatigue and exhaustion; assessment during this time needs to be sensitive to this increased potential.
6. Midline positioning is important in these early hours, yet providing support with nesting or swaddling can relax the infant and decrease the use of energy.

D. Developmental care during procedures
  1. Use nesting to promote the infant's relaxation and support positioning for umbilical line placement, IV starts, and heal sticks.
  2. Have a second person available whenever possible to support the caregiver who is providing the procedure, which can decrease stress for both the caregiver and the infant.
  3. Medicating the infant for pain prior to procedures is important to both short- and long-term developmental outcomes.
  4. Use of sucrose to support the infant should also be considered.
  5. Support the infant during potentially painful procedures; pain management in the Golden Hours is important since these events are the foundation for how an infant will react to the next painful procedure.

III. Family-centered care interventions
  A. Who is the **family** to the high-risk infant?
    1. A family is a self-defining group; it is made up of those people, related and unrelated, who provide support, structure beliefs, and define values.

2. Families provide the portal through which individuals enter and interact with society and are the means to resources and education for infants and children.
B. Parents and families most often enter the NICU exhausted, bewildered, and emotionally drained by the birth experience.
  1. At the initial moment during admission, a unique **partnership** must be formed between the family and the professionals providing care for the infant.
  2. This is often a time of acute crisis, during which the family may be unable to adequately use resources because stress decreases available coping skills.
C. Primary focus of interventions during this time
  1. Promote the parents' participation in their child's care.
  2. Facilitate parental recognition of resources and available coping strategies.
  3. Enable and empower the family unit.
D. The provision of individualized, developmentally supportive care, of which family-centered care is a core principle, is pivotal not only in the Golden Hours, but also to the long-term medical and developmental outcomes of the child.
E. Defining family-centered care
  1. Family-centered care recognizes and promotes the normal family patterns unique to that family.
  2. Within the philosophy of family-centered care, families are supported in their natural caregiving and decision-making roles by building on their unique strengths as individuals, and then as a family unit.
  3. Family-centered care begins wherever and whenever a family enters the health care system and continues through discharge; for some families, this begins during prenatal care and continues into the delivery room and into the postpartum period.
  4. Rather than expecting the family to take on the medical culture of the institution, health care professionals recognize and reinforce the family's culture through a sensitive partnership formed in the best interests of the child.
  5. Parents and professionals are equals in the partnership committed to the child and to the delivery of optimum quality in all levels of health care.
  6. Families are not replaceable at any level in the overall development of the child.
F. Assuming the parental role

1. Parenting is a major role in our society for which there is little preparation; difficulties encountered in the early stages of parenting may adversely affect all relationships within the family unit, and can be especially apparent in the relationship between the parents of the child, as well as in the parents' relationship with the child.
2. A child changes everything for a couple; in addition to being partners, there are new roles as mothers and/or fathers.
3. Many factors influence parenting: cultural background, personality, previous parenting and life experiences, available resources and support, degree of attachment to the infant, and expectations parents have of themselves and the infant.
4. Feelings of inadequacy, conflict, and fatigue are often apparent during the crisis of birth and transition to the NICU, which may adversely affect existing relationships and developing relationships between parent and child.
5. Parents faced with a crisis must modify their preconceived roles and adapt to the necessary changes encountered with the crisis; role and behavior changes can cause considerable stress, especially if these changes occur abruptly.
6. At each birth or with each interaction between a parent and child, nurses must identify adaptive and maladaptive parenting behaviors and consider strategies supporting the development of these relationships.

G. Parenting during crisis in the NICU
1. Crisis is a period of disequilibrium precipitated by an inescapable demand to which the person is temporarily unable to respond adequately.
2. Identifiable stages of grief and loss may be present.
    a. The initial response usually is overwhelming shock, often characterized by irrational behaviors and feelings of helplessness and despair.
    b. Families of a premature infant may have difficulty with organization because their lives have been disrupted by the unexpected birth.
    c. Parents may feel guilt over the premature delivery or the infant's illness; self-blame often characterizes these feelings.

- d. Parents may try to escape the situation through denial, e.g., "Everything will all be fine in just a few days."
- e. Intense feelings of resentment and anger may follow denial; parents may direct these feelings toward themselves, the infant, members of the health care team, or even each other as parents.
- f. Supporting parents through this process is an essential aspect of the attachment process that needs to occur between the parent and the child.
3. The severity of the child's illness may be a factor in how the parents display their parenting skills.

H. Creating a welcoming environment for the family during the late prenatal period, when admission to the NICU seems more likely
   1. When possible, a tour of the NICU prior to birth that includes a question-and-answer session helps the parents better understand their situation, emotionally prepare for what is to come, and develop a sense of hope for a better prognosis of their child's health.
   2. Prior to the birth of the child, examining family dynamics, roles, needs, wishes, and cultural and moral values allows for tailored prenatal education and targeted interventions to better meet the needs of the family.
   3. Developing a birth plan is important for best outcomes for the infant and family, especially if the birth is high risk or the infant is known to have problems that will require admission to the NICU.
   4. Assess for maternal depression and continue to assess throughout the Golden Hours.
   5. The health care team should establish an individualized plan of care in collaboration with the family, inviting parents to be active members of the team and respecting their cultural backgrounds, spiritual beliefs, and wishes.

I. Promoting parenting roles during delivery
   1. The delivery room is a highly charged environment for all participants; it is especially challenging for families when the delivery is characterized as high risk or things don't go as expected.
   2. Continuous and effective communication about what best to expect during the delivery process and subsequent admission to the NICU are essential parts of care.

3. Providing anticipatory guidance regarding the upcoming events has shown to decrease parental stress and fear regarding the infant's health status.
4. Studies have shown that mothers report a sense of emptiness, loss, and nonparticipation due to the shortened pregnancy and immediate separation from their newborn that often occur during the Golden Hours.
5. During the Golden Hours, it is important to acknowledge parental feelings of guilt, shame, and low self-esteem for not having a "normal, healthy baby;" the birth outcomes are seldom their fault and they often need to be reassured of this fact.

J. Assessing/acknowledging neonatal neurobehavioral development during admission
1. The attachment process between parents and their infant begins immediately after the infant is born; when the infant is transferred to the NICU or other special unit, the attachment process can be delayed or altered.
    a. For parents to attach to their infant, a welcoming, calming environment in which they feel comfortable is essential in the NICU.
    b. The environment must encourage parents to grow in their roles as primary caregivers.
    c. Parents need to be encouraged to develop skills as the advocates for their child.
2. The preterm neonate's physical appearance, disorganized behavioral responses, and variable physiologic responses to touch can cause much anxiety in the parents as they attempt to interact with their infant.
    a. Help parents understand and respond sensitively to infant cues.
    b. Point out what the infant can do for himself/herself and when the infant needs support.
    c. Communicate the maturational limits of the infant.
    d. Assess how parents interpret cues from their infant; some parents and ethnic groups may interpret touch cues differently.
    e. Provide information about the infant's approach and avoidance cues so parents learn to interact and respond appropriately.

K. Promoting family participation during the Golden Hours
1. Collaborative caregiving between the health care provider and the parents is essential.

a. Parents need support and education to understand how to interact with their infant during this time.
b. Families receiving support from the medical and nursing team will be able to become more involved in their infant's recovery process.
c. Parents who are well-integrated into the caregiving team are able to feel more in control of, and less stressed about, their child's welfare.
d. Family-centered care intervention strategies lower the degree of stress in the parents, which is beneficial to the child's development.

2. The first family meeting with the health care team should take place within 72 hours of the birth so that collaboration and planning for future care can occur.
   a. Hold regular family meetings to encourage the health care team and family to collaborate.
   b. Assemble an interdisciplinary team for family meetings to address the support needs of the infant and the family's decision-making processes.

3. Encourage developmentally supportive care, such as holding the infant, skin-to-skin holding, eye contact, or parental voice cues to increase maternal sensitivity, affectionate behaviors, bonding, and attachment as soon as the infant and family are able.
   a. Touch is important to developing attachment; provide education so the touch is appropriate to the gestation and degree of illness of the infant.
   b. Encourage and support regular skin-to-skin holding.
   c. If instituted, skin-to-skin holding should last >30 min (60–90 min is ideal) for maximum benefits.
   d. The costs vs. benefits of parent holding must always be considered, as it should be for any supportive therapy, such as medication administration and respiratory support.

4. Use every caregiving opportunity to increase parental competence by including their collaboration in the care of the infant; this builds a partnership and supports best outcomes for the family.

5. Support the provision of breast milk or breast-feeding; if appropriate, pumping must begin within 6 hours of birth and should optimally begin within the first two hours of birth.

6. Consider using the mother's own breast milk for mouth care of the infant.
7. Expanding visiting hours has had a positive influence on parents experiencing the NICU; encourage parents to be present during rounds and reports so they can provide insights about their infant and be fully incorporated into decision making about their child.
8. Communication with the family must be open and honest.
   a. Assess parent health literacy as a precursor for communication with the family about the needs of the infant.
   b. Avoid the use of medical jargon when communicating with the parents and family.
   c. Be aware of cultural sensitivities; recognize the unique needs of the parents and help guide caregiving with their infant and family.
9. Allowing siblings and other family members to visit is also beneficial. Find safe ways to increase family participation in the care of the high-risk infant, such as short visits that focus on getting to know the infant.
10. Sometimes hello is goodbye in the Golden Hours. Parents need to be able to participate in all palliative care that is put in place to support the infant during this time. Parent decision making during this time must be a priority in care delivery.
11. Health professionals need to avoid the role of "gatekeeper" of the infant patient. The baby belongs to its parents. The NICU environment must be welcoming and supportive of parents, especially in the Golden Hours.
12. Fostering healthy relationships between members of the family and the infant are important for parents in developing their role as primary caregivers. Ultimately, the development of these healthy relationships will support the infant's long-term outcomes.

References

Aita M, Snider L. The art of developmental care in the NICU: a concept analysis. *J Adv Nurs.* 2003;41(3):223-232.

Baker B, McGrath JM. Supporting the maternal experience in the neonatal ICU. *Newborn Infant Nurs Rev.* 2009;9(2):81-82. doi:10.1053/j.nainr.2009.03.002.

Baum N, Weidberg Z, Osher Y, Kohelet D. No longer pregnant, not yet a mother: giving birth prematurely to a very-low-birth-weight baby. *Qual Health Res.* 2011;22(5):595-606.

Brett J, Staniszewska S, Newburn M, Jones N, Taylor L. A systematic mapping review of effective interventions for communicating with, supporting and providing information to parents of preterm infants. *BMJ Open.* 2011;1(1):e000023. doi:10.1136/bmjopen-2010-000023.

Caeymaex L, Jousselme C, Vasilescu C, et al. Perceived role in end-of-life decision making in the NICU affects long-term parental grief response. *Arc Dis Child Fetal Neonatal Ed.* 2013;98(1):F26-F31. doi: 10.1136/archdischild-2011-301548.

Cooper LG, Gooding JS, Gallagher J, Sternesky L, Ledsky R, Berns SD. Impact of a family-centered care initiative on NICU care, staff and families. *J Perinat.* 2007;27(suppl 2):S32-S37.

Dyer KA. Identifying, understanding, and working with grieving parents in the NICU, part I: identifying and understanding loss and the grief response. *Neonatal Netw.* 2005;24(3):35-46.

Dyer KA. Identifying, understanding, and working with grieving parents in the NICU, part II: strategies. *Neonatal Netw.* 2005;24(4):27-40.

Gooding JS, Cooper LG, Blaine AI, Franck LS, Howse JL, Berns SD. Family support and family-centered care in the neonatal intensive care unit: origins, advances, impact. *Semin Perinatol.* 2011;35(1):20-28.

Hodnett ED, Gates S, Hofmeyr G, Sakala C. Continuous support for women during childbirth. Cochrane Database of Systematic Reviews 2013, Issue 7. Art. No.: CD003766. DOI: 10.1002/14651858.CD003766.pub5.

Johnson BH. Patient and family-centered care. *AHA News.* Bethesda, MD: Institute of Family-Centered Care; 2003.

Latour JM, Hazelzet JA, Duivenvoorden HJ, van Goudoever JB. Perceptions of parents, nurses, and physicians on neonatal intensive care practices. *J Pediatr.* 2010;157(2):215-220.

Lindner SL, McGrath JM. Family centered care in the delivery room environment. *Newborn Infant Nurs Rev.* 2012;12(2):70-72.

Lopez GL, Anderson KH, Feutchinger J. Transition of premature infants from hospital to home life. *Neonat Netw.* 2012;31(4):207-214.

Malusky SK. A concept analysis of family-centered care in the NICU. *Neonat Netw.* 2005;24(6):25-32.

McGrath JM. Building relationships with families in the NICU: exploring the guarded alliance. *J Perinat Neonatal Nurs.* 2001;15(3): 74-83.

McGrath JM. Strategies for increasing parent participation in the NICU. *J Perinat Neonatal Nurs*. 2011;25(4):305-306.

McGrath JM. Supporting parents in understanding and enhancing preterm infant brain development. *Newborn Infant Nurs Rev*. 2008;8(4):164-165.

McGrath JM. Touch and massage in the newborn period: effects on biomarkers and brain development. *J Perinat Neonatal Nurs*. 2009;23(4):304-306.

McGrath JM, Cone S, Samra HA. Neuroprotection in the preterm infant: further understanding of the short- and long-term implications for brain development. *Newborn Infant Nurs Rev*. 2011;11(3):109-112.

McGrath JM, Samra HA, Kenner C. Family-centered developmental care practices and research: what will the next century bring? *J Perinat Neonatal Nurs*. 2011;25(2):165-170.

Morey JA, Gregory K. Nurse-led education mitigates maternal stress. *MCN Am J Matern Child Nurs*. 2012;37(3):182-191.

Pillow M, ed. *Patients as partners: toolkit for implementing national patient safety goal 13*. Oakbrook Terrace, IL: Joint Commission Resources; 2007.

Reis MD, Rempel GR, Scott SD, Brady-Fryer BA, van Aerde J. Developing nurse/patient relationships in the NICU through negotiated partnership. *J Obstet Gynecol Neonatal Nurs*. 2010;39(6):675-683.

Samra HA, McGrath JM, Wehbe M, Clapper J. Epigenetics and family-centered developmental care of the preterm infant. *Adv Neonat Care*. 2012;12(suppl 5):S2-S9.

Treyvaud K, Doyle LW, Lee KJ, et al. Family functioning, burden and parenting stress 2 years after very preterm birth. *Early Hum Dev*. 2011;87(6):427-431.

20

Ethical Dilemmas

Margaret Conway-Orgel

I. Overview
A. Despite multiple advances in caring for the extremely premature infant, there continues to be a great deal of controversy surrounding the resuscitation of neonates at the threshold of viability.
B. This chapter serves as a guideline for members of the health care team to use when they meet with the family to formulate a plan regarding what interventions will or will not be offered to their extremely premature infant immediately following delivery.

II. Definition of viability
A. According to the Nuffield Council on Bioethics, infants born at 22–23 weeks of gestation should be considered candidates for selective resuscitation after discussion with the parents. The Neonatal Resuscitation Program (NRP) considers the appropriate age for selective resuscitation based on parental request to include infants born at 23–24 weeks of gestation.
B. Extreme prematurity — between 23 weeks and 24 weeks of gestation — is a "gray zone" or "margin of viability." Initial survival may be possible; however, the mortality and morbidity rate is high.
C. There is limited data surrounding the long-term outcomes of extremely premature infants. This makes it difficult to offer parents comprehensive information to make informed decisions regarding intervention.
   1. One source for clinicians to use is the NICHD outcomes calculator: http://www.nichd.nih.gov/about/org/der/branches/ppb/programs/epbo/Pages/epbo_case.aspx.
   2. This will help calculate known survival and associated morbidities based on gestational age, weight, gender, and use of antenatal steroids.
D. There may also be conflicts within the health care team regarding individual interpretation of viability and the use of antenatal steroids in infants below a certain gestational age.
E. Health care team members should discuss issues before proceeding with the delivery of extremely premature infants. There are two approaches, which may cause conflict within the team.

1. Vitalistic approach: All life as sacred, regardless of the quality of that life. This approach supports full resuscitation of all infants born alive, regardless of known survival or long-term outcome (life at all cost).
2. Quality-of-life approach: Intervention at the time of birth should only be initiated if there is hope for a good life quality for the infant. Defining what would constitute a good life is subjective and controversial.

F. Futility is an overriding consideration. There are several definitions of futility.
   1. Absolute futility (0% chance of cure): This is most comparable with the medical ethicist's view of futility.
   2. Low probability (less than an arbitrary number or clinical impression) of success: Health care providers often think of futility in this term.

G. When there is conflict among members of the health care team and/or the parents, a moral dilemma may occur.

H. Properly resolved, conflict may actually be beneficial and help determine ethical and unethical behaviors or practices. However, if left unresolved, conflict could result in long-term incapacitation, burnout, or ill will between team members or family and team.

I. In an effort to assist members of the health care team in dealing with ethical dilemmas surrounding the resuscitation of an extremely premature infant, it is important to be familiar with principles that are essential to providing appropriate care.

III. Ethical principles: There are four fundamental ethical principles for providing care in the NICU. These principles serve as a compass when counseling families and making decisions regarding resuscitation.

A. Autonomy: Provide the patient the necessary information to make a fully informed decision. In the case of the fetus/neonate, the parents are considered to be surrogate decision makers for the child who would make a decision in the best interest of the child. Best interest, however, is a subjective term and health team members (including families) may not agree upon what is in the patient's best interest.

B. Justice: Take actions that are fair to all involved.

C. Beneficence: Do what is good. This would suggest that the actions taken during resuscitation should be done in the best interest of the infant.

D. Non-maleficence: Most importantly, do no harm. It is the responsibility of the parents and the medical team to base their decisions on an informed assessment that balances the risk of harm with the benefits.
E. From the first communication with other members of the team caring for the mother/infant dyad, through the delivery and interventions provided to the fetus/neonate, integration of these principles will assist in formulating decisions that are grounded in ethics.

IV. Parental involvement

A. Preterm delivery is commonly unanticipated. Parents are usually not prepared (psychologically and mentally) for the critical decisions that they will be faced with in the hours or days following admission.
B. It is critical to have the neonate delivered at a level-3 NICU, despite the negative effect of maternal separation from family, friends, and other support networks. This approach places the infant's best interests first. In addition, it provides an opportunity for the health care team to discuss options and outcomes with the mother and family, often prior to the need for maternal pain or sedation medications that may be required during delivery.
C. Multiple sources in the literature support involving parents in the decision-making process as early as possible.
   1. Parents also express the importance of developing a trusting, comfortable relationship with the team members who will be involved in the resuscitation. This assists in making critical decisions before and after delivery regarding how to proceed.
   2. Ideally, parents should meet with a member of the neonatal team to discuss known survival and outcomes based on the infant's gestational age so they have time to ask questions and receive additional information. These discussions should include survival and outcome data based on gestational age specific to the institution and on regional and/or national data.
   3. Information discussed in the consultation is often forgotten or confused by the mother. This difficulty recalling may be secondary to language, literacy, or other barriers that the mother may not express at the time of the consultation.

4. If possible, present information in several formats and have nursing or family support present as well. Supplement verbal discussions with written pamphlets or pictograms that clarify what to expect following delivery, as well as some of the known risks of being delivered at this early gestational age.

V. Ethical and legal considerations

A. Most families ask for "everything to be done" following the delivery.
B. It is important to clarify what "everything" means.
C. When dealing with extremely premature neonates, there are several federal acts that the health care team needs to be aware of:
 1. Child Abuse (Baby Doe) Amendment of 1984
    a. The act described a new category of child abuse termed "medical neglect."
    b. Medical neglect is defined as withholding medically indicated treatment from a disabled infant with "life-threatening conditions."
    c. The act was tested in court and amended to protect a physician who does not initiate or withdraws medical care when he or she believes treatment is "futile" or "virtually futile" therapy, imposes excessive burdens on the infant, and prolongs dying.
 2. Born-Alive Infants Protection Act of 2002
    a. This act has been enacted by state legislatures in various forms.
    b. The act defined a born-alive infant as a "person, human being, child, or individual."
    c. This definition does not affect the applicable standard of care, but does ensure that all born-alive infants are treated as persons for purposes of federal law.
    d. The American Academy of Pediatrics (AAP) NRP Steering Committee in 2006 issued this statement: "This act does not affect the approach that physicians currently follow with respect to the extremely premature infant. At the time of delivery, the medical condition and prognosis of the newly born infant should be assessed. At that point, the decision of withholding or discontinuing medical treatment that is considered futile may be considered by the medical care providers in conjunction with the parents acting in the best interest of their child."

3. Once the decision is made to not resuscitate or to withdraw medical support, the infant should continue to be treated with dignity and respect and be provided with comfort care measures.

VI. Palliative care in the perinatal period

A. Palliative care extends beyond the immediate dying process to include the needs of the family and the baby.
   1. Provide an opportunity, if possible, for parents to spend time with their child before his/her death.
   2. Obtain meaningful mementos, such as footprints and handprints or soft plaster molds, photographs, and lockets of hair.
   3. After the infant dies, parents often find comfort in bathing their infant and dressing him/her in special outfits provided by the family or the hospital.
   4. If the infant dies while separated from family, the staff at the receiving hospital may also perform these activities.
   5. It is important for the palliative care team to follow up with parents and refer them to counseling services, if needed.
   6. If an autopsy was conducted, the family should be offered an opportunity to meet with the attending neonatologist to review results and answer any questions that may have arisen since their child's death.
B. Palliative care should add life to the infant's time, not add time to the infant's life.
C. If time permits before delivery, it is helpful to involve the palliative care team with parents and health care providers.
   1. This allows parents to discuss their hopes and desires if they choose to not resuscitate their extremely preterm infant, or in the event of an unsuccessful resuscitation.
   2. Support by a team will reduce the burdens placed on families in making difficult end-of-life decisions by converting the decision to withhold/withdraw life support to the team.
   3. Parents may develop a birth plan for their infant if they choose comfort care after delivery. The birth plan may include photographers, special music, specific rituals, or memory-making activities to mark the passage of their child's birth and death.

4. Following the delivery or the end of resuscitation, it is important to ensure that the end of the infant's life is both free of pain and met with respect.
5. Temperature and medication administration are key points that will need to be addressed.
   a. Palliative care efforts should be based on parental cultural expectations in addition to medical needs of the patient.
   b. Providing heat to dying infants is essential in both comfort terms as well as in avoiding the extension of the dying process. Extremely preterm infants lose heat quickly through their skin. Hypothermia decreases metabolic rate and prolongs the dying process.
      (1) The mother can hold the infant skin-to-skin; place a cotton cap on the baby's head.
      (2) If the mother is cold, use a heat lamp or heat pack tucked next to baby to provide warmth and comfort.
      (3) If the parents choose not to have the infant in the room with them, place the infant in a pre-warmed isolette and swaddle in plastic wrap to ensure warmth and comfort.
6. Pain medications can be administered orally or intravenously in extremely premature infants.
   a. There has been controversy about the need to provide pain medication to live-born infants who are considered non-viable (22–24 weeks gestation).
   b. However, the goal should be to provide comfort medications; providers should err on side of infant, who may be experiencing discomfort and not able to express this.
      (1) Oral or IV morphine sulfate can be administered to infant buccally. There will be absorption of medication at this site. Dose would be 0.15 mg/kg sublingual or 0.05/kg IV every 15 min as needed for agonal breathing or signs and symptoms of pain.
      (2) Intramuscular administration is not helpful; peripheral circulation is inadequate and dose will remain at administration site.
      (3) For agitation, consider the use of midazolam. Dose would be 0.5 mg/k PO or 0.1mg/kg IV every 15 min as needed to relieve agitation.

(4) Delivery of intranasal fentanyl is another method in which to provide pain relief in dying infants who do not have IV access. The dose is 0.1 mcg/kg/dose, which can be given every 5–10 min with a maximum of 3 doses in 30-min time periods.

(5) Oral sucrose (12%–50% solution) may be administered under the tongue in dosages of 0.1–0.2 mL.

VII. Conclusion

A. Extremely premature infants often present with challenges at many levels. In addition to assuring competency in resuscitation and stabilization, the neonatal health care team needs to be aware of the ethical dilemmas that may be encountered.

B. Knowledge of ethical principles as they apply to extremely premature infants — in the gray zone of viability — as well as current legal positions allow the neonatal team to be well-equipped to address issues as they arise.

C. Parents want to be involved in the decision-making process and have less moral distress when they are provided accurate information about short- and long-term outcomes.

D. Dying infants need to be treated respectfully and provided with comfort care, which includes warmth and relief from pain.

E. A palliative care team member can assist the parents in finding meaning in their child's short life.

References

Balaguer A, Marin-Ancel A, Ortigoza-Escobar D, Escribano J, Argemi J. The model of palliative care in the perinatal setting: a review of the literature. *BMC Pediatr*. 2012;12:25. doi: 10.1186/1471-2431-12-25.

Becker PT, Grunwald PC. Contextual dynamics of ethical decision making in the NICU. *J Perinat Neonatal Nurs*. 2000;14(2):58-72.

Fanaroff AA. Extremely low birth weight infants — the interplay between outcomes and ethics. *Acta Pediatr*. 2008;97(2);144-145.

Harlos MS, Stenekes S, Lambert D, Hohl C, Chochinov HM. Intranasal fentanyl in the palliative care of newborns and infants. *J Pain Symptom Manage*. 2013;46(2):265-274.

Harrison H. The offer they can't refuse: parents and perinatal treatment decisions. *Semin Fetal Neonat Med*. 2008;13(5):329-334.

International Liaison Committee on Resuscitation. The International Liaison Committee on Resuscitation (ILCOR) consensus on science with treatment recommendations for pediatric and neonatal patients: neonatal resuscitation. *Pediatrics*. 2006;117(5):e978-e988. doi:10.1542/peds.2006-0350.

Janvier A, Barrington KJ, Aziz K, Lantos J. Ethics ain't easy: do we need simple rules for complicated ethical decisions? *Acta Pediatr*. 2008;97(4):402-406.

Janvier A, Meadow W, Leuthner SR, et al. Whom are we comforting? An analysis of comfort medications delivered to dying neonates. *J Pediatr*. 2011;159(2):206-210.

Kraybill EN. Ethical issues in the care of extremely low birth weight infants. *Semin Perinatol*. 1998;22(3);207-215.

Lee HC, Bennett MV, Schulman J, Gould JB. Accounting for variations in length of NICU stay for extremely low birth weight infants. *J Perinatol*. 2013;33(11):872-876.

Lorenz JM. Ethical dilemmas and disagreement in the newborn intensive care unit. *J Arab Neonatal Forum*. 2005;2:51-56.

McHaffie HE, Lyon AJ, Fowlie PW. Lingering death after treatment withdrawal in the neonatal intensive care unit. *Arch Dis Child Fetal Neonatal Ed*. 2001;85(1):F8-F12.

Moro TT, Kavanaugh K, Savage TA, Reyes MR, Kimura RE, Bhat R. Parent decision making for life support for extremely premature infants: from the prenatal through end-of-life period. *J Perinat Neonatal Nurs*. 2011;25(1):52-60.

NICHD Neonatal Research Network (NRN): Extremely preterm birth outcome data. NICHD Web site. http://www.nichd.nih.gov/about/org/der/branches/ppb/programs/epbo/Pages/index.aspx. October 31, 2013.

Raju TN, Mercer BM, Burchfield DJ, Joseph GF. Periviable birth: executive summary of a Joint Workshop by the Eunice Kennedy Shriver National Institute of Child Health and Human Development, Society for Maternal-Fetal Medicine, American Academy of Pediatrics, and American College of Obstetricians and Gynecologists. *J Perinatol*. 2014;34(5):333-342. doi: 10.1038/jp.2014.70.

Singh J, Fanaroff J, Andrews B, et al. Resuscitation in the "gray zone" of viability: determining physician preferences and predicting infant outcomes. *Pediatrics*. 2007;120(3):519-526.

Weir M, Evans M, Coughlin K. Ethical decision making in the resuscitation of extremely premature infants: the health care professional's perspective. *J Obstet Gynaecol Can*. 2011;33(1):49-56.

Teamwork and Communication
Margaret Conway-Orgel

I. Introduction
A. Even among the most skilled resuscitation teams, outcomes during the stabilization and transport of an acutely ill infant can be poor if the communication between team members is poor.
B. Effective communication is as important as knowing the correct dose of a medication when working toward a positive patient outcome.

II. Why teamwork?
A. The development of effective teams has been shown to identify, address, and reduce errors that may compromise patient safety and potentially alter outcomes.
B. Many studies have been conducted on the value of teamwork.
   1. *To Err is Human*, a report by the Institute of Medicine, identified team communication as a key goal in health care.
   2. The Joint Commission stated that one of its safety goals was to improve communication among the health care team.
   3. The Patient Safety and Quality Improvement Act, signed in 2005, required the Department of Health and Human Services to establish a mechanism for the voluntary and confidential reporting of medical errors to patient-safety organizations.
   4. TeamSTEPPS®, a patient-safety program developed by the Department of Defense in collaboration with the Agency for Healthcare Research and Quality, applied the military's research on teamwork to the health care setting. TeamSTEPPS® takes an interrelated set of skills essential to effective teamwork which, when utilized and applied, improve patient outcomes and create a culture of safety. Leape reported a 50% reduction in poor outcomes in preterm infants when TeamSTEPPS® training was shared with labor and delivery staff.

III. Teams vs. groups
   A. Groups can achieve goals through individuals who work independently on tasks to achieve end results. This does not require coordination of tasks with others.
   B. Teams are individuals who have come together with specific functions to work interdependently with a shared vision to achieve a common goal. These groups are often time-limited and recognize that the team's mission is greater than the functions of its individual members.

IV. Team members
   A. Include anyone involved actively in caring for the patient, including the leader
   B. Have clearly defined roles
   C. Are individually accountable to the team for their actions
   D. Remain constantly aware of the situation to ensure effective team function
   E. May fail to perform effectively due to:
      1. Excessive professional courtesy or hierarchy
      2. Judgment impacted by someone's reputation (halo effect)
      3. Abdication of responsibility (just along for the ride)
      4. Hidden agendas
      5. Complacency with role (lost situational awareness)
      6. High-risk times when mistakes more likely to occur (e.g., during shift change)
      7. Becoming focused on the task without acknowledging the big picture
      8. Fatigue
      9. Lack of time
      10. Workload
      11. Lack of information-sharing
      12. Roles not clearly defined
      13. Inconsistency

V. Components of successfully functioning teams
   A. Leadership
      1. Should be assigned at start of episode of care
      2. Might transition during an event; such transition should be clearly defined and confirmed, as when an airline pilot takes control from a co-pilot during an emergency
      3. Is responsible for coordination of team activities by ensuring a clear plan of action is in place and understood
      4. Empowers team members to speak up and challenge when appropriate

5. Ensures team members are assigned roles that best use their individual skills and provide feedback as the situation dictates
6. Allows the team to see the situation as a whole, rather than as parts
7. Does not have to be an MD; can be the individual involved in the situation when it first presents
8. Can manage and resolve conflict comfortably
9. Must clearly communicate and identify changes in leadership during crisis, both between the leaders and to all team members

B. Shared awareness
1. Fosters communication to allow synchronization of care
2. Helps team members know what to expect and keep things on track
3. Creates a shared vision and common bond to achieve goals

C. Mutual support
1. Maintain positive attitude among team members.
2. Understand roles clearly going into the situation.
3. Work together to prevent individuals from becoming overwhelmed or stressed.
4. Foster a climate of trust so members will anticipate the need for help and actively seek it out when needed (got your back).
5. Encourage team members to voice concerns about patient-safety issues.
6. Provide timely feedback of performance with goal to improve outcomes.

D. Communication
1. Communication is the backbone of a successful team.
2. The Joint Commission found that ineffective communication is a root cause for nearly 66% of all sentinel events reported.
   a. Members of effective teams take the time to discuss the anticipated plan and review events after they have occurred.
   b. Communication is clear, concise, and timely.
   c. Methods such as call-out and check-back will assist in the reduction of errors and keep all team members informed.

VI. Techniques to enhance communication
A. Brief or planning phase

1. Form team, introducing members by name and specific job title.
2. Assign team roles and clarify responsibilities, if needed.
3. Establish goals.

B. Huddle or problem solving
   1. Discuss critical issues and upcoming events.
   2. Reorient group for situational awareness.
   3. Assign resources.
   4. Allow for contingency planning.
   5. Provide opportunity for team members to express concerns.

C. Debrief after event to improve and learn
   1. Reconstruct key events.
   2. Evaluate errors or communication gaps.
   3. Review workload distribution.
   4. Ask what went well.
   5. Discuss what went wrong.
   6. Identify areas to be improved.
   7. Do not recriminate any team member.

D. SBAR
   1. SBAR is a method to standardize communication about a patient's condition.
   2. SBAR may reduce errors associated with miscommunication or limited information.
   3. During the hand-off, the team members should state:
      a. **S**ituation: What is happening with the patient?
      b. **B**ackground: What is the clinical background?
      c. **A**ssessment: What do I think the problem is?
      d. **R**ecommend or **R**equest: What would I do to correct it?

E. Call-out
   1. Method to communicate important information during a critical event
   2. Helps team members anticipate and prepare for next step
   3. Benefits recorder
   4. Direct information to one individual

F. Check-back
   1. Closes communication loop
   2. Verifies and validates information exchanged
   3. Reduces communication errors

G. Hand-off
   1. Method of sharing information when a team member is relieved of duty of caring for the patient

a. Identify who is responsible for the patient and verify that the new team member is assuming responsibility.
   b. If there is any uncertainty, it is your responsibility to clear up the situation before turning the patient over to the next individual.
   c. Communicate verbally; never assume that written communication will be understood.
   d. Until next team acknowledges your hand-off, **you** are responsible for the patient.
2. Opportunity for new eyes to review a previously unresolvable challenge or problem, as well as review for safety issues
3. To assure an effective hand-off: I PASS the BATON
   a. **I**ntroduction: yourself and your role
   b. **P**atient: name, identifiers, age, sex, location
   c. **A**ssessment: present chief complaint, vital signs, symptoms, and diagnosis
   d. **S**ituation: current status/circumstances, including code status, recent changes, and response to treatment
   e. **S**afety concerns: critical lab values/reports, socioeconomic factors, alerts (e.g., isolation)
   f. **B**ackground: comorbidities, current medications, family background
   g. **A**ctions: brief rationale of actions taken or required
   h. **T**iming: level of urgency, explicit timing and prioritization of actions
   i. **O**wnership: who is responsible (nurse/doctor/team)
   j. **N**ext: next steps, anticipated changes, plans, and contingency plans

VII. Conflict resolution
A. Overview
   1. In emotionally charged situations, such as a resuscitation of a critically ill infant, there will be times when team members may not agree with each other or feel that an individual's action may cause harm to the patient. This will result in conflict.
   2. Conflict may be avoided when the team leader allows team members to speak without feeling threatened.
   3. First-name introductions and open statements asking for input are effective tools to achieve this goal.
   4. One of roles of the team leader is to prevent and, when necessary, help resolve conflicts.

5. Team members must be comfortable with speaking out when they perceive an unsafe situation.
B. Strategies to resolve conflicts
 1. Two-challenge rule
    a. Express concerns about safety assertively and offer a solution.
    b. CUS words: If a member of the team has a major concern that is not adequately addressed, CUS words can elevate the concern to the leader.
       (1) Strong phrases such as "I am **c**oncerned," "I am **u**ncomfortable," or "This is a **s**afety issue," allow the team member to communicate to the team leader that there is an unaddressed serious issue.
       (2) Leaders should take these statements seriously and analyze the concern.
       (3) Use of a CUS word twice should prompt a reevaluation of the situation with the team.
    c. All team members should be empowered to speak up or "stop the line" if they feel that patient safety is impacted.
    d. Everyone involved should stop the action in question until resolution occurs.
    e. Individuals must be prepared to take concerns to the next level if the conflict remains unresolved.
 2. DESC script: May not be appropriate during high-risk activity such as resuscitation
    a. **D**escribe the situation or behavior using concrete information.
    b. **E**xpress how the situation makes you feel, using "I" statements to avoid defensiveness.
    c. **S**uggest alternatives and attempt to achieve agreement.
    d. **C**onsequences should be stated clearly and focus on the action, not the individual.
       (1) Avoid attacking the individual.
       (2) Focus on what is wrong, not who is wrong.
 3. Other ways to resolve conflicts (some not acceptable)
    a. Compromise: Both parties "agree to disagree" and settle for less than the ideal
    b. Avoidance: Individuals avoid or sidestep issue
    c. Accommodation: Focuses on preserving relationship, not resolving conflict
    d. Dominance: Conflicts managed through authoritative manner, with directives handed down

VIII. Developing effective team communication

A. High-functioning teams do not achieve success without education and practice.
B. Across all health care disciplines, training in teamwork and communication is essential. In 2009, The American College of Obstetricians and Gynecologists (ACOG) stated: "Training in teamwork and communication techniques is increasingly being recognized as a cornerstone of a robust patient safety program."
C. Simulation is an effective way to train teams.
   1. Teams can simulate resuscitation, stabilization, and transfer of an infant to develop confidence and establish competence without the anxiety of being in a real delivery room.
   2. Debriefing and video feedback after simulation allows for communication challenges and potential for improvement to be pointed out.
   3. In areas without a simulation lab, scenarios can be performed with equipment at hand. An observer can videotape the event to use for debriefing and feedback.

IX. Additional scenarios and considerations

A. Examples of open communication statements in leadership
   1. Senior person arrives after event has begun. Senior person: "Hello everyone. Who is in charge? May I have a synopsis? OK. Please continue and I'll back you up." Current leader: "OK. Would you confirm tube position?"
   2. Senior person arrives after event has begun. Senior person: "Hello everyone. Who is in charge? May I have a synopsis? OK. If you would prepare to place lines, I will take over leading the resuscitation." Current leader: "OK. You're leading and I will place a UVC and UAC."
   3. Preparation for delivery. Leader: "We have everyone here. Let's do introductions and roles. Use first names please." Leader explains that this is to remove barriers to communication: "A team member is more likely to raise a potentially concerning comment to 'John' than to 'Dr. Smith.'"

4. Medication order and delivery. Leader: "Jan, would you give 0.3 mL/kg of 1:10,000 epinephrine — that's 0.3 mL for this 1-kg baby — via UVC please?" Jan: "Yes. 0.3 mL of 1:10,000 epinephrine — 1 kg is 0.3 mL by UVC." Leader: "Yes — 0.3 mL of 1:10,000 epi." Jan: "Epi in." Leader. "Thank you. Epi in."
    5. Resuscitation failing: Leader: "Let's review. We have [reviews situation]. Does anyone have additional suggestions?"
  B. Questions for huddle before team event
    1. Employ SBAR statements (or alternative communication tool).
    2. What do we expect as we enter this event? (Ask for a range of possibilities from best case to worst.)
    3. Are we prepared for the worst-case situation?
    4. Does anyone else need to be present or available? Are there too many people for the event?
    5. Do we need any additional equipment specific for this situation?
    6. What is our planned sequence of intervention? Who does what?
  C. Questions for debriefing
    1. What were we expecting at the start of the event?
    2. Did the course unfold as expected?
    3. What unfolded that was unexpected? Were we prepared?
    4. What worked?
    5. What could we have done differently?
    6. If we could improve one aspect of this team event, what would it be?
    7. If we could rehearse one aspect of this team event, what would it be?

X. Conclusion
  A. Communication is crucial in every aspect of health care, but perhaps most importantly in an emotionally charged arena such as a delivery room.
  B. Medical professionals have vital knowledge and skills, but without teamwork and seamless communication, the ultimate outcome of an infant in distress may be less than optimal.

References

American College of Obstetricians and Gynecologists Committee on Patient Safety and Quality Improvement. ACOG committee opinion no. 447: patient safety in obstetrics and gynecology. *Obstet Gynecol.* 2009;114(6):1425-1427.

Committee on Quality of Health Care in America. *To Err is Human: Building a Safer Health System.* Washington, DC: National Academy Press; 2000.

Deering S, Johnston LC, Colacchio K. Multidisciplinary teamwork and communication training. *Semin Perinatol.* 2011;35(2):89-96.

Edwards S, Siassakos D. Training teams and leaders to reduce resuscitation errors and improve patient outcome. *Resuscitation* 2012;83(1):13-15.

The Joint Commission. Improving America's hospitals: The Joint Commission's annual report on quality and safety – 2007. http://www.joint-commission.org/assets/1/6/2007_Annual_Report.pdf. Accessed December 18, 2013.

Leape LL, Berwick DM. Five years after to err is human: what have we learned? *JAMA.* 2005;293(19):2384-2390.

Norris EM, Lockey AS. Human factors in resuscitation teaching. *Resuscitation.* 2012;83(4):423-427.

TeamSTEPPS Fundamentals Course: Module 6. Agency for Healthcare Research and Quality Web site. http://www.ahrq.gov/teamsteppstools/instructor/fundamentals/module6/slcommunication.htm#sl4. Accessed September 11, 2013.

Thomas EJ, Williams AL, Reichman EF, Lasky RE, Crandell S, Taggart WR. Team training in the neonatal resuscitation program for interns: team and quality of resuscitations. *Pediatrics.* 2010;125(3):539-546.

22

Neonatal Transport

Fran Byrd

I. Introduction
A. Optimal outcomes for transported very low birth weight (VLBW) infants begin with detailed, advanced planning and preparation so that the level of care experienced within the NICU walls can be delivered over distance.
B. Transport can be a challenging and unpredictable environment; but experienced, vigilant, and compassionate team members with the correct equipment can make the process flow more smoothly.

II. Essential points to ponder
A. Care of the VLBW infant in the transport setting should reflect the same principles and evidence-based practice standards expected in a tertiary level NICU.
B. Numerous studies have shown that transport teams with experience in the care of sick infants decrease the morbidity and mortality of infants born in a non-tertiary level facility, where an estimated 14%–30% of VLBW infant births occur.
C. Optimal outcomes are supported when specialized neonatal teams take time at the referring facility to assess, perform essential management, and "package" the VLBW infant to avoid the need for procedures and interventions during the motion of transport.
D. Communication is a critical element in the overall transport process, including the following:
   1. Initial exchange between referring hospital and tertiary center
   2. Intra-transport communication between the referring and receiving physicians and the team for problem resolution and/or plan of care
   3. The team's interaction with staff upon arrival to receive, report, and review referring hospital assessments, diagnostics, and interventions
   4. Follow-up communication from the tertiary center to the referring hospital to provide updates to staff and family
E. In-house transport of the VLBW infant requires meticulous pre-transport preparation, followed by monitoring the infant's clinical status in transit and providing appropriate hand-off.

III. General considerations for transport of the VLBW infant
A. Patient safety
1. Patient safety begins with selection of the appropriate team and transport mode to initiate and maintain the optimal level of care for each infant.
2. Prior to actual transport use, evaluate equipment function under motion and vibration conditions.
   a. If planning to transport in aircraft at altitude, pay attention to ventilator calibration and proper function of flow meters and infusion pumps.
      (1) Ventilators are generally calibrated at sea level, and changes in barometric pressure have been shown to decrease the actual respiratory rate delivered vs. the desired rate set on the ventilator and to increase tidal volumes (Tv) at altitude in a variety of ventilator models.
      (2) Infusion pump rates and gas flow may vary with altitude changes in flight.
   b. Equipment to accompany any transport should be appropriately secured at an assigned location to avoid injury to patient/personnel or equipment failure.
   c. All federal, state and system regulations in place must be followed to ensure that the judgment and performance of air and ground team members are maximized for patient safety.
   d. Positioning of infant(s) and crew must allow for unimpeded access to all patients and equipment.
3. Infection control should follow standard procedures used in the NICU.
   a. Hand hygiene (hand washing and/or the use of approved hand sanitizers) is critical in the much larger and potentially contaminated areas encountered during the transport process.
   b. All equipment and non-disposable supplies used in transport should be cleaned according to hospital standards to reduce the chance of nosocomial infections.
4. Allow for thorough drying and dissipation of cleaning-agent odors prior to equipment use.
5. At any time an infant is in a transport incubator, the unit should be "on" and powered by wall outlet (AC) or battery power (DC) — otherwise, the incubator becomes a closed plastic box.

6. All modes of transport generate mean sound levels that exceed recommendations for NICU sound-level limits.
7. To minimize the impact of noise, use earmuffs or other approved forms of hearing protection for the VLBW infant.
8. Restraining the VLBW infant for safety purposes can be difficult based on size; however, it is important to utilize an approach that provides the maximum degree of body stabilization without impeding airway, circulation, or visibility.
9. When positioning the incubator and/or infant, consider the potential gravitational effects on blood flow created by sudden stops/starts or changes of direction during transport, such as sudden acceleration/deceleration in ambulances and takeoffs/landings in fixed-wing aircraft.
    a. When the head is toward the front of the vehicle or aircraft, there is a tendency for blood to move to the lower body during acceleration or takeoffs and toward the head during sudden stops or landings.
    b. When the head is toward the rear of the vehicle or aircraft, there is a tendency for blood to move to the head and upper body during acceleration or takeoffs and toward the lower body during sudden stops or landings.
    c. Although positioning cannot always be changed, a side-lying (crossways) position to the forces of acceleration and deceleration should be considered.
    d. For ground transport, set the expectation that vehicle stops/starts will be as smooth as possible and that the return to the receiving facility will be accomplished without lights and sirens, if possible.
    e. The infant's head should be maintained in a neutral position during transport. To prevent intraventricular hemorrhage (IVH), it should be level or slightly elevated, but never in a down position.
B. Monitoring the VLBW infant in transport
    1. At minimum, the ability to monitor temperature, heart rate, respiratory rate, oxygen saturation, and blood pressure is required.
        a. Continuous monitoring is preferable.
        b. Monitoring devices should have visual alarms in addition to any audible alarms.

c. Based on noise, vibration, and potential signal interference during transport, continuous visual assessment is essential.
2. For intubated or mechanically ventilated infants, a method of monitoring end-tidal CO_2 levels is indicated. End-tidal CO_2 levels can be reliably measured in intubated infants down to 1,000 g. If a continuous setup is unavailable for transport of the VLBW infant, an appropriately sized disposable adaptor for confirmation of tube placement and intermittent checks should be available.
3. Continuous oximetry monitoring is essential.
4. Point of care (POC) testing
   a. Obtain the infant's blood glucose level and temperature immediately before transport departure.
   b. Monitor glucose levels during transport.
   c. If available, use of approved POC systems to monitor blood gases and electrolytes can provide valuable information for addressing changes in oxygenation/ventilation and/or fluid and electrolyte balance on extended transports.

C. Family support
   1. It is essential for the team to project a sense of experience, as well as a caring, compassionate nature that is reflected in their approach to care of the VLBW infant and their concern for the family.
   2. Provide an opportunity for the mother and other significant family members to see and touch the infant prior to transport, which may require moving the infant to the mother after stabilization is complete or bringing the mother to an unstable infant's bedside if necessary.
   3. If the infant's condition is such that survival during transport is deemed unlikely, the team should have a plan that involves discussion between the referring facility and tertiary center staff, and with the infant's family, to determine if the best approach is to avoid separating the infant from the family unnecessarily.
      a. It is crucial that staff of the referring hospital, tertiary center, and transport team be in agreement as to the plan of care and communication with the family to facilitate the best possible bonding and/or grieving processes.

b. If the decision is made to transport an infant whose survival during or immediately following transport is extremely doubtful, it is important to provide pre-transport support options for the family, such as:
    (1) Encouraging and supporting the family's presence during stabilization
    (2) Obtaining photographs of the family with and touching the infant
    (3) Providing a small sample of the infant's hair for the mother, if feasible and approved by the family
    (4) Facilitating the performance of religious rites as requested by the family
    (5) With the help of the referring facility, selecting a route out of the facility that allows the extended family (including siblings, if desired) a private viewing of the infant in the incubator prior to transport departure
4. Describe how the infant will be transported, where the infant will be admitted, and the name of the receiving provider, if known.
    a. For separate informed consents for transport obtained by the transport team, the potential risks of transport in general and of the specific mode of transport should be discussed with the parent or guardian signing the consent.
    b. Provide written information about the receiving NICU, pertinent telephone numbers, and a detailed map for locating both the facility and the NICU.
    c. If possible, brochures should have a separate map with a perforated page that can be removed and used immediately by family coming to the regional center, while the brochure with pictures and information should be left for the mother if she must remain hospitalized.
5. Obtain telephone numbers from significant family members.
6. Assure the mother that if she remains hospitalized, she will receive a call from the transport team as soon as her infant is admitted to the NICU — **it is very important to follow up on this promise.**
7. Take a photograph that can be printed and left with the mother prior to departure.

8. If transporting in a specialized ambulance, consider having small pictures available that the transport team can give to the infant's mother on the occasion of discharge from the NICU for inclusion in the baby book under "first ride or trip".
D. Transport documentation
1. Should include copies of maternal and infant records, lab reports and imaging provided by the referring facility, and all consents for referral and transport.
2. Transport team documentation should contain information that outlines the continuum of care, including the infant's status at the time of arrival at the referral hospital, through stabilization, transport, and hand-off to the receiving NICU staff.
    a. Any medications administered should be recorded as dictated by policy.
    b. Any interventions performed should be documented, along with the infant's response.
E. Standard supplies and medications
1. Supplies and medications carried for transport of the VLBW infant should mimic as closely as possible those available within the NICU.
2. Medications such as surfactant, which requires refrigeration, will need to be transported in appropriate carriers with cool packs.
3. Supply and medication bags should be assembled for transport based on the neonatal populations stabilized and transported by the individual facility, using national standards as guidelines.

IV. Factors exerting physiologic impact on the VLBW infant
A. Noise and vibration
1. Both noise and vibration are aspects of transport that are **very** difficult to address in ground and air transport.
    a. Use of a stethoscope for auscultation is generally not an option in ambulances and rotor-wing aircraft, based on noise levels.
    b. Use clinical assessment of the infant's oximetry, perfusion, chest rise, and changes in respiratory rate/depth.
    c. Note EKG, blood pressure (BP), pulse oximetry oxygen saturation (SpO_2), and end-tidal carbon dioxide monitoring trends.

2. Noise levels in transport that exceed the recommended levels for the NICU setting can increase respiratory rate, heart rate, BP, and anxiety levels; use earmuffs or a thermal cap with a padded lining that can be pulled down over the infant's ears.
3. Vibration at moderate levels has been shown to increase metabolic rate and oxygen demands.
   a. It is preferable to leave gel mattresses or similar cushioning in the transport incubator at all times so that the mattress or padding is pre-warmed.
   b. Provide safety restraints that also incorporate padding measures around the infant for stabilization.
B. Laws of flight physiology — **e**ffects of Boyle's law
   1. As altitude increases, atmospheric pressure decreases, resulting in:
      a. An increase in gas volume
      b. Additional impact (not generally emphasized for Boyle's law) — a wider spread of molecules
   2. Physiologic impact of increased gas volume in closed cavities:
      a. Clinical implications include worsening of pulmonary air leaks and increase in abdominal and intestinal distention, with potential for rupture or worsening pneumatosis intestinalis.
         (1) Consider insertion of a vented orogastric tube for every VLBW infant transported, with specific attention to those with a suspected gastrointestinal anomaly or disorder or those being transported at altitude.
         (2) Confirm that any chest tubes or endotracheal (ET) tubes are clear and patent; suction ET tube as indicated to maintain patency.
         (3) Assess for and/or manage any air leaks prior to flight.
      b. Equipment implications include potential for gas expansion in any non-vented device or supplies, e.g., IV drip chambers, BP cuffs, ventilators, non-vented incubator mattresses.
         (1) If using external BP cuffs, do not leave connected between readings.
         (2) If special circumstances require a cuffed ET tube or tracheostomy tube; use water, rather than air, to inflate the cuff for flights at altitude.

3. Physiologic impact of more widely spread molecules, including water vapor:
   a. A decrease in the number of molecules of oxygen available per volume of inspired gas
      (1) Clinical implication includes hypoxia.
      (2) Close assessment for signs of hypoxia with immediate action as indicated in transport-specific airway approaches is required.
   b. Wider dispersion of molecules of water vapor
      (1) Clinical implications include drier air and less humidification of ambient gases.
      (2) All inspired gases should be heated and humidified.
4. Under Boyle's law, as altitude decreases, atmospheric pressure increases, resulting in a compression of gas molecules and leading to a decrease in gas volume.
   a. Physiologic impact of gas compression — contraction of air/soft tissues in closed cavities
   b. Clinical implication — small size of Eustachian tube in VLBW infants can lead to collapse and pain
      (1) Assess infant for indications of pain or stress.
      (2) Offer non-nutritive sucking option, if feasible.

C. Laws of flight physiology — effects of Dalton's law
   1. At any given altitude, total barometric pressure equals the sum of all the partial pressures of the gases within a mixture.
   2. Oxygen remains 21% of the atmospheric pressure; however, coupled with Boyle's law, fewer oxygen molecules are present per volume of gas, thereby exerting decreased partial pressure.
   3. Physiologic impact of decreasing arterial oxygen tension at increasing altitude:
      a. Clinical implication includes hypoxia.
      b. A modest decrease in the partial pressure of alveolar oxygen results in neonatal hypoxia.
      c. Hypoxia is a greater risk for neonates than adults, as there is a larger alveolar-oxygen difference: 25 mmHg in neonates vs. 10 mmHg in adults.
      d. For infants on supplemental oxygen, anticipate the need for an increase in the fraction of inspired oxygen (FiO_2) and closely follow pulse oximeter readings with response as indicated by SpO_2.

e. Formula to adjust:
$$\text{New FiO}_2 = (\text{FiO}_2 \times P_{B1})/P_{B2}$$
Where:
P_{B1} = Current barometric pressure
P_{B2} = Barometric pressure anticipated at highest flight altitude

D. Laws of flight physiology — effects of Charles' law (some attribute to Gay-Lussac's gas law)
  1. Following the volume effects of Boyle's law, the more widely molecules are spread within an increased volume of gas, the less often they collide, thereby generating less heat.
  2. Physiologic impact of decreased molecular collision is a decrease in ambient temperature.
  3. Clinical implications include hypothermia/increased metabolic rate and oxygen consumption.

V. Transport-specific aspects of care
A. Thermoregulation
  1. One of the most critical and challenging aspects of transport.
     a. Advanced planning and preventive approaches are critical to successful thermal regulation.
     b. Transport incubators on standby for use should be under AC power with a preset temperature of 35°C–36.1°C (95°F–97°F) to provide immediate warmth. For the extremely low birth weight (ELBW) infant, the preset temperature should be 37°C (98.6°F), with the goal of maintaining the infant's temperature at 36.5°C–37.5°C (97.7°F–99.5°F).
     c. Mattresses and other items for contact with the infant must be pre-warmed in the transport incubator or by other means prior to application.
     d. Any IV fluids to be administered should be pre-warmed, if possible.
  2. All heat-loss mechanisms pose an even greater risk in the transport environment.
     a. Double-walled transport incubators should always be used, if available, for this population.
     b. Radiant heat losses are markedly increased if attention is not paid to the ambient temperature of ambulance compartments, aircraft cabins, or location of the incubator in radiology and surgery areas of the hospital.

(1) Aim for an ambient environmental temperature between 24°C and 27°C (75°F and 80°F); for ELBW infants, environmental temperatures may need to be even higher.

(2) If the incubator needs to be opened during transport (beyond use of the portholes) or the external environmental temperature is very cold, increase the ambient temperature to compensate for major increases in heat loss.

(3) All infants <29 weeks should be wrapped in polyethylene plastic wrap, bubble wrap (air-caps), or bowel bags to reduce evaporative losses.

   (a) Once the infant is wrapped, assessments and care should be done without removing the wrap, including obtaining a weight prior to final placement on the NICU bed at the tertiary center.

   (b) A hat should be used on all infants since there is major heat loss through the head.

c. Use pre-warmed gel or chemical thermal mattresses to avoid conductive losses if wrap is not available or if hypothermia persists despite the wrap.

   (1) Be cautious of any uncontrollable source of heating in contact with the VLBW infant's skin — use padding between the device and the infant and frequently monitor skin appearance.

   (a) Use of chemical thermal mattresses and wrap can cause hyperthermia, which should be avoided.

   (2) Reduce evaporative and convective losses.

   (3) Heat and humidify all medical gases delivered to the infant.

   (4) May not be able to achieve target humidity levels with some setups available for transport; however, maximum effort should be made to provide humidity.

3. To combat extremes in cold or hot environmental conditions, cover the transport incubator with a blanket or quilt during movement in and out of vehicles, aircraft, and/or buildings.

4. Maintain the ability to provide close visual assessment during these transitions, which increase the risk for unanticipated changes in condition.

5. If temperature is not on continuous monitoring:
   a. Obtain a baseline axillary temperature prior to any major change with potential thermal impact, e.g., a move from radiant warmer to incubator, from inside facility to outside vehicle, after opening main incubator hood/door; and obtain another temperature determination following such events.
   b. During rewarming of any hypothermic infant, obtain temperature every 15 min with minimal disruption of heating interventions.
   c. Monitor to avoid iatrogenic hyperthermia caused by aggressive or inappropriate heating or rewarming interventions.
   d. Hyperthermia increases metabolic rate, oxygen demands, vasodilation, and insensible water loss (IWL).
   e. Observe for apnea, hypotension, dehydration, and possible seizure activity.

B. Airway — with focus on supporting oxygenation and ventilation during transport
   1. Depending upon available resources and mode of transport, VLBW infants can be transported with respiratory support ranging from supplemental oxygen to continuous positive airway pressure (CPAP) to high frequency ventilation (HFV).
      a. It is important to ensure that the equipment/supplies to be used are "transport worthy", meeting national standards for use in a transport environment.
      b. Select the airway option based on the individual infant's needs and the approach that is most likely to provide a secure airway and to maintain or improve respiratory status during transport.
      c. If nasal CPAP is planned for transport, keep in mind that it is more difficult to maintain and requires careful attention to infant positioning, prong stabilization, and use of all available airway monitoring devices, as well as increased visual assessment.
      d. At least one transport team member should be knowledgeable about the placement and maintenance of an ET tube and the operation and troubleshooting of any ventilator to be used.
      e. Approximately 10% of transports experience a ventilator- or ET tube-related problem.

f. Meticulous attention should be given to securing the ET tube prior to moving the infant.
2. Recognize that hypoxia is an increased risk during transport, secondary to the VLBW infant's underlying condition, physiologic responses to fluctuations in temperature, barometric pressure at altitude, and as a potential response to increased vibration; therefore, evaluate and act accordingly.
   a. Observe for signs of increasing respiratory rate if spontaneous respirations are present.
   b. Trend heart rate for any evidence of subtle-onset tachycardia.
   c. Maintain close visual attention to SpO_2 monitor, as audible alarms may not be heard.
   d. Anticipate the need to increase FiO_2 levels and/or increase positive end-expiratory pressure (PEEP) if mechanically ventilated.
3. Surfactant use
   a. A number of referring hospitals do not stock surfactant.
   b. Develop a system to remind team members to obtain the medication prior to departure on any transport in which its use is anticipated.
   c. Provide an approved method of refrigerating this medication for transport.
   d. If surfactant is administered by the referring hospital just prior to transport team arrival, or is administered by the team upon their arrival:
      (1) Additional bedside stabilization time may be warranted (~20–30 min) following administration to:
         (a) Confirm that the ET tube does not become obstructed or dislodged
         (b) Allow for early changes in pulmonary compliance that impact optimal ventilator settings for transport
         (c) Detect any potential air leaks
      (2) A pre-departure arterial blood gas to establish new baseline is recommended; repeat 15–30 min into transport if POC testing and an arterial line are available.

4. Assess/manage pneumothorax
   a. Rule out the presence of an existing air leak prior to moving any VLBW infant to the transport incubator.
   b. Evacuation of a pneumothorax is critical prior to air transport at altitude.
   c. Chest tube placement is indicated for mechanically ventilated infants.
   d. With limited ability to monitor during ground transport, consideration should be given to needle aspiration of any existing pneumothorax.
   e. For unstable or mechanically ventilated infants, have an appropriately trained provider place a chest tube prior to departure from the referring facility if return transport time will be prolonged.
   f. For any infant with increased risk factors for pneumothorax, a portable transilluminator and needle aspiration setup should be readily available on the transport incubator.
   g. Attention to pain and sedation needs should not be overlooked in the transport setting.
      (1) Consider transport mode, monitoring capabilities, and potential impact on infant's current diagnosis/status when selecting drugs and dosing.
      (2) Recommend use of tertiary center protocols and/or direct communication to ensure infant's comfort with minimal undesirable effects.

C. Cardiovascular status
   1. Key to successful transport management is establishing an acceptable baseline prior to departing from the referring facility.
   2. If possible, acceptable pulses, perfusion, BP, and acid/base status should be achieved; or actions should be initiated to address any unacceptable parameters that may occur during transport.
   3. If the infant remains unstable or if stability is difficult to achieve, prepare volume solutions or pressors before transport so they are ready for use if necessary.
   4. There is high variability in monitor function and difficulty in clinically assessing cardiovascular status under circumstances of motion.

5. Whenever possible, avoid invasive or repeated interventions during the transport process to minimize disruption in thermal measures and to avoid increasing the infant's stress level.
6. Once an acceptable baseline is achieved, close monitoring for changes in transport are indicated, with appropriate measures taken as necessary.

D. Metabolic — with focus on glucose homeostasis
1. Obtaining baseline labs at the referring facility is highly desirable so that pre-departure stabilization can be individualized to address any major deviations in values and a maintenance plan for the transport period can be developed.
   a. A repeat glucose value is recommended just prior to departure.
2. Fluid and glucose requirements are based on the VLBW infant's gestational age, weight, chronologic age, current clinical status, and the anticipated transport environment.
3. At minimum, determination of the infant's glucose status is critical prior to selection of fluid and IV rate for transport to achieve/maintain target glucose levels and appropriate fluid balance.
4. If possible without delaying transport team departure, obtain a parenteral nutrition solution so that increased protein losses can be addressed during stabilization and return transport.
5. Transport factors that may increase fluid needs or alter the ability to achieve/maintain target glucose levels include:
   a. Current thermal status and availability of a double-walled incubator
   b. Expected outside temperatures and number of vehicle or aircraft transfers required
   c. Vibration level of transport, which may increase the metabolic rate
   d. Level of ability to provide humidity in the infant's environment and inspired gases

VI. Key points regarding in-house transports within the birth facility

A. Pre-transport preparation of equipment/supplies
1. Pre-warmed transport incubator with thermal support supplies for the infant

2. Portable equipment and supplies capable of providing all necessary support of the infant's needs while moving from one area of the facility to another
   a. At a minimum, this would include oxygen and air with blender capability; airway supplies to handle supplemental oxygen administration, bag/mask ventilation, CPAP and ET intubation; portable suction; EKG monitor; pulse oximeter capable of reliable display of saturation and heart rate; and medications appropriate for VLBW resuscitation.
   b. In addition, battery-powered equipment, including an appropriate transport ventilator to support ongoing or anticipated treatment is recommended.
3. Equipment checklist that includes power status, temperature setting, adequate medical gas pressure, appropriate gas connectors
4. Assigned schedule to confirm devices secured to the incubator are clean, charging, and ready for immediate use
   a. The availability of additional supply and/or medication bags to accompany the incubator should be confirmed during checks to avoid delays.
   b. Medical gas and battery supplies should be adequate to support unexpected delays.

B. Transport from the delivery area to the nursery
   1. In-house transports present an increased risk for adverse events.
   2. Adult studies of in-house transports between the emergency department and ICU documented 68% with unanticipated events, with 5% of those events being serious in nature.
   3. Any infant whose status excludes transport from the delivery area with the mother should be transported to the nursery in a pre-warmed incubator with readily available, blended medical gases and support supplies, as previously noted.
   4. Application of a heat-conserving head covering and polyurethane plastic or bubble wrap (air caps) blanket is essential.
   5. Adjustments to the incubator temperature for appropriate response to the infant's current thermal status should be made prior to departure from the delivery suite.
   6. Maintain close attention to the infant's appearance and SpO_2 readings throughout the transfer.

7. Do not hesitate to pull aside and address any signs of deterioration.
8. Provide a hand-off report to the receiving nursery staff that includes pertinent maternal history, intrapartum events, infant's condition at birth, Apgar scores, and the infant's response to any interventions performed after birth, as well as any changes in condition and/or interventions performed in transit.
9. Obtain baseline vital signs to include axillary temperature prior to moving the infant from the incubator to the radiant warmer or other nursery location for admission.

VII. Transport from the NICU to another area of the hospital

A. Commonly done to access advanced imaging or interventional radiology or surgical interventions.
B. These infants generally require more support, so preparation prior to leaving the unit is critical.
C. Personnel trained in the care of the VLBW infant should accompany and remain with the infant during imaging procedures and in the surgery area until the definitive transfer of the infant to the surgical suite.
D. The incubator should be AC-powered any time it is immobile to conserve batteries.
E. The incubator should be positioned away from cold interior walls during any waiting periods.
F. Standard transport supplies/equipment, as well as any specific to the individual infant, should accompany the transport.

VIII. Inter-facility transport aspects

A. Recognize that successful outcomes in neonatal transport are often attributed more to the expertise of the transport team than to the specific mode of transport chosen.
   1. All team members providing transport to the VLBW infant should be experienced in the assessment and care of VLBW infants and skilled in providing this level of care in a mobile environment.
   2. Plan to be completely self-sufficient.
   3. The team should not expect that the referring facility will have equipment, supplies, medications, or additional experienced staff to support the transport needs of the VLBW infant, and should prepare and proceed accordingly.
   4. Medical gas supplies should be adequate to cover double the expected time for a given transport.

5. If the infant is not in the transport incubator (e.g., being stabilized prior to moving from the referring hospital equipment), medical gas supplies on the incubator should be turned off to avoid risk of inadvertent depletion.
6. Medical gas connectors should be compatible to provide quick connections between incubator and ambulance/aircraft or wall outlets in referral facilities.
7. Battery support for all necessary equipment should be provided to meet twice the expected time anticipated in transport.
8. Plug the transport incubator into an AC-power outlet while the infant is being stabilized prior to moving from the referring hospital equipment.

B. Selection of transport mode is multifactorial and includes:
 1. Current clinical status of the VLBW infant and any anticipated changes in condition
 2. Ability of the referring facility to initiate recommended stabilization and perform urgent interventions
 3. Readily available modes of acceptable transportation
 4. Equipment and number of personnel indicated for care of the infant
 5. Distance to be traveled and geography involved
 6. Current and short-term weather patterns

C. Comparison of modes of transport for the VLBW infant
 1. Ground (surface)
    a. Most common form of transport for sick neonates
    b. Depending on terrain and traffic, can be useful up to 100 miles from home base or travel times of 60–90 min
 2. Rotor-wing (helicopter)
    a. Consider for transports from 100 to 200 miles away and/or if travel time is >90 min
    b. May be indicated in congested or hard-to-reach areas for much shorter distances
 3. Fixed-wing aircraft — generally considered for distances >150 miles

D. Advantages of ground transport
 1. Provides "door-to-door" service, which reduces multiple moves of the infant and exposure to external temperature extremes
 2. Generally more spacious, allowing for fewer weight constraints, increased number of personnel, and more room to manage the infant

3. Environmental lighting usually better
4. Vehicle can be pulled over and stopped for emergent stabilization needs
5. Less impacted by effects of weather and aspects of flight physiology
6. Fuel, parts, and backup vehicles more easily accessed if needed

E. Limitations of ground transport
1. Much slower than other modes of transport
2. Ride can be rough, depending on construction of vehicle
3. Subject to traffic congestion, unanticipated highway delays/closures, weather

F. Advantages of rotor-wing transport
1. Possible to decrease one-way travel time by 75% over ground transport
2. Able to avoid traffic delays in congested locations and/or at congested times of day
3. Can be valuable resource when rapid acquisition of the unstable infant is needed
4. Useful to deliver team to site for initiation of stabilization and await ground transport for return

G. Limitations of rotor-wing transport
1. Not pressurized; VLBW infants may experience physiologic problems at lower altitudes
2. Noise and potential for significant vibration in hover or takeoff mode
3. Require landing zone and often some form of transport to the hospital
4. Can be severely limited by weather
5. Size of aircraft can restrict ability to perform interventions in flight
6. Weight restrictions limit number of team members and equipment

H. Advantages of fixed-wing transport
1. Much faster to reach distant locations
2. Generally able to carry more personnel and equipment than rotor-wing
3. Usually have pressurization to decrease impact of physiologic concerns
4. Less noise and vibration than rotor-wing and some ambulances

I. Limitations of fixed-wing transport
   1. Require an airport for landing and ground transport to the hospital, increasing the number of high-risk transfers required for the infant
   2. Usually the most costly transport option

References

Felmet K. Transport medicine. In: Vincent JL, Abraham E, Moore FA, Kochanek PM, Fink MP, eds. *Textbook of Critical Care*. 6th ed. Philadelphia, PA: Saunders Elsevier; 2011:1627-1632.

Felmet K, Orr RA, Han YY, Roth KR. Pediatric transport: shifting the paradigm to improve patient outcome. In: Fuhrman BP, Zimmerman JJ, eds. *Pediatric Critical Care*. 4th ed. Philadelphia, PA: Mosby Elsevier; 2011:130-138.

Guidelines for Air and Ground Transport of Neonatal and Pediatric Patients. 3rd ed. Elk Grove Village, IL: American Academy of Pediatrics; 2007.

Jaimovich DG, Vidyasagar D, eds. *Handbook of Pediatric and Neonatal Transport Medicine*. 2nd ed. Philadelphia, PA: Elsevier Health Sciences; 2002.

Melton K, Pettett G. Transport of the ventilated infant. In: Goldsmith JP, Karotin EH, eds. *Assisted Ventilation of the Neonate*. 5th ed. St. Louis, MO: Saunders Elsevier; 2011:531-541.

Rodenberg H, Blumen IR, Thomas SH. Air medical transport. In: Marx J, Hockberger RS, Walls R, eds. *Rosen's Emergency Medicine: Concepts and Clinical Practice*. 8th ed. Philadelphia, PA: Saunders Elsevier; 2014:2442-2448.

Stroud MH, Trautman MS, Meyer K, et al. Pediatric and neonatal interfacility transport: results from a national consensus conference. *Pediatrics*. 2013;132(2):359-366.

Woodward GA, Kirsch R, Trautman MS, et al. Stabilization and transport of the high-risk neonate. In: Gleason CA, Devaskar S, eds. *Avery's Diseases of the Newborn*. 9th ed. Philadelphia, PA: Saunders Elsevier; 2012:341-358.

Procedural Review

Cheryl A. Carlson

I. Intubation

A. Indications
   1. Need for initial stabilization or resuscitation
   2. Need for continued mechanical ventilation
   3. Administration of medications such as surfactant or epinephrine
B. Equipment
   1. Laryngoscope handle and appropriately sized blade (size 0 blade for preterm infants, size 00 for extremely low birth weight infants)
   2. Endotracheal tube (ETT) with 2.5- or 3-mm internal diameter
   3. Stylet that fits into ETT (may be optional)
   4. Flow-inflating bag with adjustable pop-off or self-inflating bag with reservoir
   5. Oxygen source with blender to adjust oxygen administration
   6. Suction source with various-sized catheters for suctioning oropharynx and ETT
      a. 5 or 6 Fr for 2.5-mm ETT
      b. 6 or 8 Fr for 3-mm ETT
   7. Stethoscope
   8. Carbon dioxide detector for ETT
   9. Personal protective equipment, including mask and gloves
C. Procedure
   1. Place the infant in supine position with the head slightly extended and the body aligned straight (**Fig 23-1**).
   2. Holding the laryngoscope in the left hand, pass the blade into the right side of the infant's mouth, advancing to midline and sweeping the tongue out of the way.
   3. Advance the blade into the vallecula and raise the handle to visualize the vocal cords (**Fig. 23-2**).
   4. Carefully lift the laryngoscope handle; do not rock or lever the blade once in place.
   5. Applying cricoid pressure on the larynx with the fourth or fifth finger of the left hand, or with the help of an assistant, may help to visualize the cords and displace the trachea posteriorly.

6. Hold the ETT in the right hand and advance between the vocal cords ~1–2 cm below the glottis; insertion length is generally at 6–7 cm for the very low birth weight (VLBW) infant.
7. Once in place, hold the tube against the plate and gently remove the laryngoscope blade.
8. Use auscultation and a carbon dioxide detector to verify tube placement while ventilating the infant by hand; confirm correct placement with chest x-ray.
9. Secure the tube in place with tape or an ETT holder.
10. Nasal intubation is not generally performed on VLBW infants during resuscitation due to the size of their nasal passages (see **Table 23-1**).

II. Umbilical line placement
A. Indications
 1. Umbilical arterial catheter
    a. Continuous blood pressure monitoring
    b. Frequent blood gas and laboratory monitoring
    c. The Centers for Disease Control and Prevention (CDC) recommends removal as soon as possible (within 5 days) with any sign of vascular insufficiency

FIGURE 23-1
Infant Positioning with Laryngoscope

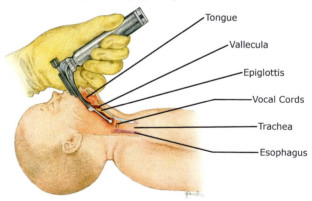

©2014 The National Certification Corporation

Intubation may be indicated for initial stabilization or resuscitation, for continued mechanical ventilation, or to administer medications such as surfactant or epinephrine. Place the infant in a supine position with the head slightly extended and the body aligned straight.

2. Umbilical venous catheter
   a. Emergency access for administration of resuscitation medications
   b. Fluid administration
   c. Parenteral administration
   d. Administration of continuous infusion medications
   e. The CDC recommends removal when no longer needed; should not remain >14 days
B. Equipment
   1. Sterile tray, sterile drapes, additional syringes, sterile flush, stopcocks
   2. Umbilical catheters
      a. Single- and double-lumen catheters, 3.5 and 5 Fr

FIGURE 23-2
View of Airway Through Laryngoscope

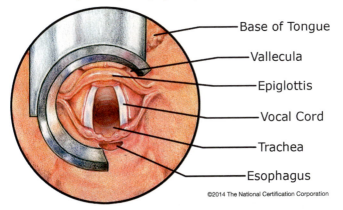

©2014 The National Certification Corporation

Holding the laryngoscope in the left hand, pass the blade into the right side of the infant's mouth, advancing to midline and sweeping the tongue out of the way. Advance the blade into the vallecula and raise the handle to visualize the vocal cords.

TABLE 23-1
Endotracheal Tube (ETT) Size and Insertion

Weight	Gestational Age	ETT size	Depth of Insertion
<750 g	23–25 weeks	2.5 mm	6.0–6.5 cm
1 g	25–29 weeks	3.0 mm	7 cm

b. Size and type of catheter depends on clinical condition of infant; e.g., infant may need vasopressors, continuous pain medication, or may benefit from having double-lumen umbilical venous catheter in place
c. Full personal protection equipment: sterile gown, gloves, mask, hat for all personnel present and in the immediate area
3. Skin-cleansing solution and full sterile barriers to prep and protect umbilical site per hospital policy

C. Procedure
1. Maintain sterile technique at all times.
2. Several methods can be used to calculate catheter insertion length:
   a. High placement of umbilical artery catheter (see **Table 23-2**)
      (1) Calculation:
         [(3 x weight in kg) + 9] + length of umbilical stump = cm to place line
      (2) Measurement:
         Umbilicus-to-shoulder length in cm + 2 cm + length of stump = cm to place line
      (3) Place at thoracic vertebrae T6–T9.
      (4) Low umbilical arterial line placement is not recommended; if essential, place tip of catheter between the third and fourth lumbar vertebrae.
   b. Placement of umbilical venous catheter (optimal placement through ductus venous and at junction at inferior vena cava and right atrium)

TABLE 23-2
Umbilical Placement Measurement

Umbilical Arterial Line	Umbilical Venous Line
High placement at T6–T9	Optimal placement through ductus venous and at junction of inferior vena cava and right atrium
[(3 x weight in kg) + 9] + length of umbilical stump = cm for line	[(3 x weight in kg) + 9] / 2 + length of umbilical stump = cm for line
Measure umbilicus-to-shoulder length in cm + 2 cm + length of stump	Measure xiphoid-to-umbilicus in cm + 0.5 to 0.01 cm
Low placement with tip of catheter between L3 and L4	**Low placement for emergency use: Insert 2–5 cm**

(1) Calculation:
[(3 x weight in kg) + 9] / 2 + length of umbilical stump = cm to place line
(2) Measurement:
Xiphoid-to-umbilicus length in cm + 0.5 to 0.01 cm
3. Wash hands with surgical scrub and put on sterile gown and gloves.
4. Prepare umbilical cord and skin with hospital-recommended cleansing agent.
5. Prepare catheters by flushing with sterile saline solution, including stopcocks and syringes for each stopcock port.
6. Have assistant use forceps to hold up stump.
7. Cleanse stump per hospital protocol.
   a. To prevent chemical burns, do not leave excess on skin or allow pooling under infant.
   b. For VLBW infants, wipe off excess with sterile water.
8. Drape infant with sterile drape to completely cover the surgical field.
9. Place umbilical tape around the base of the cord, avoiding the skin.
   a. It may be necessary to place tie around umbilical skin if the cord is too short.
   b. If so, loosen tie after catheter placement to avoid necrosis of the umbilical skin.
10. Stabilize the cord using sterile 4 x 4 gauze pads and forceps to expose the vessels.
11. Identify the vessels in the cord (two arteries and one vein).
12. Umbilical arterial catheterization: See **Table 23-2** for insertion calculations.
    a. Carefully dilate the arterial opening.
       (1) Gently insert iris forceps into the lumen.
       (2) Allow forceps to open.
       (3) Repeat this procedure until artery is dilated.
    b. Once dilated, gently insert the umbilical catheter and advance.
       (1) Initial resistance, if met, can usually be overcome with gentle pressure to allow further dilation; the catheter will pass through the base of the cord.
       (2) Advance the catheter to the desired length and withdraw blood for lab studies.
       (3) Suture in place and further secure with umbilical bridge.

c. Possible problems with umbilical arterial line placement:
  (1) Catheter may not pass through into the aorta; may be due to an occurrence of a false tract out of the arterial lumen.
  (2) Catheter may not advance into the abdominal aorta.
  (3) Catheter may pass into the aorta and then loop back on itself.
  (4) To correct, it may be possible to pass another catheter past the blocked catheter.
13. Umbilical venous catheterization
  a. Identify umbilical vein.
  b. Prepare site as described in Section II.C.4.–11.
  c. Determine length of insertion (**Table 23-2**).
    (1) For emergency administration of medication, insert 2–5 cm.
    (2) For continuous infusion of fluids, advance catheter to position as determined in **Table 23-2**.
    (3) Prepare site and catheter as with umbilical arterial catheter placement, if not already done.
    (4) Insert catheter into umbilical vein while exerting gentle traction on the umbilical cord; resistance may be met if catheter does not enter the ductus venous.
14. Confirm placement of umbilical arterial and venous catheters with chest and abdominal x-ray (babygram); adjust and reconfirm with x-ray as needed.

III. Thoracentesis
A. Needle aspiration
  1. Indication: Emergency evacuation of air from pleural space
  2. Equipment
    a. 24-gauge butterfly needle or 24-gauge IV catheter
    b. 10- or 20-cc syringe
    c. 3-way stopcock
    d. T-connector for use with IV catheter
    e. Sterile gloves and mask
    f. Skin-cleansing agent per hospital protocol
  3. Procedure
    a. Wash hands and use sterile gloves.
    b. Attach syringe to stopcock.

- c. Identify insertion site at second or third intercostal space, mid-clavicular line.
- d. Prepare insertion site per hospital protocol.
- e. Insert the needle into the intercostal space at a 45-degree angle over the top of the third rib.
- f. Hold the needle firmly in place.
    (1) Butterfly needle:
        (a) During insertion, have assistant exert continuous pressure to the syringe with the stopcock open to the infant.
        (b) When air is obtained, stop advancing the needle to avoid injury to the lung.
    (2) 24-gauge IV catheter:
        (a) Attach stopcock to T-connector.
        (b) Insert IV catheter as described in Section III.A.3.b.–f.
        (c) Once in the pleural space, remove the needle and have assistant attach the T-connector to the IV catheter and exert continuous pressure on syringe with the stopcock open to the baby.
- g. Remove the needle once air has been evacuated.
- h. The butterfly needle or IV catheter and stopcock setup may remain in place to allow for repeated aspirations for a continuous air leak and while preparing for chest tube insertion.

B. Chest tube insertion
  1. Indication: Evacuation of air from pleural space in infants receiving positive-pressure ventilation
  2. Equipment
     a. Sterile gown, gloves, hat, and mask
     b. Morphine sulfate or pain medication
     c. 1% lidocaine for local anesthesia: 1 mL with 25-gauge needle
     d. Skin-cleansing agent per hospital policy
     e. Sterile drapes
     f. Sterile transparent dressing
     g. Chest tube drainage system
        (1) Negative-pressure drainage system set to wall suction
        (2) Amount of negative pressure in the VLBW infant generally between 10 and 15 cm
     h. Chest tube options: Other equipment and procedures depend on type of chest tube used

(1) Thoracotomy tube (10 Fr for VLBW), sterile tray including curved hemostat, curved Kelly clamp, scissors, needle holder, 3-0 or 4-0 silk suture
(2) Percutaneous chest tube insertion set (8 or 10 Fr), sterile field, 10- or 20-mL syringe
(3) Pigtail insertion set (6.5 or 8.5 Fr)
3. Standard procedure
   a. Maintain sterile technique at all times.
   b. Administer pain medication.
   c. Wash hands and put on sterile gown and gloves.
   d. Position infant on side with side of pneumothorax up.
   e. Place sterile drapes on the surface around infant and insertion site.
   f. Prep chest area with antiseptic solution as defined by hospital policy.
      (1) Determine insertion site, usually the fourth or fifth intercostal space in the mid-anterior axillary line (as a reference, the nipple lies in the fourth intercostal). See **Fig. 23-3**.

FIGURE 23-3
Determination of Insertion Site

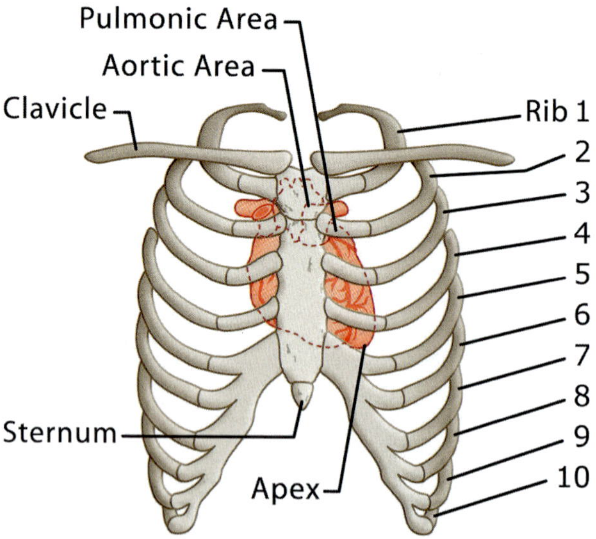

©2014 The National Certification Corporation

For standard-procedure chest tube insertion, the insertion site is usually the fourth or fifth intercostal space in the mid-anterior axillary line (as a reference, the nipple lies in the fourth intercostal space).

(2) Infiltrate subcutaneous tissue around insertion site with 1% lidocaine, if time permits.
4. Procedure for placement of standard thoracotomy tube (**Fig. 23-4**)
   a. Open sterile tray.
   b. Make small incision through the skin in the sixth intercostal space, parallel to the rib, at mid-axillary line.
   c. Place chest tube (without trocar) within the tip of the curved hemostat; position the chest tube on the underside of the hemostat.
   d. With curved hemostat and chest tube, dissect subcutaneous tissue overlying the rib.
   e. Make a track in the subcutaneous tissue to the fourth intercostal space.
   f. Enter the pleural space at the intersection of the nipple line, just anterior to the mid-axillary line.
   g. Push the hemostat through the intercostal muscles into the pleural space.
      (1) Always puncture just over the rib to avoid injury to the nerve and bleeding from the artery or vein (**Fig. 23-5**).

FIGURE 23-4
Placement of Standard Thoracotomy Tube

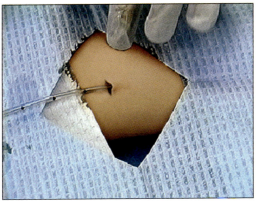

Make a small incision through the skin in the sixth intercostal space, parallel to the rib, at the mid-axillary line. Enter the plural space at the intersection of the nipple line, just anterior to the mid-axillary line.

h. Once in the pleural space, open the hemostat and advance the chest tube anteriorly into position with all holes within the pleural space; the chest tube may steam up, indicating placement within the pleural space.
i. Attach the chest tube to the chest drainage system.
j. Secure the chest tube using a purse-string suture around the tube.
   (1) Clean the cleansing solution from the site and pat dry.
   (2) Use small piece of Vaseline or petrolatum gauze around the insertion site; cover with a split 2 x 2 gauze and a transparent dressing.
   (3) Dressing does not need to be routinely changed unless it becomes non-occlusive.
   (4) Place a chevron style of tape around the chest tube below the dressing site to secure to infant.

5. Procedure for placement of percutaneous chest tube insertion catheter or pigtail catheter
   a. Prepare sterile field.
   b. Open package and attach 10- or 20-ml syringe to insertion needle.
   c. Determine insertion site at the fourth or fifth intercostal space, mid- to anterior-axillary line.

FIGURE 23-5
Choosing the Site

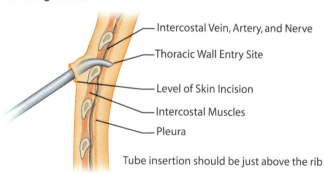

- Intercostal Vein, Artery, and Nerve
- Thoracic Wall Entry Site
- Level of Skin Incision
- Intercostal Muscles
- Pleura

Tube insertion should be just above the rib

©2014 The National Certification Corporation

Always puncture just over the rib to avoid injury to the nerve and bleeding from the artery or vein.

d. Using the needle with syringe attached, place needle tip at entrance site, insert over the underlying rib, and enter the intercostal space.
e. Withdraw syringe until air is obtained; a stopcock may also be used with the syringe.
f. Hold the needle in place and remove the syringe and stopcock, if used.
g. Place the tip of the guide wire on the needle hub and advance to target distance.
h. Hold the guide wire in place and remove the needle.
i. Depending on the size of the percutaneous chest tube, one or two dilators may need to be advanced over the guide wire to enlarge the pleural opening.
j. Once dilated, advance the chest tube or pigtail catheter over the guide wire and into place.
k. Remove the guide wire while holding the chest tube/catheter in place.
l. Secure the tube.
    (1) Clean prep solution from insertion site with sterile water and pat dry.
    (2) Pigtail catheter may be secured with a transparent dressing.
    (3) Dressing does not need to be routinely changed unless it becomes non-occlusive.
    (4) Place a chevron style of tape around chest tube below dressing site to secure to the infant.
    (5) If using a purse-string suture to secure the pigtail catheter, be careful not to suture too tightly; the catheter is very soft and flexible; place dressing on site as above.

IV. Lumbar puncture
A. Indications
1. Diagnose central nervous system infection (meningitis, encephalitis).
2. Diagnose TORCH (toxoplasmosis or other, e.g., syphilis, rubella, cytomegalovirus, or herpes simplex).
B. Equipment
1. Neonatal lumbar puncture tray
2. Spinal needle with short-bevel, 22- to 24-gauge x 1.5-inch with stylet
3. Sterile gown, gloves, hat, and mask
4. Morphine sulfate or pain medication

5. 1% lidocaine for local anesthesia: 1 mL with 25-gauge needle (optional)
6. Skin-cleansing agent per hospital policy; chlorhexidine not recommended for use in lumbar puncture
7. Sterile drapes

C. Procedure
1. Maintain sterile technique at all times.
2. Administer pain medication as indicated.
3. Wash hands and put on sterile gown and gloves.
4. Prepare tray and check needle.
5. Have assistant position infant in lateral decubitus position, holding the infant securely so that the lower part of the infant's spine is curved (assistant should wear hat and mask for procedure).
6. Place sterile drapes on the surface around the infant and insertion site.
7. Prep lower lumbar area with antiseptic solution as defined by hospital policy.
8. Insertion site of needle is in the midline space between the fourth and fifth lumbar processes.
9. Slowly advance the needle in the direction of the umbilicus.
10. Withdraw the stylet frequently to detect presence of spinal fluid.
11. Collect spinal fluid in 3–4 sterile tubes, ~0.5- to 1-mL per tube.
    a. Tube 1: Gram stain and culture
    b. Tube 2: glucose and protein
    c. Tube 3: cell count and differential
    d. Tube 4: other tests, such as polymerase chain reaction (PCR) for herpes
12. Once fluid is obtained, replace stylet and withdraw needle.
13. Hold pressure on site until there is no bleeding or leakage of fluid.
14. Clean any remaining skin prep from the area.

V. Pericardiocentesis – needle aspiration
A. Indications
1. Treatment of life-threatening cardiac tamponade
2. Consult pediatric cardiology, as use of echocardiogram is preferable

B. Equipment
1. Skin-cleansing agent per hospital policy

2. 22- or 24-gauge IV catheter connected to T-connector and 3-way stopcock and 10- or 20-mL syringe
   3. Sterile gown, gloves, hat, and mask
   4. Sterile drape
C. Procedure
   1. Maintain sterile technique.
   2. Wash hands and put on sterile gown and gloves.
   3. Have assistant position infant in supine position (assistant should wear hat, mask, and sterile gloves).
   4. Prepare subxiphoid-area insertion site with cleansing agent.
   5. Insert the IV catheter at a 30- to 45-degree angle into the subxiphoid space, toward the infant's left shoulder.
   6. While holding the needle in place, remove the stylet and connect the T-connector and stopcock with syringe to the IV catheter.
   7. With the stopcock open to the baby, have assistant aspirate air with the syringe.
   8. Once the air is evacuated, remove the catheter.

VI. Abdominal paracentesis
A. Indications
   1. Improvement of cardiorespiratory function in infants with massive abdominal ascites
   2. Removal of abdominal fluid to reduce intra-abdominal pressure
B. Equipment
   1. Skin-cleansing agent per hospital policy
   2. Sterile gown, gloves, hat, and mask
   3. Sterile drape
   4. 1% lidocaine for local anesthesia: 1 mL with 25-gauge needle (optional)
   5. 24- or 25-gauge IV catheter
   6. 3-way stopcock
   7. 10- to 20-mL syringes
   8. Collection tubes for specimen collection
   9. Sterile 2 x 2 gauze and transparent dressing
C. Procedure
   1. Maintain sterile technique.
   2. Wash hands and put on sterile gown and gloves.
   3. Have assistant position the infant in supine position with a soft support under the infant's left flank (assistant should wear hat, mask, and sterile gloves).

4. Prepare lower abdominal-area insertion site with cleansing agent and place sterile drape.
5. Infiltrate subcutaneous area of insertion site with local anesthetic agent when possible.
6. Position the IV catheter immediately lateral to the rectus sheath or at a level one-third of the distance between the umbilicus and the anterior superior iliac spine; avoid midline insertion.
7. Insert the catheter at a 45-degree angle toward the infant's back. Once the needle tip is below the skin, remove the stylet and connect the T-connector and stopcock with syringe to the IV catheter while holding the needle in place.
8. With the stopcock open to the baby, have assistant aspirate fluid with the syringe.
9. Once fluid is evacuated, remove the catheter and apply sterile dressing.

References

Cloherty JP, Eichenwald EC, Hansen AR, Stark AR. *Manual of Neonatal Care.* 7th ed. Philadelphia, PA: Wolters Kluwer Health/Lippincott Williams & Wilkins; 2012.

Donn SM, Sinha SK, eds. *Manual of Neonatal Respiratory Care.* 3rd ed. New York, NY: Springer; 2012.

Gomella TL, Cunningham MD, Eyal FG, eds. *Neonatology: Management, Procedures, On-Call Problems, Diseases, and Drugs.* 7th ed. New York, NY: McGraw Hill/Lange; 2013.

Healthcare Infection Control Practices Advisory Committee. *Guidelines for the Prevention of Intravascular Catheter-Related Infections.* Centers for Disease Control and Prevention Web site. http://www.cdc.gov/hicpac/BSI/BSI-guidelines-2011.html. Updated April 1, 2011. Accessed November 11, 2013.

MacDonald MG, Ramasethu J, Rais-Bahrami K eds. *Atlas of Procedures in Neonatology.* 5th ed. Philadelphia, PA: Lippincott Williams & Wilkins; 2012.

Textbook of Neonatal Resuscitation. 6th ed. American Academy of Pediatrics and American Heart Association; 2011.

Appendix A: Resource Toolbox

This Resource Toolbox supports and builds on the information provided throughout *Golden Hours: Care of the Very Low Birth Weight Infant*. Though some of the information is repeated in-depth in the individual chapters, this Toolbox is designed as a handy, quick reference that practitioners can use to help prioritize the assessment and management of common situations encountered in the NICU. The goal, as it is throughout the book, is to reduce risks and improve outcomes associated with the care of this very vulnerable population.

NICU professionals can apply these resources and tools in real time. Topics include:
- Cardiovascular system
- Fetal assessment
- Fluids and electrolytes
- Neurological system
- Procedures
- Respiratory system
- Thermoregulation
- Web resources

The American Academy of Pediatrics (AAP) and the American Heart Association (AHA) have developed standards for neonatal resuscitation. Their guidelines are based on the International Liaison Committee on Resuscitation consensus and are used within the Neonatal Resuscitation Program (NRP) that is a national standard for all heath care providers who attend deliveries. These principles are stressed throughout this book.

It is imperative that you always follow your facility's protocols, guidelines, and dosage plans.

I. Fetal Assessment

I-A Fetal Lung Maturity

Test	Normal	Abnormal
L/S ratio	>2: normal	1.5–2: immature, incidence of RDS low <1: incidence of RDS high
PG	Present	Absent
TDx-FML II	≥55 mg/g: likelihood of RDS small	40–54 mg/g: intermediate risk for RDS <39 mg/g: likelihood of RDS high

L/S ratio = ratio of lecithin to sphingomyelin; PG = phosphatidylglycerol; RDS = respiratory distress syndrome

I-B Reference Values For Umbilical Cord Blood Gas Values

	pH	Base Excess	PCO_2	PO_2
Umbilical arterial blood (reflects fetal status)	7.26 [0.07]	-4.0 [3.0]	53 [10]	17 [6]
Umbilical venous blood (reflects maternal and placental status)	7.34 [0.06]	-3.0 [3.0]	41 [7]	29 [7]

Values are expressed as mean and standard deviation.

(Adapted from Helwig JT, Parer JT, Kilpatrick SJ, Laros RK Jr. Umbilical cord blood acid-base state: what is normal? *Am J Obstet Gynecol*. 1996;174(6):1807-1812.)

I-C Umbilical Sampling

Umbilical Gas	Reflects	Sampling
Umbilical artery	Most accurate regarding fetal and newborn acid-base status; represents fetal metabolic condition at moment of birth	• 10- to 20-cm section of cord double-clamped on ice at birth • Assess accurately up to 60 min • Utilize heparinized blood gas syringe; obtain 1 cc of blood • Sample umbilical artery or both artery and vein • Label samples carefully
Umbilical vein	Reflects maternal acid base status and placental function	
Paired arterial and venous umbilical	Magnitude of difference between umbilical artery gas and umbilical venous gas can be predictor of encephalopathy	

Appendix A: Resource Toolbox 379

II. Respiratory System

II-A Targeted Saturation Goal in the First 10 Min of Life

Time	Saturations	Provide or Increase Oxygen
1 min	60%–65%	If <60% at 1 min
2 min	65%–70%	If <65% at 2 min
3 min	70%–75%	If <70% at 3 min
4 min	75%–80%	If <75% at 4 min
5 min	80%–85%	If <80% at 5 min
10 min	85%–95%	If <85% at 10 min

Note: Once a decision is made to provide oxygen, wean or discontinue it as tolerated to keep saturations in acceptable ranges after they reach 85%.

(Adapted from MacDonald MG, Mullett MD, Seshia MMK, eds. *Avery's Neonatology: Pathophysiology and Management of the Newborn*. 6th ed. Philadelphia, PA: Lippincott Williams & Wilkins; 2005.)

II-B Apgar Scoring at Birth

Sign	0	1	2	1 min	5 min	10 min	15 min	20 min
Color	Blue or pale	Acrocyanotic	Completely pink					
Heart Rate	Absent	<100 bpm	>100 bpm					
Reflex Irritability	No response	Grimace	Crying or active withdrawal					
Muscle Tone	Limp	Some flexion	Active motion					
Respirations	Absent	Weak crying, hypoventilation	Good, crying					
TOTAL								
Support Provided at Time of Apgar Score (check box)								
Oxygen								
PPV/NCPAP								
ETT								
Chest compressions								
Epinephrine								

bpm = beats/min; ETT = endotracheal tube; NCPAP = nasal continuous positive airway pressure; PPV = positive-pressure ventilation

II-C Initial Positive-Pressure Ventilation (PPV)

Type of Device	Setting Flow	Setting Positive End-Expiratory Pressure (PEEP)	Setting Peak Inspiratory Pressure (PIP)	Rate
Self-inflating bag	5–10 lpm		20–25 cm H_2O	40–60 breaths/min
Flow-inflating bag	5–10 lpm	5 cm H_2O		
T-piece	5–15 lpm	2–5 cm H_2O		

lpm = liters/min

II-D Intubation Guidelines

Weight (g)	Gestational Age (weeks)	Tube Size Inside Diameter (mm)	Blade Size to Consider	Suction Catheter Size	Securing Tube (lip to tip)
<1,000	<28	2.5	00–0	5–6 Fr	6–7
1,000–2,000	28–34	3.0	0–1	6 or 8 Fr	7–8
2,000–3,000	34–38	3.5	0–1	8 Fr	8–9
>3,000	>38	3.5–4.0	1	8 or 10 Fr	9–10

III. Thermoregulation

III-A Recommended Axillary Temperatures in Infants ≤1,500 Grams

Ranges	Temperature	Action Needed
Normal	36.5°C–37.5°C (98°F–100°F)	Continue
Potential cold stress	36°C–36.5°C (97°F–98°F)	Cause for concern
Moderate hypothermia	32°C–36°C (90°F–97°F)	Danger; immediate warming of baby needed
Severe hypothermia	<32°C (90°F)	Outlook grave; skilled care urgently needed

Note: The American Heart Association and the American Academy of Pediatrics in 2006 stated that the goal (of the first temperature) should be an axillary temperature of 36.5°C (98°F). Goal is to achieve normothermia and avoid hyperthermia, which is associated with progressive cerebral injury.

(Adapted from Bhatt DR, White R, Martin G, et al. Transitional hypothermia in preterm newborns. *J Perinatol*. 2007;27(suppl 2):S45-S47.)

III-B Recommended Stabilization Room Temperatures Based on Post-Menstrual Age and Birth Weight

Estimated Post-Menstrual Age (weeks)	Estimated Birth Weight (g)	Delivery Room/Stabilization Area Temperature
≤26	≤750	27°C (80°F)
27–28	751–1,000	27°C (80°F)
29–32	1,001–1,500	≥22°C (72°F); goal 24°C (75°F)
33–36	1,501–2,500	≥22°C (72°F); goal 24°C (75°F)
37–42	≥2,501	≥21°C (70°F); goal 24°C (75°F)

Based on the American Society of Heating, Refrigerating and Air-Conditioning Engineers (ASHRAE) and World Health Organization recommendations for delivery room temperatures.

(Adapted from Bhatt DR, White R, Martin G, et al. Transitional hypothermia in preterm newborns. *J Perinatol*. 2007;27(suppl 2):S45-S47.)

III-C Example of Humidity Guidelines

1. Have humidified incubator ready on admission.
2. Consider the use of humidified incubator care for infants 32 weeks gestation and/or 1,200 g to decrease transepidermal water loss (TEWL), maintain skin integrity, decrease fluid requirements, and minimize electrolyte imbalance. Strict equipment cleaning protocols should be utilized while providing humidified air.
3. The recommended relative humidity (RH) is 75%–80% for the first seven days, decreasing to 50%–60% RH, **if possible**, during the second week until 30–32 weeks postmenstrual age.
4. The table below shows sample guidelines. Every unit should review the literature and develop guidelines appropriate for their unit.
5. Infants >1,500 g do not require humidity; use should be based on clinical assessment.
6. Continue moderate humidity for infants who remain critically ill until 34 weeks gestation.
7. Change incubator and porthole sleeves every 7 days or if visibly dirty.
8. Porthole sleeves should be used to avoid loss of humidity during patient care.
9. Portholes should be used for all primary access to maintain temperature and humidity. If door access is needed, use a boost-air curtain. Canopies should only be raised during emergencies.

Gestational Age	Initial Humidity	Time Frame	Secondary Humidity	Time Frame	Discontinue Humidity
≤28 weeks	80%	2 weeks	50%	2 weeks	32 weeks
29–30 weeks	80%	1 week	50%	2 weeks	32–33 weeks
31–34 weeks	50%	1 week	0	0	32–35 weeks

Note: Skin maturation occurs after birth; therefore, infants born at 28 weeks of gestation can tolerate removal of humidity at 32 weeks (after 4 weeks of maturation), vs. infants during the first week of life born at 32–34 weeks.

Appendix A: Resource Toolbox

IV. Cardiovascular System

IV-A Treatment of Hypotension

Cause of Hypotension	Volume	Dopamine	Dobutamine	Epinephrine	Hydrocortisone
Acute blood loss or hypovolemia	**1st choice (blood may be preferred)**	Consider if volume is not effective			
Myocardial dysfunction		Add if dobutamine is not effective alone	1st choice	If both dobutamine and dopamine do not work in combination, discontinue dopamine and add epinephrine	
Chorioamnionitis or sepsis/sudden inflammatory response syndrome (SIRS)		1st choice		Consider 2nd if dopamine doesn't work	If refractory hypotension, consider low dose (obtain baseline serum cortisol)
Unknown		1st choice	Add as 2nd choice	If adding dobutamine is ineffective, consider switching to epinephrine	If refractory hypotension, consider low dose (obtain baseline serum cortisol)

IV-B Recommended Volume Expanders in the Delivery Room

Volume Expander	Dosage	Repeat	Notes
0.9% NaCl	10 mL/kg	Once	Give over at least 5–10 min or slower if possible
Ringers lactate	10 mL/kg	Once	Give over at least 5–10 min or slower if possible
Blood – maternal crossmatch	10 mL/kg	Once	Use judiciously in infants with *in utero* anemia; rapid administration may cause heart failure
Blood – type O, Rh-negative	10 mL/kg	Once	Use judiciously in infants with *in utero* anemia; rapid administration may cause heart failure

Note: In critically unstable infants with evidence of large blood loss, additional volume may be considered.

V. Fluids And Electrolytes

V-A Suggested Response to Blood Glucose ≤45 mg/dL or Symptomatic (Example of a Protocol)

• Bolus: 200 mg/kg (2 mL/kg) D10W if IV fluids have not been initiated yet and start IV fluids.
• Bolus: 200 mg/kg (2 mL/kg) D10W and increase GIR to 6–8 mg/kg/min if IV fluids are already infusing at an adequate rate and GIR.
• Monitor blood glucose every 20–30 min until stable, then every 1–2 hours (if stable), then every 4–6 hours.
• Adjust GIR to maintain blood glucose >50 mg/dL.
• Monitor blood glucose for the first 24–48 hours or until stabilized, especially those infants at risk of hypoglycemia.
• Infants who require high infusion rates or a dextrose concentration >12.5% require placement of a central venous catheter (UVC, PICC).

GIR = glucose infusion rate; PICC = peripherally inserted central catheter; UVC = umbilical venous catheter

VI. Neurological System

VI-A Grading of Intraventricular Hemorrhage (IVH)

Grade	Defined
Grade I IVH	Germinal matrix hemorrhage with no or minimal intraventricular blood
Grade II IVH	Hemorrhage with intraventricular blood
Grade III IVH	Hemorrhage with intraventricular blood occupying >50% of ventricular volume
Grade IV IVH	Periventricular hemorrhagic infarction

VII. Procedures

VII-A Umbilical Line Measurements and Placement

Postion	Measurements	Catheter Size
Umbilical Arterial Catheter (UAC)		
High: T6–T9	1. Shoulder-to-umbilicus length + length of umbilical stump and skin at base of stump in cm 2. UAC distance in cm = (birth weight in kg x 3) + 9	<1,200 g: 3.5 F
Low: L3–L4	1. Birth weight in kg + 7	>1,200 g: 5F *(never use 8F)*
Umbilical Venous Catheter (UVC)		
Tip above the diaphragm (in the inferior vena cava, above the level of the ductus venosus and below the level of the right atrium)	1. Shoulder-to-umbilicus length in cm x 0.6 2. (UAC length in cm/2) + 1 3. (1.5 x birth weight in kg) + 5.5	<1,500 g: 3.5F >1500-3,500 g: 5F

VIII. Web Resources

Neoknowlege Web Site (www.neoknowledge.org)
The Neoknowledge web site contains tools to help neonatal health care professionals estimate and calculate important clinical parameters in the field:

- 22–25 week outcomes
- A-a gradient
- Acid-base calculator
- BiliTool
- Early-onset sepsis risk
- Lactation and medications
- NICU tools
    Body surface area
    Endotracheal tube and umbilical line measurements
    Gestational age
    Glucose delivery
    Partial exchange transfusions

Neonatology on the Web (www.neonatology.org)
Neonatology on the Web is dedicated to support the relationships that exist between neonatal practitioners, their patients, and their patients' families. The site includes links to clinical resources for various neonatal conditions, tests, treatments, procedures, and medications.

Appendix B: Glossary of Acronyms

A
AAP	American Academy of Pediatrics
ABCO	Airway, breathing, circulation, other
ABG	Arterial blood gas
ACOG	American College of Obstetricians and Gynecologists
AFP	Alpha-fetoprotein
AFV	Amniotic fluid volume
AHA	American Heart Association
AIDS	Acquired immunodeficiency syndrome
AML	Acute myelocytic leukemia
ANC	Absolute neutrophil count
ANP	Atrial natriuretic peptide
APRs	Acute phase reactants
AS	Aortic stenosis
ASD	Atrial septal defect
AV	Atrioventricular

B
BAT	Brown adipose tissue
BMI	Body mass index
BP	Blood pressure
bpm	Beats per minute (beats/min)
BPP	Biophysical profile
BUN	Blood urea nitrogen

C
CAH	Congenital adrenal hyperplasia
CaO$_2$	Arterial oxygen content
CBC	Complete blood count
CBF	Cerebral blood flow
CCAM	Congenital cystic adenomatoid malformation
CDC	Centers for Disease Control and Prevention
CDH	Congenital diaphragmatic hernia
CHARGE syndrome	A disorder that affects multiple systems: coloboma (C), heart disease (H), choanal atresia (A), retarded growth and development (R), genital hypoplasia (G), and ear abnormalities (E)
CHD	Congenital heart disease
CHF	Congestive heart failure
CMV	Cytomegalovirus
CNS	Central nervous system
CoNS	Coagulase-negative *Staphylococci*

lpm	Liters per minute (liters/min)

M
MAP	Mean airway pressure (chapter 8)
MAP	Mean arterial pressure (chapter 3)
MBV	Maternal blood volume
MD	Medical doctor
MoM	Multiples of mean
MRSA	Methicillin-resistant *Staphylococci aureus*
MV	Minute ventilation

N
NAIT	Neonatal alloimmune thrombocytopenia
NCPAP	Nasal continuous positive airway pressure
NICHD	National Institute of Child Health and Human Development
NICU	Neonatal intensive care unit
NIH	National Institutes of Health
NIPPV	Nasal intermittent positive-pressure ventilation
NIRS	Near infrared spectroscopy
NRP	National Resuscitation Program
NST	Non-stress test

O
17-OHP	17-hydroxyprogesterone

P
ΔP	Delta P PIP-PEEP
PAC	Premature atrial contractions
PaCO$_2$ (also PCO$_2$)	Partial pressure of carbon dioxide
PaO$_2$ (also PO$_2$)	Partial pressure of oxygen
PAPP-A	Pregnancy-associated plasma protein-A
PCO$_2$ (also PaCO$_2$)	Partial pressure of carbon dioxide
PCR	Polymerase chain reaction
PDA	Patent ductus arteriosus
PEEP	Positive end-expiratory pressure
PFO	Patent foramen ovale
PG	Phosphatidylglycerol
PGE$_2$	Prostaglandin E2
PHH	Posthemorrhagic hydrocephalus
PHI	Periventricular hemorrhagic infarction
PICC	Peripherally inserted central catheter
PIE	Pulmonary interstitial emphysema
PIP	Peak inspiratory pressure
PIV	Peripheral intravenous catheter
PMI	Point of maximal impulse
PMN	Polymorphonuclear

PNA	Postnatal age
PO dose	Per oral dose
PO$_2$ (also PaO$_2$)	Partial pressure of oxygen
POC	Point of care
PPROM	Preterm premature rupture of the membranes
PPV	Positive-pressure ventilation
PVC	Premature ventricular contractions
PVL	Periventricular leukomalacia
PVR	Pulmonary vascular resistance

R

RBCs	Red blood cells
RDS	Respiratory distress syndrome
RH	Relative humidity
RhD	Rh blood group, D antigen
ROM	Rupture of membranes
RPR	Rapid plasma reagin
RR	Respiratory rate
RVOT	Right ventricular outflow tract

S

S2	Second heart sound
SaO$_2$	Oxygen saturation
SC	Subcutaneous reservoir
SEM disease	Skin, eyes, and mouth disease
SGA	Small for gestational age
SIRS	Sudden inflammatory response syndrome
SpO$_2$	Pulse oximetry oxygen saturation
SSA antibodies	Anti-Ro antibodies
SSB antibodies	Anti-La antibodies
SVR	Systemic vascular resistance
SVT	Supraventricular tachycardia

T

T4	Thyroxine
TAPVR	Total anomalous pulmonary venous return
TBW	Total body water
TE	Tracheo-esophageal
TEWL	Trans-epidermal water loss
TGA	Transposition of great arteries
TORCH syndrome	Toxoplasmosis (T), other e.g., syphilis, varicella (O), rubella (R), cytomegalovirus (C), herpes simplex (H)
TRALI	Transfusion-associated lung injury
TRH	Thyrotropin-releasing hormone
TSH	Thyroid-stimulating hormone
Tv	Tidal volume

U

UAC	Umbilical arterial catheter
UAs	Umbilical arteries
UV	Umbilical vein
UVC	Umbilical venous catheter

V

V/Q	Ventilation-perfusion
VACTERL syndrome	A disorder that affects multiple systems: vertebral defects (V), anal atresia (A), cardiac defects (C), trachea-esophageal (TE) fistula, renal anomalies (R), and limb abnormalities (L)
VDRL	Venereal Disease Research Laboratory
VON	Vermont Oxford Networks
VLBW	Very low birth weight
VP	Ventriculoperitoneal
VSD	Ventricular septal defect
$V_T e$	Expired tidal volume
VZV	Varicella-zoster virus

W

WC-MS	Whole-cell mass spectrophotometry

Index

A

ABCO (airway, breathing, circulation, and other), 80
  breathing/respiratory rate, 81
  circulation, 82
    hemorrhage, 83
    hypotension, 83, 177-179
  evaluation
    initial, 80
    secondary, 84
  skin color, 83
  upper airway patency, 80
Abdominal distention, 173
  intra-abdominal pressure, 173
Abdominal wall defects, 281-283
  bladder exstrophy, 282
  gastroschisis, 283
  omphalocele, 281
ABO incompatibility, 269
Air leak syndromes, 161
  clinical presentation, 163
  etiology, 162
  management, 164
  pathophysiology, 162
Ambiguous genitalia, 308-310
Amniotic banding, 293-294
Anal anomalies, 297
Anemia, 265
  causes, 265-266
  signs, 265
Antenatal fetal screening
  first trimester, 43
    maternal serum markers, 43
    nuchal translucency, 43
    ultrasound, 43
  second trimester, 44
    alpha-fetoprotein (AFP), 44
    triple screen, 44
Antenatal steroids, 54
Antibacterials, 238
Apnea, 51, 106, 131
Apnea of prematurity, 152
  definition, 152
  diagnosis, 152
  management, 155
  pathophysiology, 153
Arterial blood gas assessment, 114-115
Arthrogryposis, 295-296
Asphyxia, 105
  perinatal, 187
Aspiration syndrome, 159
  clinical presentation, 159
  etiology, 159
  management, 159
  pathophysiology, 159
Assisted ventilation, 106
  continuous positive airway pressure (CPAP), 106-107, 156-157
  failure to respond, 109
  intubation, 109
  positive-pressure ventilation (PPV), 107-108
Atrial flutter, 203, 205-206
Autoimmune neonatal thrombocytopenia, 276-277
Autonomy, 326
Axillary temperatures, 125

B

Beckwith-Wiedemann syndrome, 225, 273, 282, 305-306
Beneficence, 326
Biophysical profile (BPP), 15-17, 41, 63
Bladder exstrophy, 282, 286
Born-Alive Infants Protection Act of 2002, 328
Breast-milk feedings, 218

C

Cardiac arrhythmias, 203
  fetal, 203
  neonatal, 204
Care bundles, 243
CHARGE syndrome, 298-300
Child Abuse (Baby Doe) Amendment of 1984, 328
Choanal atresia, 171
  clinical presentation, 172
  etiology, 171
  management, 172
  pathophysiology, 171-172
Chronic fetal hypoxia, 272
Cleft lip/palate, 307-308
Coagulation disorders, 277
  secondary, 278

Coarctation of the aorta, 197-198
Communication, 335-340
   call-out, 336
   check back, 336
   debrief, 336, 340
   during intra- and inter-facility transport, 343
   hand-off, 336
   huddle, 336, 340
   SBAR, 336
Complete atrioventricular block, 204, 206-207
Conduction, 128
Conflict resolution, 337-338
Congenital anomalies, 47, 48, 52, 289
   definitions, 289
   incidence, 291
   multiple, 290
Congenital diaphragmatic hernia (CDH), 169
   clinical presentation, 170
   etiology, 169-170
   incidence, 170
   management, 171
   outcomes, 171
Congenital heart disease (CHD), 189
   diagnostic evaluation, 191
   evaluation, 190
   physical examination, 190
   types, 191
      cyanotic, 191-192
      left-sided obstructive lesions, 197-200
Contraction stress testing (CST), 13
Convection, 127
Cyanosis, 139

D

Dehydration, 212, 213
Developmental care
   family-centered interventions, 316-322
   supportive strategies, 315-316
Ductal-dependent structural heart defects, 187
Ductus arteriosus, 90-91
Ductus venosus, 92

E

Electrolyte requirements, 215
   chloride, 216
   potassium, 216
   sodium, 215
Enteral feedings, 218
Esophageal atresia, 297
Essential fatty acid deficiency (EFAD), 216
Ethics, 325
   legal considerations, 328
   palliative care, 329-330
   parental involvement, 327
   principles, 326-327
Evaporation, 129
Exchange transfusion, 270

F

Factor deficiencies, 277
Fetal circulation, 8, 89, 90, 185
   ductus arteriosus, 8
   foramen ovale, 8
   placenta, 89
   pulmonary blood flow, 89
   umbilical arteries (UAs), 8, 89, 90, 98
   umbilical vein (UV), 8, 89
   ventricular output, 89
Fetal circulatory failure, 98
Fetal growth, factors affecting, 34-37
Fetal hyperinsulinemia, 46, 47
Fetal movement counting, 11
Fetal neuroprotection, 41
Fetal surveillance, 3, 10
Fluids and electrolytes
   factors that decrease, 209, 213
   factors that increase, 209
   insensible water loss (IWL), 209, 212
   thermal-neutral environment, 212
   total body water (TBW), 209
Fungal infections, 241
   clinical presentation, 241
   treatment, 242
Futility, 326

G

Gastroschisis, 283
Gestational age (GA) assessment, 85
   definitions, 4
   ultrasonic measurements, 5
Gluconeogenesis, 221

Glucose requirements, 214
Glucose-6-phophsate dehydrogenase (G6PD), 271
Glycogenolysis, 221
Grunting, 139

H

Head-to-toe physical examination, 85
Heat loss, 127
  factors affecting, 129-130
Heat loss mechanisms, 126
  conduction, 128
  convection, 127
  evaporation, 129
  radiation, 128
Heat production, 123
  brown adipose tissue (BAT) metabolism, 125
  non-shivering thermogenesis, 124-125
  role of norepinephrine, 125
  shivering, 126
  thyroid surge, 126
Hemolysis, 268
  ABO incompatibility, 269
  immune mediated, 268
  Rh incompatibility, 268
Hemorrhagic disease of the newborn, 277
  classic presentation, 278
  early presentation, 277
  late presentation, 278
  prophylaxis, 278
HIV testing, 66
Humidity, 210
  humidity guidelines, 211
Hyperbilirubinemia, 55, 270
Hyperglycemia, 214-215
Hyperthermia, 135
  causes, 136
  management, 137
  prevention, 136
  signs and symptoms, 136
Hypo-caloric/trophic feedings, 218
Hypoglycemia, 6, 53, 131, 214, 221
  clinical presentation, 222
  defined, 214, 221
  etiology, 223
    persistent, 224, 226
    transient, 224
  incidence, 222
  management, 224-225
  pathophysiology, 221
  potential outcomes, 228
  risks, 222
Hypoplastic left heart syndrome, 198-199
Hypothermia, 131
  causes, 131
  definition, 131
  prevention and management, 132
  recommended room temperatures, 133
  rewarming, 135
  signs and symptoms, 131
Hypovolemia, 176
Hypoxia, 154

I

Infection control, 242-243, 344
Intrapartum fetal monitoring, 19-20
  baseline rate, 21-22
  baseline variability, 23-24
  categories, 23-24
  periodic/episodic changes, 24
    accelerations, 24-25
    arrhythmias, 30-31
    early accelerations, 25-26
    late decelerations, 26-28
    variable decelerations, 28-30
  uterine activity, 20
Intravenous (IV) lipids, 216-217
Intraventricular hemorrhage (IVH), 247
  complications, 254
  diagnosis, 251
  grading, 250, 252-253
  incidence, 251
  management, 253-260
  pathophysiology, 247
  predictors of outcomes, 261
  prevention, 261

J

Justice, 326

K

Kleihauer-Betke (KB), 266

L

Laryngeal masks, 109
Law of Laplace, 140
Laws of flight physiology, 349-351
Leukocytosis, 274
Lung maturity tests, 38-40

M

Maintenance fluid requirements, 213-214
Maternal risk factors
  chlamydia, 75-76
  congenital syphilis, 74-75
  diabetes, 45-51
  gonorrhea, 72-73
  hepatitis, 69-72
  herpes, 67-69
  human immunodeficiency virus (HIV), 65
  preeclampsia and HELLP syndrome, 60-63
  thyroid disease, 55-59
Mechanical ventilation, 111-112, 148
Methylxanthines, 155
Multiple gestation, 1
  twin-twin transfusion syndrome, 267, 272
Myocardial dysfunction, 187

N

Nasal flaring, 80, 139
Neonatal alloimmune thrombocytopenia (NAIT), 276
Neutropenia, 273-274
Noise and vibration during transport, 348-349
Non-maleficence, 327
Non-stress test (NST), 11
Nutrition, 146, 209
  amino acids, 216
  lipids, 216
  protein, 216

O

Omphalocele, 281
Open neural-tube defects, 44
Over-hydration, 212

P

Palliative care, 329
Parenteral nutrition, 216
Patent ductus arteriosus (PDA), 183, 201-202
  clinical presentation, 201
  diagnosis, 202
  management, 202
Patient Safety and Quality Improvement Act, 333
Periodic breathing, 153
Peripheral vasodilation, 188
Periventricular leukomalacia (PVL), 256
Phototherapy, 270
Physical assessment of the neonate
  approach, 78
  during the Golden Hours, 79
  evaluation, 78-79
Physiologic weight loss, 209, 213
Pierre Robin syndrome, 172
  clinical presentation, 173
  etiology, 172
  management, 173
  pathophysiology, 172-173
Placenta, 6
  abnormalities, 7
  implantation, 6
  maternal circulation, 9
  normal development, 7
Placental abruption, 175, 187, 266-267
Platelets, normal values, 275
Pneumatosis intestinalis, 349
Pneumomediastinum, 164-165, 168
Pneumonia (congenital), 160
  clinical presentation, 160
  etiology, 160
  management, 161
  pathophysiology, 160
Pneumopericardium, 163, 166, 168
Pneumoperitoneum, 163, 167, 168
Pneumothorax, 162, 163, 165, 168
Polycythemia, 54, 272
  causes, 272-273
  clinical presentation, 272
  definition, 272
  management, 273
Posthemorrhagic hydrocephalus (PHH), 257
Potter's sequence, 291-292
Pregnancy, 1
  duration, 1
  trimesters, 1-4
Premature beats, 207
Preterm labor and delivery, 37
Procedures, 363
  abdominal paracentesis, 375-376
  intubation, 363
  lumbar puncture (L/P), 373-374
  pericardiocentesis, 374-375

thoracentesis, 368
   chest tube insertion, 369-370
   needle aspiration, 368
umbilical line placement, 364-368
Pulmonary hypoplasia, 168
  clinical presentation, 169
  etiology, 168
  management, 169
  pathophysiology, 169
Pulmonary interstitial emphysema (PIE), 163-164, 166

R

Red blood cells (RBCs), normal values, 265
Renal vein thrombosis, 54
Respiratory distress syndrome (RDS), 54, 139
  diagnosis, 141
  management, 143
  pathophysiology, 140
  risk factors, 139
  ventilation weaning protocols, 145
Restraints during transport, 345
Resuscitation and stabilization, 101
  equipment, 101-102
  oxygen needs during resuscitation, 103-104
  preparation, 101
  sequence of interventions, 102
  targeted oxygen saturation, 105
Retractions, 139
Rh incompatibility, 268
Robin sequence/complex, 292-293

S

Sacral agenesis, 47
Sepsis, 231
  antibiotic therapy, 237
  clinical presentation, 233
  definitions, 231
  diagnostic and laboratory tests, 234-236
  early-onset sepsis (EOS), 231
  hospital acquired infection (HAI), 231
  predominant organisms, 232
Shock, 175, 186-187
  assessment, 179
  treatment, 180-183
  types, 175

Spherocytosis, 271
Stratum corneum, 130, 210
Suctioning the airway, 110
  meconium, 110
  procedure, 110
  setup, 110
Supraventricular tachycardia (SVT), 203, 204
Surfactant replacement therapy, 147
  use in transport, 354

T

Teams
  components, 334
  members, 334
  vs. groups, 334
TeamSTEPPS®, 333
Tetralogy of Fallot, 191-192
Thermoregulation, 123
  after birth, 124
  fetal, 123-124
  pathophysiology, 123-126
Thrombocytopenia, 275
  causes, 275-276
  definition, 275
To Err is Human, 333
Total anomalous pulmonary venous return (TAPVR), 195-196
Transient tachypnea of the newborn, 148
  diagnosis/clinical presentation, 150
  management, 151
  pathophysiology, 148
Transition to extrauterine life, 89
  alveolar oxygen tension, 90
  cardiac adaptation to extrauterine life, 185
  ductus arteriosus, 90-91, 200-201
  ductus venosus, 92
  fetal shunts, 90-92
  foramen ovale, 92
  oxygen as a pulmonary vasodilator, 90
  pulmonary vascular resistance (PVR), 90
  removal of the placenta, 91
  systemic vascular resistance (SVR), 90

Transport of neonates, 353-356
  airway management during transport, 353
  documentation, 348
  equipment and supplies, 348
  family support, 346-348
  general considerations, 344-345
  inter-facility transport, 358-361
  monitoring during transport, 345-346
  physiologic impact, 348-351
  thermoregulation during transport, 351-353
  transport within the birth facility, 356-357
Transposition of great arteries (TGA), 191
Tricuspid atresia, 194-195
Triglycerides, 217
Trisomy syndromes, 37, 44, 276, 300-305
Truncus arteriosus, 193-194

U

Umbilical cord
  cord clamping, 90
  cord compression/occlusion, 96-98
  cord gas values, 94-95
  factors that affect cord gas interpretation, 94-97
  sample collection and labeling, 92-94
Umbilical Doppler velocimetry, 18
Umbilical line placement, 364
Urine, 212
  creatinine, 212
  oliguria, 212
  output, 212
  serum blood urea nitrogen (BUN), 212
  serum sodium, 212
  urine specific gravity, 212

V

VATER/VACTERL anomalies, 296-297
Ventilation-perfusion (V/Q), 141
  matching, 147, 148

Ventilators, 111
  considerations with transport, 344
  high-frequency, 113-114
  pressure-controlled, 111
  synchronized intermittent mechanical, 112
  volume-controlled, 112
Ventricular septal defect (VSD), 199-200, 297
Ventricular tachycardia, 206
Vertebral anomalies, 297
Very low birth weight (VLBW) infant
  effects of maternal thyroid disease, 58, 60
  effects of maternal hypertensive disorders, 63
  infants of diabetic mothers (IDMs), 51
  resuscitation and stabilization, 111
  shock, 175
  special needs during transport, 343
  thermoregulation, 123-127
  water imbalance, 210
Viability defined, 325
Viral infections, 239
  diagnosis, 240
  presentation and classifications, 240
  treatment, 240-241
Volume expansion, 176, 183, 188

W

Water loss
  extracellular water, 209
  trans-epidermal water loss (TEWL), 130, 210
White blood cells, 273
  normal values, 273

Z

Zidovudine, 65-66